Paediatric Cochlear Implantation
Evaluating Outcomes

ED Thoutenhoofd
Moray House School of Education, University of Edinburgh

SM Archbold
Education Co-ordinator, The Ear Foundation;
Advisor, Nottingham Cochlear Implant Programme

S Gregory
Consultant Clinical Psychologist

ME Lutman
Institute of Sound and Vibration Research, University of Southampton

TP Nikolopoulos
Professor in Otorhinolaryngology, Athens University

TH Sach
University of Nottingham

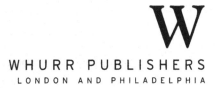

WHURR PUBLISHERS
LONDON AND PHILADELPHIA

© 2005 Whurr Publishers Ltd
First published 2005
by Whurr Publishers Ltd
19b Compton Terrace
London N1 2UN England and
325 Chestnut Street, Philadelphia PA 19106 USA

British Library Cataloguing in Publication Data

A catalogue record for this book
is available from the British Library.

ISBN 1 86156 366 3

Typeset by Adrian McLaughlin, a@microguides.net

Contents

Acknowledgement   vi
Preface   vii

Chapter 1   **Reviewing research on outcomes of paediatric cochlear implantation**   1

Chapter 2   **A summary of outcome measures**   19

Chapter 3   **The research reviews**   48

Chapter 4   **Outcomes and factors: a discussion**   241

List of abbreviations   269
Glossary of health economic terms   272
Papers reviewed   279
Additional references   287
Further reading   288
Index   289

Acknowledgement

The authors are grateful for the support of Cochlear Europe which made this literature review possible. The work was carried out entirely independently and the project was managed by The Ear Foundation.

Preface

Cochlear implantation is a major innovation in the area of deafness and has had a significant effect on the lives of many deaf children and their families. It is necessarily a medical and surgical intervention, but one where successful long-term outcomes are largely seen in social, educational and linguistic outcomes. The rapid development in this complex area has led to a wide range and number of research studies published in a variety of journals and books. For this reason it was timely to review these studies, their methodologies and conclusions, and assess the current state of the art.

The range of outcomes reported in the literature has included specific measures of functional outcome such as auditory performance and speech perception and intelligibility, as well as broader measures of outcome, such as educational issues, social interaction and quality of life. However, specific measures have tended to receive more attention than broader ones. Over the past ten years, the procedure and its outcomes have been the subject of evaluation, partly due to the need to justify its development and cost and partly to influence practice and decisions. Because the research has been reported in a wide range of contexts and professional journals, this has made accessibility and comparability difficult. Any researcher studying cochlear implantation would have this difficulty; it is hoped that this review will assist future researchers in evaluating the literature and planning further research. No such comprehensive review of the literature has been undertaken until now; previous reviews have either had a very tight and restricted focus, or have been confined to the medical literature. The implications of paediatric cochlear implantation are much broader than this, and an analysis of outcomes should be seen in this broader context. Therefore this review deals specifically with the areas of language and communication, speech production and perception, family and social life, educational attainments and the health economics literature.

The aim of this book therefore can be summarized as a systematic litera-ture review of key research findings on outcomes associated with paediatric cochlear implantation. Two subsidiary aims are:

- to summarise the current knowledge on this topic and identify gaps in the literature
- to make recommendations for future research in the area, identifying aspects of benefit not previously taken into account.

Chapter 1

Reviewing research on outcomes of paediatric cochlear implantation

Introduction

This volume presents a review of the research on outcomes of cochlear implantation for children. It considers outcomes in the areas of language and communication, speech production and perception, family and social life, and educational attainments. It also reviews the health economics literature with respect to cochlear implants. It does not consider the extensive literature that deals specifically with medical outcomes or detailed audiological outcomes, unless they relate to the more general use of audition.

Implantation is a comparatively new process and not without controversy. This chapter introduces the review by looking at the development of cochlear implantation. It also examines audiological and medical issues, which are included to provide background about the process of implantation. For the reader who would like more detail we provide a suggested reading list. The chapter goes on to consider the context in which implantation occurs by reviewing our understanding of the impact of childhood deafness on the language and communication of the child, on the family, on social life, and on education. The final part of the chapter introduces the review and describes the process of the literature review itself.

The development of paediatric cochlear implantation

Cochlear implantation for young deaf children, providing useful hearing to those unable to benefit significantly from conventional hearing aids, is a comparatively recent development. Implantation was first carried out on children in the 1980s and the technique developed more rapidly through the 1990s. Initially, implants were used only for deafened adults, but the results led surgeons and parents alike to consider cochlear implantation for children. At first, only those children who were deafened, rather than born deaf, were considered. The results were encouraging, although such an operation on children was not accepted by all. Attention then turned to those children who are born profoundly deaf. However, this resulted in further controversy, particularly from the deaf community, who viewed it as the imposition of the medical model of deafness. Cochlear implantation was perceived as treating deafness as a deficit rather than recognizing it as a difference, through trying to 'normalize' deaf children by 'curing' their deafness. The controversy has continued to a greater or lesser degree, and the pace of progress has varied from country to country, often influenced by the prevailing philosophy of educating deaf children, for example whether it should be by sign language or through spoken language, and attitudes to deafness. Influences in moving cochlear implantation forward include individual endeavours and pressure from parents; those that have hindered progress include financial pressures and lack of experienced staff.

In spite of the continuing controversy and concerns about making a lifelong decision involving an elective surgical procedure on behalf of a young child, cochlear implantation has grown rapidly, and worldwide there are now almost 40,000 children under the age of 16 with cochlear implants. As outcomes have exceeded initial expectations, children with increasing levels of hearing are currently being implanted, together with those at increasingly young ages, including those under the age of 12 months, and children with complex needs. Interestingly, given the controversy, there are also increasing numbers of deaf parents considering cochlear implantation for their deaf children.

Audiological issues

The developing technology

The earliest commercially available devices had only a single channel and their use was confined almost entirely to adults. Implantation of children in large numbers began in the late 1980s, when multi-channel devices became commercially available, and was accelerated by the approval given by the US Food and Drugs Administration (FDA) to the Nucleus-22 device, now sold under the trade name Cochlear. The two other major devices are produced by Advanced Bionics and MED-EL. Systematic evidence for outcomes of implantation in children is now based entirely on multi-channel devices. One of the most basic outcomes of cochlear implantation is an increase in the ability to hear sound. In cases of profound or total hearing loss, there is a change from a situation where most everyday sounds are not heard at all to one where most everyday sounds, including speech, can at least be detected.

There has been substantial further development of multi-channel devices and the pace of technological advance shows no sign of slowing down at the time of writing. Such developments have led to gradual improvements in the overall performance of cochlear implant systems and presumably the corresponding outcomes. Therefore, evaluation of evidence on outcomes must be tempered by an appreciation of the changes that have occurred. This has implications when comparing cross-sectional studies reported in different years, where apparent improvements may be related either to explicit differences between the studies or to intrinsic improvements in technology over time. Similar confounding may occur with longitudinal studies that involve different cohorts or where participants may have received upgrades to their system over the study period.

Tuning the system

While the effect of the implant is to increase the audibility of sounds, this is not straightforward. It is the process of adjustment of the cochlear implant system, which entails mapping an input range of sound frequencies and intensities on to the available range of perceptible electrical stimulation levels, that ensures that audibility occurs. In a real sense, this outcome is not a meaningful measure of the performance of the implant, because it is entirely under the control of the audiologist who adjusts the system. While many publications present data on aided hearing threshold levels with the implant, this has limited value as an outcome measure. The information is useful, however, as an indicator of quality control. Clearly, if the system is not adjusted properly, performance may be degraded. Adjustment, or mapping, of systems for adults is straightforward in principle. They are able to tell the audiologist when sounds are detectable and when they are too loud. However, this process is more difficult for young children and is particularly difficult for infants. With implantation occurring in younger and younger children, the notion of accurate adjustment may become an ideal rather than a realizable goal. The existence of cognitive disability additional to deafness, which may occur in a number of cases of post-meningitis deafness and in a number of forms of congenital deafness, makes the likelihood of accurate adjustment lower.

Hence, evaluation of outcomes of cochlear implantation should recognize that young age can influence outcomes indirectly through the audiological fitting process, as well as possibly directly. Similarly, additional disabilities may have this dual impact.

Discrimination of sounds

In addition to audibility of everyday sounds, audiological assessment of cochlear implant performance may focus on discrimination between differing sounds. For meaningful differences to be recognized, for example between environmental sounds or speech sounds, it is essential that they can be discriminated. The nature of operation of cochlear implant systems means that some sounds may give similar electrical stimulation. Therefore, performance depends on the detailed characteristics of the implant sound processor, which in turn may depend on choices made by the audiologist in setting it up. The skills of the implant team therefore have a bearing on outcomes. Children with implants are also likely to differ in their intrinsic discrimination abilities, and these will affect outcomes.

Candidacy issues

When children were first considered for cochlear implantation only those with virtually total deafness were included. They had little useful hearing to lose and the risks of implantation to residual hearing were small. Moreover, it was unknown whether children could learn spoken language entirely from electrical stimulation. Therefore, only children who had experienced spoken language through hearing were included. The vast majority of acquired hearing loss cases were as a consequence of meningitis. As further experience was gathered, it became apparent that congenitally deaf children could benefit just as well and that benefits were often better than had been anticipated. Hence, criteria for implantation gradually changed from having little or no potential for auditory stimulation to being likely to benefit more from an implant than a hearing aid. Corresponding audiometric guidelines have followed this rationale and changed from having aided hearing thresholds in the range of 90–100 dB to having aided thresholds in the range 50–55 dB in the upper speech frequencies (2–4 kHz). Hence, some candidates who are selected according to current criteria may be classified as having severe rather than profound deafness. In the early 1990s, virtually all candidates would have had profound or almost total deafness.

These changes in candidacy criteria almost certainly have a material effect on outcomes. Not only does severe rather than profound deafness imply that the surviving auditory system is in a better state, but also in many cases of congenital deafness the child will probably have had some useful experience of hearing prior to implantation. Furthermore, there is a greater possibility of benefit from hearing aids. While the benefit from hearing aids worn from soon after birth until implantation may be limited, the consequences for the early developing auditory system may be great. Without meaningful auditory stimulation, areas of the central nervous system become available for different tasks. Once the neural resources intended for hearing have been reallocated, there is a reduced likelihood that they will be allocated again to hearing. The use of hearing aids, however limited in their benefit, may reduce or slow down such consequences of plasticity on auditory potential. For these reasons, residual hearing capacity prior to cochlear implantation may be one of the most important factors governing outcomes in relation to audition. It is important that evidence on outcomes is accompanied by information on residual hearing prior to implantation and that evaluation of the outcomes takes this into account.

Decisions about which ear to implant

Residual hearing may be present in one or both ears before implantation. This raises the question of which ear to implant and also the issue of simultaneous use of a cochlear implant on one side and a hearing aid on the other. Some centres have tended to implant the worse hearing ear based on the rationale that there is less to lose. Other centres have argued that the better hearing ear has the greater potential for benefit and have implanted the better ear. (The advent of bilateral implantation may make this debate redundant.) Where the poorer ear is implanted, there is greater potential for wearing a hearing aid on the opposite ear, with the aim of achieving some binaural benefit. Binaural benefits may include reducing adverse head shadow effects when listening to sounds from the side opposite the implant, improved separation of speech from noise and improved localization of sound sources. These factors complicate the interpretation of outcomes from cochlear implantation substantially, particularly when evaluating benefits expressed in general terms from everyday experience of implant use. Ideally, evidence on outcomes should be accompanied by information on hearing aid use before and after implantation, as well as residual hearing abilities in both ears.

Implant performance

As with all technology, there is the possibility that cochlear implants may not perform continuously to specification and may even break down entirely. While currently available devices are generally reliable, there are instances of failure of the internal device and more numerous instances of breakdowns of the sound processor and ancillary cables and coils. Failures of the internal devices have received greatest attention because replacement entails revision surgery. There is less systematic evidence on breakdowns of external parts. The important issue for the present review is that many children will have experienced some instances of reduced performance or breakdown of the equipment. Because it is not possible for other people, such as parents, to try out the system, many performance degradations probably go undetected until they become more obvious. These degradations presumably have an impact on outcomes and are more likely to go unreported with infants than with older children. The perceptiveness of parents, teachers and other professionals in regular contact with the child may be a factor in how quickly such faults are rectified. Hence, there may be complex confounding effects that include the age of the child and ability to detect or indicate problems, the quality of parental and other support, and the intrinsic reliability of the device the child has received. In practice, it is unlikely that the consequences of these confounding factors can be separated out.

Medical and surgical issues

Paediatric cochlear implantation, maybe more than any other surgical procedure, has led doctors to realize the importance of multidisciplinary team work, not only in the assessment phase but also during surgery and in the long follow-up and rehabilitation of deaf children. Audiological evaluation is normally the basis of the preliminary assessment of a deaf child. At this stage some children will be deemed unsuitable for implantation, either because their hearing is better than that considered appropriate for implantation or because of the lack of an adequate trial of appropriate hearing aids. Once the child has undergone audiological assessment and has been found appropriate for further investigation, medical evaluation and radiological imaging will be carried out.

Surgical issues

The various factors that the surgeon will take into account in assessing any child for implantation may be summarized as follows:

- aetiology of deafness (including investigation of whether the cause of deafness is inherited or syndromal)
- age at onset of deafness and whether progressive or not
- confirmation of the degree and nature of hearing loss
- otological assessment (including the exclusion of a conductive disorder and, if found, the management of a disease such as otitis media with effusion)

- radiological imaging (including modern magnetic resonance imaging (MRI) techniques)
- general medical evaluation, including assessment and management of other underlying general medical problems
- general developmental assessment, including psychological evaluation where appropriate.

Although these factors of themselves rarely lead to the exclusion of cochlear implantation as a choice of management in profoundly deaf children, they may highlight surgical difficulties or modify short- and long-term parental expectations.

Deaf children with additional needs

In the early stages of cochlear implantation, difficult surgical cases and children with additional needs were not considered as candidates for implantation. However, an increasing number of children with complex needs or inner-ear malformations have now been implanted, revealing that these children may derive benefit from cochlear implantation. This benefit, even variable and in some cases limited, may lead to substantial improvements in the quality of life of these children and their families. Children with craniofacial syndromes and deafness may need higher levels of electrical stimulation of the implant compared to other children with implants, and stimulation of the facial nerve may be a problem that needs special attention. The pre-implant assessment of these children requires detailed radiological investigation and extensive interdisciplinary discussion, and parents need to receive realistic counselling about outcomes. After implantation, these children continue to require well-coordinated medical and interdisciplinary management tailored to their specific needs.

The results of the pre-implant assessments and the input from all specialists involved (including teachers of the deaf, speech and language therapists, etc.) will determine if a deaf child is suitable for cochlear implantation or not. However, if the child is suitable, the parents make the final decision as to whether to go ahead and their role in all phases, including the long (re)habilitation of their children, is crucially important, and they should have realistic and well-founded expectations.

Implanting very young children

The whole process becomes more complex with the current pressure for implantation of very young deaf children identified in the neonatal hearing screening programmes. Although there is evidence for the safety and feasibility of surgery in children under 2 years of age and the early results are encouraging, there is no consensus on the most appropriate age for implantation of deaf children identified at birth. Moreover, long-term results concerning outcomes and complications in very young children were inevitably still limited at the end of the search.

Surgical complications

Surgical techniques for cochlear implantation have evolved over the past 15 years. Incisions have become smaller and minimally invasive surgery is now a reality. However, surgical complications, although relatively few and more frequently minor, are still a matter of concern as they may cause serious morbidity and even mortality in the case of meningitis. Therefore, several studies in the literature have reported on surgical outcomes, the majority of which report major complications. Large centres report between 3 and 4% complications in implanted children. However, most of these studies have a relatively short follow-up and this is an important shortcoming as it may be that long-term complications are underestimated.

The role of follow-up care

While it has been recognized that it is important to monitor the outcomes from paediatric cochlear implantation, the importance of long-term follow-up care of these children has also increasingly been recognized. The children continue to require technical and audiological support for the use of their implant systems and, as has been explained, the functioning and tuning of the implant system will have an influence on their progress following implantation.

There has also been debate about the amount and type of rehabilitation (or habilitation) support they require following implantation. A range of follow-up services has evolved, ranging from provision mainly within a clinical setting to provision provided solely by the local educational services. The contact between the cochlear implant service and the family and local service varies widely, from little or none, to regular close cooperation with shared personnel. In addition to the quantity and organization of varying levels of support, the support may differ greatly in emphasis, for example whether an oral approach is emphasized or whether sign language is used, to whatever degree. The influence of this wide range of follow-up care inevitably adds to the complexities of comparing outcomes from implantation, and the subtleties may be lost to the researcher who is clinic based or unfamiliar with the diversity of provision for deaf children.

Deafness in children

In reviewing the outcomes of paediatric cochlear implantation and the role of rehabilitation, it is important to consider the impact of childhood deafness on the language and communication of the child, on the family, on social life and on education.

Deaf children: the development of language and communication

For children, a major impact of deafness is on the ability to acquire, use and overhear spoken language, and thus there is a need for extra attention to be given to language development. Deaf children differ from those with speech and language problems as it is not a difficulty with language acquisition itself, and virtually all deaf children are able to acquire sign language if provided with appropriate input. Some deaf children do acquire and use sign language as a first or preferred language, while for others the focus is on developing their spoken language competence. Some may be bilingual in sign language and spoken language.

However, as the majority of deaf children are born into hearing families, providing access to appropriate sign language communication during the early years is not always straightforward, as the language of the family will be spoken language. Difficulties can emerge in the early months when the child is developing those prelinguistic skills necessary for the later acquisition of language and communication. It may be more difficult for parents to establish such behaviours as turn taking, following a point and naming with a child who is deaf.

As a deaf child starts to acquire spoken language, their deafness can mean that they may have a smaller spoken language vocabulary and have difficulty with some grammatical constructions that can be taken for granted with hearing children. Deaf children may have difficulty in understanding the speech of others and in making themselves understood. Some deaf children will find one-to-one interaction using speech problematic, and their deafness may often mean that they will find conversation in group situations difficult.

Additional consequences of deafness can include limited access to incidental knowledge, which is typically acquired through taking part in or overhearing general conversation, and through incidental learning from the media. There can be difficulties in developing literacy skills, due to limited access to sound and/or spoken language. Both limited language competence and poorer understanding of the nature of a story may make it difficult to guess the next word or phrase when reading. In addition, word-building skills can also be limited by poor phonological awareness. This will, of course, vary for different deaf children. Also, deaf pupils who use sign language may not experience difficulties in the same areas, although there are other issues for this group.

Deaf children: family and social life

The vast majority of deaf children are born into hearing families. The diagnosis of deafness for these families is often devastating and the implications complex. Early decisions concern amplification and the use of hearing aids and/or cochlear implants. Families also need to consider the communication that is used in the family and whether or not to use sign. Signing provides a visual form of language which is usually easier for deaf children to acquire, but more difficult in terms of involvement of the whole family, and thus can often limit the number of family members with whom the child can communicate. Later decisions relate to the educational placement of the child and the approach to be used.

It is difficult to generalize about social factors and deafness, given the heterogeneity of deaf children in terms of degree of deafness, ability and other factors, and the vast range of family situations in which deaf children live their lives. While many deaf children have very good relationships with their families and beyond, and enjoy active social lives, a significant number of deaf children do experience problems. In particular, the incidence of emotional disturbance in school-age deaf children is higher than for hearing children.

For that minority of deaf children born into families where the parents are deaf, the situation may be different. Many deaf people, usually members of the deaf community, do not see their deafness as a disability but rather as a difference. They see deafness as a positive aspect of their lives. Many research reports suggest that deaf children of deaf parents do better than those with hearing parents, both socially and academically, although it is not clear whether this is due specifically to the early use of sign language or to other factors.

Attention to the quality of life of deaf children and their families would seem to be important, and yet for deaf children in general it is an under-researched area. However, in the context of paediatric cochlear implantation, it has become significant because of the medical context of the intervention, and the need to evaluate the benefits of implantation, particularly in the context of health economics.

Deaf children: issues in education

The main debates in deaf education have traditionally been concerned with the language that should be used in education and the setting for the education of deaf children.

The debate over language use with deaf children concerns the use of an oral approach with spoken language or the use of signs. In the UK, this relates mainly to British Sign Language (BSL) and English. (For convenience, the discussion here describes the situation with respect to English and BSL, but clearly equally applies to spoken and sign languages as used throughout the world.) BSL is a language in its own right with a different syntax and vocabulary. It is the language of choice of many deaf adults. Some argue that as the natural language of deaf people it should have a place in the education of deaf children in order to provide better access to the curriculum and not to disadvantage children who find it difficult to access spoken language. They argue that children should be educated bilingually, through both English and BSL (or multilingually for children using additional other languages). Others argue that English should be given priority and the approach to education should be oral, or oral-aural using only English in both its spoken and written forms. They feel this is necessary in order for deaf children to take their place in the hearing world. A third approach uses the signs from BSL simultaneously with English, thus using English syntax rather than that of sign language. This gives a visual representation of English (known variously as Sign Supported English, simultaneous communication, manually coded English or Total Communication, a term also sometimes used to include the sign bilingual approach and over which there is much confusion). These debates impact on cochlear implantation, where the aim is to provide access to hearing and spoken language and hence spoken language approaches to education.

The essence of the debate over placement is whether deaf children should be educated in mainstream schools alongside their hearing peers, or whether they should be in specialist provision, either a mainstream school resourced for deaf pupils or a special school. Currently the trend for all pupils with special needs is towards inclusion, and thus a growing number of deaf children are being educated in mainstream schools.

The worldwide move towards inclusion, where deaf children have increasingly tended to be placed in mainstream schools rather than in special provision for deaf pupils, has meant that in some instances it has been more difficult to collect and collate data on deaf children as a separate group. Studies tend to be small scale and often relate to a particular educational context or approach. Currently, there is not a clear and coherent picture of the educational achievements of deaf children, and although there is a significant amount of data it is difficult to give a comprehensive account of deaf children's attainments. However, some general conclusions can be drawn. Research does suggest that deaf children do not achieve as much as their hearing counterparts, despite the fact that overall non-verbal intelligence is similar. Assessment of reading ability, in particular, consistently shows a delay in attainment that could be expected to affect other curriculum areas.

Evaluating outcomes of cochlear implantation

Cochlear implantation is an expensive procedure, and involves lifelong maintenance by an unusually wide range of professionals. As such, it has demanded assessment of outcomes, placed as it is in increasingly accountable healthcare services. Assessment of outcomes has a number of purposes:

- information for healthcare purchasers and referrers
- information for parents on which to base their decision
- ongoing assessment to monitor progress and identify any changes in management required, any problems with the device or any difficulties which the child may have in addition to deafness.

Cochlear implantation is a surgical procedure, and one that involves a lifelong decision by parents for their child. On what basis is this decision made? What outcomes are necessary to inform this decision? Although the outcomes are seen mainly in the areas of speech, language, education and social issues for children, the procedure has largely been set in a scientific and medical context, and this has influenced the ways in which it has been evaluated.

However, much healthcare research is based on large-scale studies and with a limited number of variables; research with deaf children has long been known to involve a large range of variables, including age at onset, aetiology, cognition, the presence of other learning difficulties and management itself. Cochlear implantation has introduced a number of other variables, including numbers of electrodes inserted, age at implantation, and the functioning and tuning of the system. The interaction of these variables inevitably poses challenges to those requiring rigorous research; in addition, outcomes from cochlear implantation become apparent over years rather than months, during which time the technology used itself may have changed significantly. The traditional purest form of research, that of randomised controlled trials, may not be ethically appropriate, or possible, and the inclusion of qualitative methods may be important.

Differing perspectives of outcomes

In addition to the complex picture outlined above, there may be different perspectives on outcomes. It is possible to divide outcomes from cochlear implantation into: primary outcomes, such as changes in auditory perception, including environmental sounds and spoken language; and those that arise out of these changes, the secondary outcomes.

These secondary outcomes include the development of spoken language, changes in behaviour and educational outcomes. Inevitably, research into outcomes initially focused on the former, as these are the first to appear. The secondary outcomes only become apparent over years, making the collection of long-term data important, but lengthy. Secondary outcomes from implantation have been largely looked for in the educational field, and for many clinicians this involves a new way of looking at deafness. The medical model of deafness, as something to be remedied, is far removed from the educational and sociological models of deafness, where deafness may be seen as a cultural or linguistic difference, rather than a deficit. These differences may have a significant influence on the way in which outcomes from implantation are viewed and how they are evaluated. The medical model of research may not fit comfortably within an educational context, and deaf education in particular, with all its complexities. For example, if speech perception is seen as a primary outcome from implantation this may be evaluated relatively easily in the clinic, but many assumptions may be made by a non-specialist clinician about the interaction of the many variables involved and the complexity of language acquisition in young children, particularly young deaf children. The more complex assessments of secondary outcomes such as language itself demand particular expertise with young deaf children.

In addition, the relative importance of differing outcomes from cochlear implantation may be viewed differently by parents, the range of professionals involved, the deaf community and by the children themselves as they grow up. The emphasis on medical and scientific views of research and of what constitutes important outcomes from cochlear implantation may lead to certain differences in approach. For example, the scientist in the clinic may view outcomes solely in terms of changes in auditory perception, while for the teacher of the deaf working with the child in the classroom, the child's ability to acquire reading skills via audition may be a critically important change brought about by cochlear implantation.

The major criticisms of cochlear implant research have been that it has been carried out by those with a vested interest – the cochlear implant centres or manufacturers; that the groups studied have been heterogeneous and carefully selected; and that there has been selective reporting on a small group. In spite of the difficulties, it is vital that research and ongoing audit into the provision of cochlear implants for children is continued, and that outcomes are provided which are meaningful and accessible to parents and a wide range of professionals, and that they are collected as rigorously as possible.

The literature search

The aim of this literature review is to consider recent research on outcomes of paediatric cochlear implantation. The review process involved a literature search to identify published work in this field that met particular criteria, described below. It was conducted in two ways. We invited active researchers, in the UK and beyond, to contact the project and provide us with bibliographies of their research output published in English, and fliers were handed out at an international meeting early in 2002. From submitted reading lists, only those articles that fell within the restrictions of the project were entered into the database. Some researchers were contacted on an individual basis in a follow-up request for additional information. Second, an extensive electronic literature search was conducted on a number of appropriate and available bibliographic databanks. These searches were conducted early in the project, in February 2002.

The literature search on which the present analysis is based concerns 145 articles from the 248 that were initially located. This final number is based on a few restrictions and characteristics in the selection process. Before detailing the restrictions, we will detail the journals identified by the collection of search engines.

Key journals for research on outcomes in paediatric cochlear implantation

Below is a list of the journals which account for all the output published in journals contained in our sample (only a few book chapters were included in the review). For ease of reference and future follow-up they are arranged in alphabetical order. The medical journals are by far the most densely covered, in the journals of otology, otolaryngology and otorhinolarynogology. Other titles were located in journals on hearing, audiology and deafness in general. A minority were found in journals with language, education or medical technology as a topic. A few of the journals listed have since been amalgamated into a single title.

Table 1.1 Journal Listing

Acta Oto-Laryngologica
Acta Oto-Rhino-Laryngologica Belgica
Advances in Cochlear Implants
Advances in Oto-Rhino-Laryngology
American Annals of the Deaf

Table 1.1 Journal Listing contd.

American Journal of Audiology
American Journal of Otology
Annals of Otology, Rhinology and Laryngology
Archives of Otolaryngology
Archives of Otolaryngology, and Head and Neck Surgery
Archives of Otorhinolaryngology, and Head and Neck Surgery
Audiology
Audiology and Neuro-Otology
Audiology–Journal of Auditory Communication
British Journal of Audiology
British Medical Journal
Caeddh Journal/La Revue Acesm
Cerebral Cortex
Cochlear Implants International
Deafness and Education
Deafness and Education International
Developmental Psychology
Ear and Hearing
European Archives of Oto-Rhino-Laryngology
Hearing Research
International Journal of Audiology
International Journal of Language and Communication Disorders
International Journal of Otorhinolaryngology
International Journal of Pediatric Otorhinolaryngology
International Journal of Technology Assessment in Health Care
Journal of the Acoustical Society of America
Journal of the American Medical Association
Journal of American Speech, Language and Hearing Research
Journal of the British Association of Teachers of the Deaf (BATOD)
Journal of Communication Disorders
Journal of Deaf Studies and Deaf Education
Journal of Early Intervention
Journal of Laryngology and Otology
Journal of Otorhinolaryngology
Journal of Speech and Hearing Research
Journal of Speech, Language and Hearing Research
The Lancet
Laryngoscope
Medical Progress through Technology
Otolaryngologic Clinics of North America
Otolaryngology – Head and Neck Surgery
Otology and Neurology
Otology and Neurotology
Psychological Science
Scandinavian Audiology
Special Educational Needs
Volta Review
Volta Voices

Search restrictions

First, searches were restricted to publications in the English language but not limited to English-speaking countries, so that some English language articles on 'foreign language' implanted children are included. The initial return included articles on Dutch, French, German, Polish, Spanish and Swedish children. However, despite publication in English being part of the search criteria, a number of foreign language articles turned up, mostly because either their abstract or their title was included in a database in English translation.

Second, we defined a cut-off date at 1994 for the start of the review. This was done not so much to limit the number of returns, but to eliminate articles based on children with single-channel implants. As a consequence, all articles here concern populations with multi-channel implants, which became commonplace in the early 1990s. This is significant, because the results reported here therefore pertain almost entirely to the current generation of devices, although one or two articles may include a post hoc comparison population predating the published article. Such a comparative population may or may not have been described demographically in sufficient detail, and therefore some single-channel use may have entered into the data through the back door.

And third, it was agreed to include only reports based on sample sizes of at least 12 children (or parents in the case of parent interviews). There is a good reason for limiting the minimum sample size: the literature contains any number of case studies, which, although of interest, have low validity for the purpose of comparisons, while no generalizations can be made from findings on one or a few individuals. On the whole, as with the quantitative research reviewed here, qualitative case studies and small sample studies are of great value if methodologically sound, and they have a perfectly legitimate place among the available research. Qualitative research often contains a sense of reality and proximity, of bearing witness to the messiness of 'real life', and paying close attention to individual variation. For this reason, where smaller-scale research turned up in our searches and was deemed of special interest, we have included it and noted the reason.

One exception was agreed to the minimum sample size of 12: because some child characteristics or outcome measures might be of special interest, we agreed to allow smaller sample sizes if articles contributed something important to the overall emerging picture that otherwise would be lacking. An example is an outcome measure shared by relatively few individuals in a given population. Where a report on a sample smaller than 12 individuals is included in the review, we provide our reasons for including it.

Database search results

All searches were conducted in early 2002, on electronic search engines. Since most databases run with a backlog of a few months, the results are likely to be exhaustive up to mid-2001. Of course, a significant number of search results in any one of the databases listed below overlapped with those of another. In the brief summary below, these have not been filtered out. Search results across the databases overlapped, in particular with the results of Medline searches, an observation that reflects the types of journal in which articles on paediatric implantation most frequently appear (i.e. in medical journals rather than education journals), but which also reflects the generous scope of Medline. Therefore the figures in Table 1.2 are a rough guide to the returns within each database on a list of search words detailing non-medical outcomes in paediatric cochlear implantation.

Subsequent checking of reference lists in the texts located and increasing reduplication of search results (as should be expected) together suggest that the searches became largely circular. Therefore, within the criteria specified, we are relatively certain that the bulk of work published between 1994 and summer 2001 concerning paediatric implantation, detailing samples of 12 subjects and over, and certainly most of those commonly cited in that publication period, are included in this review. We regret any inadvertent exclusions.

General outcomes and issues

Table 1.2 lists the issues and topics that have found some form of representation in the sample of articles reviewed. It is by no means the case that all of the elements below have been deliberately measured and analysed. Most of those that have been represent issues that were raised in the course of the research, or concerns expressed as part of findings or conclusions.

Table 1.2 List of concerns and measures in the review sample

adolescents	cochlear implant non-use
adult role models	cochlear implant on and off
aetiology	cochlear implants and tinnitus
age	cognition
age at implantation	communication mode
audiological performance	communicative behaviour
audiovisual speech cues	communicative development
behaviour	comparison of children versus adults
choice	comparison of congenitally deaf with
cochlear implant evolution	prelingually deaf
cochlear implant candidacy	comparison with tactile vocoders

Table 1.2 List of concerns and measures in the review sample contd.

comparison with hearing aids
comparison with hearing peers
comparison with non-cochlear implant
   deaf
cost benefits
cost-effectiveness
cost utility
deaf child of deaf parents
deaf culture
developmental plasticity
device failure
early communicative behaviour
early diagnosis and neonatal screening
early education
educational placement
educational resources
equivalent hearing loss
feature identification
future performance
grammar
health economics
health technology
home environment
human resources
identity
individual variance
inclusion
interaction attitude
interscorer reliability
interviews
language delay
language development
language processing
literacy
mainstream
meta-analysis
minimal skills
mismatch negativity
mode of communication
morphology
motor and cognitive delays
multi-handicap

multilingualism
music
narrative ability
natural oral/aural approach
neurophysiology
parents' perspectives
patient factors
peer relationships
phonology
post-implantation period
preschool
preconditions
prediction
prior performance
professional collaboration
personal and social development
psychological factors
psychological wellbeing
quality of life
reimplantation
reading and writing
rehabilitation
resources
sign language
signal processing
social integration
speech intelligibility
speech perception
speech production
speech recognition
speech therapy
stress
teachers' perspectives
temporal versus spatial sequencing
test development
test evaluation
test reliability
training
verbal and spatial working memory
video analysis
visual attention
working memory

Chapter 2

A summary of outcome measures

Introduction

This chapter aims to provide a brief overview of the research in the field of paediatric cochlear implantation available at the time of writing; the reviewed papers are presented individually and in alphabetical order in Chapter 3. A number of key areas of research are discussed briefly to facilitate access to the more detailed review. Some papers here cover a number of areas and thus appear under more than one heading.

This chapter does not offer a critical review of the papers; this is given for individual publications in Chapter 3, and for the research in general in Chapter 4, where there is a detailed consideration of outcomes themselves and the emphasis of the research. Chapter 4 also includes a consideration of the various factors that contribute to the effectiveness of cochlear implantation.

Speech recognition

Since the aim of cochlear implantation is to restore some functional hearing, research measuring the effects of the intervention focuses mainly on spoken language, and in particular, on the ability to hear speech – referred to as speech recognition.

Speech recognition is one of the most researched outcomes in the available literature. One of the most common findings in research measuring speech-recognition skills in cochlear-implanted children is the wide variation in individual performance. A number of characteristics common in the research itself may significantly account for this key finding. First, the age distribution in the sampled populations is often very wide, although in some instances attempts were made to control for the effect of age on results. For example, the population reported in Gantz et al. (1994) ranges in age from 20 months to 15 years, but even in 2001, Hildesheimer et al. reported on a population of 81 with an age range between 1.6 and 16 years, while also including 39 adults.

Second, the demographic reporting focuses mostly on audiological, implant and placement criteria to the exclusion of others. Relative to the huge range of factors that may affect outcome (comparable to those in deaf education, cf. Powers et al. 1998: 19), there is a more general under-analysis of demographic sample characteristics and few attempts at factoring out intervening variables. Hence any number of outside factors might help to explain individual variation. Indeed, some research reporting on speech recognition measures does so with this in mind. For example, Pyman et al. (2000) focused on delayed milestones in cognitive and motor development, Dawson et al. (2000) on electrode discrimination. Lesinski et al. (1995) and Hamzavi at al. (2000) report on outcomes in multi-handicapped cochlear-implanted children, while Gordon et al. (2000) targeted professionals supporting cochlear-implanted children who attained below-average speech-perception outcome scores in a survey on likely factors involved in underperformance.

Third, varying preoperative performance may account for variation postoperatively (Zwolan et al. 1997) and research effort here is therefore relevant to issues in cochlear implant candidacy.

Speech recognition and age at implantation

Meyer et al. (1995) report in an investigation on 71 cochlear-implanted children that younger implanted children outperformed older implanted children; the research concerns limited measures at a single point in time. Tye-Murray et al. (1995) concluded that children implanted before the age of 5 years may well show greater benefit than those implanted aged over 5. In their sample of 28 children, the implant age ranged from 31 to 170 months (average 85 months). Fryauf-Bertschy et al. (1997) found no significant differences in performance for children implanted before the age of 5 years, at either 36- or 48-month test intervals among their sample of 34 children implanted between the ages of 3 and 5 years. Lesinski et al. (1997) split their substantial sample of 359 cochlear-implanted children implanted at the University of Hannover into those implanted below age 4 and those implanted later – an arbitrary disaggregation. They note greater performance increases for those implanted younger.

In Tait and Lutman's work on early communicative behaviour (1997), the effect of age at implantation is illustrated in case studies rather than enumerated. In Tyler et al. (1997b), the 'implanted young' group (2–4 years) outperformed the 'implanted old' (4–9 years) group in the 36 months post-implantation test measures. The sample size is not recorded, but reference is made to the Fryauf-Bertschy et al. (1997) population of 34 children. Waltzman et al. (1997b) broke down their sample of 38 implanted children into two groups – those implanted below age 3 (*n* = 15) and those implanted between the ages of 3 and 5 (*n* = 23). They observed that speech-perception scores of all children improved over time, up to 5-year post-implantation data, and concluded that cochlear implants provide significant and usable speech perception for children implanted before the age of 5. Illg et al. (1999) concluded that younger implanted children make more rapid gains than older implanted children, who tend to plateau between 12 and 18 months post implantation; they comment that deaf children aged 1–5 can benefit most from implantation. Their sample comprised 167 children, with age at implantation ranging from 15 months to 15 years (average 6.5 years).

Lenarz et al (1999) report speech-perception findings relating to a population of nine children implanted before the age of 2, and reported encouraging outcomes in a summary fashion. Miyamoto et al. (1999) observed that age at implantation correlates significantly with speech-perception measures. Their sample of 33 children is divided into three groups: those implanted before the age of 3 years (n = 14), those implanted between age 3 and 3.11 years (n = 11) and those implanted between 4 and 5 years (n = 8). Nikolopoulos et al. (1999) concluded that prelingually deaf children implanted before the age of 8 years will develop significant auditory perception. Allum et al. (2000) note that children implanted at a very young age (below 3 years) improved little in the first 6 months, but thereafter improved much faster than those implanted at a later age – these later-implanted children were more susceptible to an adaptation effect of renewed auditory stimulation. The sample's age range at implantation is broken down per cochlear implant device, a breakdown that is less helpful in the context of the other variables recorded.

Dorman et al. (2000) recognized that the deaf child with a cochlear implant must deal with an auditory signal that is seriously degraded – they note that the use of at least eight active electrodes is required for a less excessively prolonged period of language acquisition post implantation. In distinguishing between 43 'late-implanted' children (mean 5.4 years of age) and 13 'early implanted' children (mean 3.3 years of age), they observed that the distribution of scores for early- and late-implanted children differed, but not their overall performance. Gordon et al. (2000) report that all of the participating children who ultimately achieved no open-set word recognition skills were implanted at ages beyond 5 years, with over five years of deafness. Nevertheless, they concluded that these factors alone cannot account for speech-perception performance, and should not be used in isolation to make predictions of post-implant performance.

Lesinski et al. (2000) report summary details of speech-perception outcomes for a population of 70 and, based on an arbitrary subdivision on the basis of age at implantation (above or below 4 years), they concluded that group mean outcome performance was greater for those implanted below age 4. McDonald Connor et al. (2000) observed that although younger age at implantation positively affects the overall outcomes according to their complement of measures, there is no such effect for receptive vocabulary development, where the group of implanted children reflected an overall growth rate increasingly behind that of the (hearing) test standardization data.

Nikolopoulos et al. (2000) report, for a population of 130 unselected children with cochlear implants, that 36- and 48-month post-implantation CAP (Categories of Auditory Performance) scores were significantly associated with age at implantation. O'Donoghue et al. (2000) report that age at implantation is an important co-variate, with post-implant speech-perception test score improvements measured for up to five years in a sample of children implanted at a mean age of 52 months (range 30 months to 7 years). Tyler et al. (2000a) suggest that a minimum of three years' worth of post-implantation test score data are needed to demonstrate that children implanted below age 3.5 years generally obtain higher post-implantation speech-perception scores; their conclusion resets that age to below 3 years.

Tyler et al. (2000b) report that prelingually deafened children may obtain speech-perception scores as high as, or even higher than, those of adults. Harrison et al. (2001) noted that out of a sample of 70, the PB-K scores of children implanted below (exactly) 8.4 years are significantly better than the scores of those implanted later – theirs is a study design characterized by a particularly powerful statistical measure for this correlation. Although they find overall robust differences in performance based on age at implantation, they nevertheless insist that the complexity of an overall outcome assessment significantly moderates considerations of age at implantation. Hildesheimer et al. (2001) replicated the general study design (comparing child with adult implantees) of Tyler et al. (2000b), and arrived at a similar conclusion: implanted children do not achieve lower outcomes than implanted adults.

Nakisa et al. (2001) report that age at implantation correlated positively with functionally equivalent age (implanted below age 4 years), with functionally equivalent hearing level and functionally equivalent aided thresholds, in a study reporting on 31 cochlear-implanted children. Baumgartner et al. (2002) split their sample into those implanted below the age of 3 years and those implanted later, and reported outperformance by those implanted earlier. But although the two group sizes are similar, the overall age range at time of implantation was 0.9–9 years; therefore there is a much wider chronological age distribution in the 'older' implanted group. Hence the correlation will borrow some of its effect from the artificial disaggregation for age at implantation, a recognized problem with randomly split sample subdivisions.

Speech recognition and cochlear implant experience

Ideally, implant experience should be investigated over time. Experience is something that builds up slowly in individuals, and is therefore not well measured by recording one single point-in-time measure in a population with varying individual experience, and then disaggregating by the level of experience. Furthermore, this measure in particular is sensitive to sample size falling significantly over time, and reduced statistical effect over time as a result.

Kiefer et al. (1996) report that the percentage of children in their sample (n = 19) scoring above chance, and the level of scores, both improved as a significant effect over time. Implant experience, as well as duration of deafness and age at onset, correlated strongly with test scores of the four-year period. In Boothroyd's (1997) investigation, implant experience explained 7% of variance in test performance. In his sample of 50 children, the implant age ranged from 0.9 to 5.3 years (mean 2.6 years). Fryauf-Bertschy et al. (1997) measured a significant correlation between amount of daily use of a cochlear implant and speech-perception test performance, repeated at 36- and 48-month intervals. Their sample of 34 children have 3–5 years of cochlear implant experience. Experience of the cochlear implant significantly correlated with IPSyn scores in the sample of 29 in a study by Tomblin et al. (1999), outperforming chronological age as a factor in a comparison with deaf children using hearing aids. By contrast, Dawson et al. (2000) concluded that cochlear implant experience did not account for significant variance in speech-perception scores in their sample of 17 children with implant experiences ranging between 1.5 and 7 years in their study on active electrode discrimination. Nakisa et al. (2001) did find significant interaction between cochlear implant experience and speech-perception scores for the sample of 31 children in their modelling of functionally equivalent age, hearing level and aided thresholds.

Speech recognition and age at onset

Age at onset is differentiated at two levels, one medical and one linguistic. The first differentiation is between those children born deaf (congenital deafness) and those children deafened after birth (acquired deafness) – this is primarily a medical assessment. This differentation is often linked to aetiology. Second, a distinction is made between those children deafened before the onset of language development (prelingual deafness) and those children who became deaf later (postlingual deafness) – this is primarily a linguistic assessment. Note that prelingually deaf children, more commonly interpreted as those children who became deaf before their third birthday, may also be congenitally deaf, and so on. The differentation between pre- and postlingual onset of deafness is particularly problematic because linguistic evidence is divided on the nature of language triggers and critical periods for language development (see in particular Szagun 2001).

In their 1994 study, Gantz et al. compared the over-time (four-year) speech-perception scores of congenitally deaf children with those of prelingually deaf children deafened by meningitis. They concluded that congenitally deaf children outperformed the prelingually deaf group, and noted that any prior auditory stimulation the prelingually deaf children may have enjoyed prior to the onset of meningitis was negated by the adverse effects of that illness. Shea et al. (1994) report that postlingually deaf children outperformed prelingually deaf children in their study, but the postlingual deaf group included only four subjects, while there was great migration across tests and over time in their study. Kiefer et al. (1996), however, noted a strong correlation between test scores over time (four years) and age at onset; the latest age at onset in their sample of 19 was 14 years, while the sample contained 14 prelingually deafened children (age at implantation range 3–18 years).

In Boothroyd's (1997) study, age at onset of deafness did not account for any variance in test scores, in either the cochlear implant group ($n = 50$, range of age at onset 0–14 years) or in the deaf children using hearing aids. Nikolopoulos et al. (1999) noted significant increases in outcome scores over time (six years) in 103 prelingually deafened cochlear-implanted children, all implanted before age 8. In their survey of support professionals, Gordon et al. (2000) noted a predominant concern for the combinatory factor of duration of deafness and chronological age, and reported a correlation between these and depressed speech-perception outcome scores for their small population of five cochlear-implanted children.

Speech recognition and long-term findings

Although many reports make reference to long-term findings, the length of time is on a continuum across the reports, starting at just two years post implantation. The earliest research to report five-year post-implantation data included in this review is that by Gantz et al. (1994). Their concern was with issues of candidacy, and much of the comparison is between prelingually and congenitally deaf children. The clear ceiling effects noticeable on some outcome measures might reflect the relatively early (in this review) publication date, but also raise issues about the appropriateness of existing speech-perception measures and tests. Tye-Murray et al. (1995) report on 28 total communication children, and noted that sign language does not disappear from the communication of postoperative children. The paper is included here because of its reference to 'prolonged experience' in the title; the average experience among the sample is 36 months. Kiefer et al. (1996) report on data up to five years postoperatively, but the distribution of the population size at the different intervals remains unclear, while the overall low number reduces the statistical power of the findings.

Fryauf-Bertschy et al. (1997) report on 34 children with 3–5 years' experience; their analysis concerns the effect of age at implantation on outcome performance, but some findings are weakened by the significant age range of the population (2–15 years at implantation). Mondain et al. (1997) report on 64 French cochlear-implanted children, but their over-time measure (up to four years postoperative) was an artificial construct, since it concerned a single point-in-time measure of children with varying levels of cochlear implant experience. Tyler et al. report four-year (1997a) and five-year (1997b) data of the Fryauf-Bertschy (1997) population – all of whom were in total communication settings – but the lack of demographic description complicates interpretation of findings. Waltzman et al. (1997b) report up to five years' postoperative data, but the population size dropped dramatically over time, from 38 in year 1 to three in year 5. However, all children were implanted below age 5, making for an unusually homogeneous sample. Waltzman et al. (1997a) report data up to four years post implantation, but their confused reporting does not present a clear set of findings, while their sample size dropped to just three children at the four-year test interval.

Illg et al. (1999) report data for up to two years postoperatively, and the initial sample size was considerable, with 167 children. However, for unexplained reasons the sample size dropped to ten children at the two-year interval, while the absence of demographic description or comparison with other deaf children leaves the findings wanting for a valid interpretation. Nikolopoulos et al. (1999) report speech-perception outcomes of 103 children up to six years post implantation, attesting to the great value of the detailed follow-up programme in situ. Allum et al. (2000) report three-year data (single point-in-time) for 71 children, against a hypothesis involving maturation of the audiology cortex and a 'catching-up' period following implantation. Gstöttner et al. (2000) report three-year postoperative data on German cochlear-implanted children; the population size of 31 at the first test interval dropped dramatically over time.

Hamzavi et al. (2000) report on speech performance in a population of ten multi-handicapped, cochlear-implanted children out of direct concern with issues of cochlear implant candidacy; in their view, not all multi-handicapped children should be contraindicated for implantation. Tyler et al. (2000a) report no less than seven-year data for the Fryauf-Bertschy (1997) cohort, and also report on a comparison between prelingually deafened children and postlingually deafened adults (Tyler et al. 2000b). Baumgartner et al. (2002) report that up to two years of experience were required for their sample of 33 implanted children to attain 'adequate' speech-perception skills; analysing data for three years post-implantation they noted that children implanted below age 3 years outperformed those implanted at a later age.

Speech recognition and comparisons with other aided populations

Comparisons between cochlear implant users and deaf children using other types of hearing aids are commonplace in the literature. More usefully it has resulted in the notion of 'equivalent hearing loss': an assessment of the (aided) level of hearing loss at which the outcome performance of hearing-aided children is roughly equivalent to that of cochlear implant users. Boothroyd and Eran (1994) report on such a direct comparison with the purpose of establishing an unaided hearing loss threshold for a working notion of equivalent hearing loss, and they found a direct correlation between IMSPAC scores and assessments of equivalent hearing loss as an effect of age at implantation.

Geers and Brenner (1994) report on an element of the CID study, and compare speech-perception outcomes of CID children with cochlear implants with deaf children using other hearing aids but enrolled in the same oral programme, concluding that cochlear-implanted subjects outperformed those using other hearing aids. Eilers et al. (1996) observed that cochlear-implanted children did not significantly outperform children using tactile vocoders, but the comparison drew on cochlear implant data published five years earlier.

Miyamoto et al. (1995) report on a direct comparison between the speech-perception outcomes of cochlear-implanted children and those of hearing-aided children, but their findings are weakened by the recombination of data from different time intervals. The theme of equivalent hearing loss is emergent within their account, which groups hearing aid users according to functional performance. Boothroyd (1997) applied the notion of equivalent hearing loss in the assessment of the value of the IMSPAC test. Geers (1997) reported on CID research, which had dropped the tactile aided children but included a five-year over-time assessment of a hearing aid group matched with cochlear-implanted children. Meyer et al. (1998) contribute a comparison between cochlear-implanted and hearing aid children in an assessment of the notion of equivalent hearing loss using a significant-sized population of 74 children. In their 1998 study, Osberger et al. (1998) suggested that cochlear-implanted children outperform hearing-aided children in an assessment more driven by placement concerns. Spencer et al. (1998) contribute a single point-in-time comparison between cochlear implant and hearing aid users, focusing on sublexical performance indicators.

Truy et al. (1998) contribute a small-scale study on French cochlear-implanted children compared with hearing aid users, and in their conclusions remained unusual in demonstrating a keen awareness that speech is but one communication option available to cochlear-implanted deaf individuals. Svirsky and Meyer (1999) report on a comparison of 221 cochlear-implanted children with smaller samples of hearing aid users in a single point-in-time measure that also reported on communication mode. Tomblin et al. (1999) report a single point-in-time speech-perception measure contrasting the three-year post-implantation performance of 29 cochlear-implanted children (age range 2–13 years) with that of non-implant children. They suggested that cochlear implant experience correlated with performance for cochlear-implanted children, but chronological age correlated with performance for non-implanted children.

Dorman et al. (2000) made a valuable contribution in a comparison between cochlear-implanted children and hearing children being given an impoverished (cochlear implant equivalent) input signal. Blamey et al. (2001) contribute a carefully balanced and analysed set of findings on 40 cochlear-implanted children compared with 40 hearing aid users, and drew on natural language development to compare the relative contributions of each type of aid. Their general account provides significant detail for the notion of equivalent hearing loss. Lachs et al. (2001) tested cochlear-implanted children for communication mode against the hypothesis involving knowledge of the vocal tract and the presence of both visual and motor skills. Nakisa et al. (2001) report on the value of a computer-based test design, while comparing cochlear-implanted children with both normally hearing children and deaf children with hearing aids.

Speech recognition and candidacy

Cowan et al. (1997) report on a study using speech-perception performance indicators to correlate with preoperative residual hearing levels, arguing for a loosening of implant candidacy criteria. Gantz et al. (1999) investigated the speech-perception scores of a subset of implanted children, focusing on those with prior residual hearing. They noted that this subpopulation, who had prior limited word understanding using hearing aids, attained higher outcome scores than did profoundly deaf non-implanted children. Blamey et al. (2001) differed on such findings, arguing instead that language performance behaves independently of residual hearing. Zwolan et al. (1997) report on a comparison between children with some versus children with no preoperative speech-perception skills, suggesting that cochlear implantation may be appropriate for children with some prior speech-perception skills.

Speech recognition and educational placement

Osberger et al. (1994) report on a comparison between implanted oral programme children and total communication children, with outcomes that replicated the research on oral children of the previous decades. Hodges et al. (1999) investigated a range of placement and communication mode-related factors using speech-perception performance in 40 children, but their research findings are invalidated by auditory mode-only test administered to total communication children. Miyamoto et al. (1999) report on 33 children according to placement, aggregated according to age at implantation, all within a narrow chronological age range (all were 4 years old at the time of testing).

Svirsky and Meyer (1999) report on communication mode in 221 cochlear-implanted children using speech-perception tasks. Daya et al. (2000) report changes in placement following cochlear implantation, motivated by improved speech-perception outcome. McDonald Connor et al. (2000) contribute a highly significant study of 147 cochlear-implanted children. Their study is statistically detailed, but their performance measures concerned spoken language exclusively, which weakens their findings in relation to placement. O'Donoghue et al. (2000) report on a study of 40 children, which included analysis of a number of key variables (including placement as well as inserted electrodes and socio-economic status); the authors recognize the value of disaggregation for age, but the study would have lost statistical power. Diller et al. (2001) report on 103 cochlear-implanted children in a much larger study on placement for deaf children in Germany. They noted that the speech performance of some cochlear-implanted children reflected normal rates of language acquisition.

Speech recognition and other factors

Purdy et al. (1995) used speech-perception data of 6–12 months post implantation as a variable correlating with parental stress. Given the low population size ($n = 6$) and the short time interval post implantation, their results are likely to prove tentative. Tait and Lutman (1997) used postoperative speech-perception performance to assess the predictive validity of pre-verbal communicative behaviour assessments, an exercise repeated in Tait et al. (2000) for 33 children. Dawson et al. (1998, 2000) used speech-perception measures to assess the value of a language-independent feature discrimination test. Kirk (1998) did the same to assess the LNT test. In a further study, Kirk et al. (2000) showed that lexical difficulty and talker variability affect outcomes. Young et al. (1999) used speech-perception measures to compare different cochlear implant manufacturers' devices;

serious test design weaknesses and small overall numbers characterize their assessment. Frisch and Pisoni (2000) focused on speech-perception tasks to clarify the relative contribution of different theories of speech-perception strategy. Davidson et al. (2000) showed that the better the growth of loudness across the intensity scale, the better the speech-perception score suggesting an effect of the match between the user and the working of the device.

Gordon et al. (2000) focused on a subsample of cochlear-implanted children scoring low on speech-perception measures, to identify possible influencing factors in a survey design. Kirk et al. (2000) observed that lexical difficulty, stimulus variability and word length were significant test factors in speech-perception outcomes among 28 implanted children tested. Pyman et al. (2000) measured speech-perception performance in a subsample of 75 children characterized as having suffered 'delayed milestones' in cognition or motor skills, in an attempt to explain some of the individual variation of outcome performance. Harrison et al. (2001) report on 70 cochlear-implanted children using a variety of tests and subjected the results to a binary partitioning algorithm to divide the dataset on the basis of age at implantation. One of their significant findings is that tests have a varying 'optimum' age at their maximum performance point – in other words, tests outcomes vary with age distribution.

Huang and Huang (1997) report on eight Mandarin-speaking implanted children, with data limited to one year post implantation. The study, which is mainly of interest because Mandarin is a tone language, found clear speech-perception gains across their population, but no effect for tone itself. Hildesheimer et al. (2001) report a study on Hebrew children that compared speech-perception scores of cochlear-implanted children with those of cochlear-implanted adults; the findings are limited by the overall lack of description. Finally, Parisier et al. (2001) report on a study focused on speech-perception performance after reimplantation necessary because of device failure, reporting mainly that speech-perception performance generally improved following reimplantation.

Reviewed material on speech recognition

Allum JH, Greisiger R, Straubhaar S, Carpenter MG (2000)
Archbold SM, Nikolopoulos TP, Tait M, O'Donoghue GM, Lutman ME, Gregory S (2000)
Baumgartner WD, Pok SM, Egelierler B, Franz P, Gstöttner W, Hamzavi J (2002)
Blamey PJ, Sarant JZ, Paatsch LE, Barry JG, Bow CP, Wales RJ, Wright M, Psarros C, Rattigan K, Tooher R (2001)
Boothroyd A (1997)
Boothroyd A, Eran O (1994)
Cowan RS, DelDot J, Barker EJ, Sarant JZ, Pegg P, Dettman S, Galvin KL, Rance G, Hollow R, Dowell RC, Pyman B, Gibson WP, Clark GM (1997)
Davidson L, Brenner C, Geers A (2000)

Dawson PW, McKay CM, Busby PA, Grayden DB, Clark GM (2000)

Dawson PW, Nott PE, Clark GM, Cowan RS (1998)

Daya H, Ashley A, Gysin C, Papsin BC (2000)

Diller G, Graser P, Schmalbrock C (2001)

Dorman MF, Loizou PC, Kemp LL, Kirk KI (2000)

Eilers RE, Cobo-Lewis AB, Vergara KC, Oller D et al. (1996)

Frisch SA, Pisoni DB (2000)

Fryauf-Bertschy H, Tyler RT, Kelsay DM et al. (1997)

Gantz BJ, Rubinstein JT, Tyler RS, Teagle HFB, Cohen NL, Waltzman SB, Miyamoto RT, Kirk KI (1999)

Gantz BJ, Tyler RS, Woodworth GG, Tye-Murray N, Fryauf-Bertschy H (1994)

Geers AE (1997)

Geers A, Brenner C (1994)

Gordon KA, Daya H. Harrison RV, Papsin BC (2000)

Gstöttner W, Hamzavi J, Egerlierler B, Baumgartner WD (2000)

Hamzavi J, Baumgartner WD, Egelierler B, Franz P, Schenk B, Gstöttner W (2000)

Harrison RV, Panesar J, El-Hakim H, Abdolell M, Mount RJ, Papsin B (2001)

Hildesheimer M, Teiltelbaum R, Segal O, Tenne S, Kishon-Rabin L, Kronenberg Y, Muchnik C (2001)

Hodges AV, Dolan Ash M, Balkany TJ, Schloffman JJ, Butts SL (1999)

Huang WH, Huang TS (1997)

Illg A, von der Haar-Heise S, Goldring JE, Lesinski-Schiedat A, Battmer RD, Lenarz T (1999)

Kiefer J, Gall V, Desloovere C, Knecht R, Mikowski A, von Ilberg C (1996)

Kirk KI (1998)

Kirk KI, Hay-McCutcheon M, Sehgal ST, Miyamoto RT (2000)

Lachs L, Pisoni DB, Kirk KI (2001)

Lenarz T, Lesinski-Shiedat A, von der Haar-Heise S, Illg A, Bertram B, Battmer RD (1999)

Lesinski A, Battmer RD, Bertram B, Lenarz T (1997)

Lesinski A, Hartrampf R, Dahm MC, Bertram B, Lenarz T (1995)

Lesinski A, von der Haar-Heise S, Battmer RD, Cords S, Goldring J, Lenarz T (2000)

McDonald Connor C, Hieber S, Arts HA, Zwolan TA (2000)

Meyer V, Hertram B, Lenarz T (1995)

Meyer TA, Svirsky MA, Kirk KI, Miyamoto RT (1998)

Miyamoto RT, Kirk KI, Svirsky MA, Sehgal ST (1999)

Miyamoto RT, Kirk KI, Todd MA, Robbins AM, Osberger M (1995)

Mondain M, Sillon M, Vieu A, Tobey E, Uziel A (1997)

Nakisa MJ, Summerfield AQ, Nakisa RC, McCormick B, Archbold S, Gibbin KP, O'Donoghue GM (2001)

Nikolopoulos T, Archbold SM, Lutman ME, O'Donoghue GM (2000)

Nikolopoulos TP, Archbold SM, O'Donoghue GM (1999)

O'Donoghue G, Nikolopoulos TP, Archbold SM (2000)

Osberger MJ, Fisher L, Zimmerman-Phillips S, Geier L, Barker MJ (1998)

Osberger MJ, Robbins AM, Todd SL, Riley Al (1994)

Parisier SC, Chute PM, Popp AL, Suh GD (2001)

Purdy SC, Chard LL, Moran CA, Hodgson SA (1995)

Pyman B, Blamey P, Lacy P, Clark G, Dowell R (2000)

Shea JJ, Domico EH, Lupfer M (1994)

Spencer LJ, Tye-Murray N, Tomblin JB (1998)

Svirsky MA, Meyer TA (1999)

Tait DM, Lutman ME (1997)

Tait DM, Lutman ME, Robinson K (2000)

Tomblin JB, Spencer L, Flock S, Tyler R, Gantz B (1999)

Truy E, Lina-Granade G, Jonas AM, Martinon G, Maison S, Girard J, Porot M, Morgon A (1998)

Tye-Murray N, Spencer L, Woodworth GG (1995)

Tyler RS, Fryauf H, Gantz BJ, Kelsay DMR, Woodworth GG (1997a)
Tyler RS, Fryauf-Bertschy H, Kelsay DMR, Gantz BJ, Woodworth GP, Parkinson A (1997b)
Tyler RS, Gantz BJ, Woodworth GG, Fryauf-Bertschy H, Kelsay DMR (1997c)
Tyler RS, Kelsay DMR, Teagle HFB, Rubinstein JT, Gantz BJ, Christ AM (2000a)
Tyler RS, Rubinstein JT, Teagle H, Kelsay DMR, Gantz BJ (2000b)
Tyler RS, Teagle HFB, Kelsay DMR, Gantz BJ, Woodworth GG, Parkinson AJ (2000c)
Waltzman SB, Cohen NL, Gomolin RH, Green J, Shapiro W, Brackett D, Zara C (1997a)
Waltzman SB, Cohen NL, Gomolin RH, Green JE, Shapiro WH, Hoffman RA, Roland JT (1997b)
Young NM, Gorhne KM, Carrasco VN, Brown C (1999)
Zwolan TA, Zimmerman-Phillips S, Ashbaugh CJ, Hieber SJ, Kileny PR, Telian SA (1997)

Speech production

Speech production and the intelligibility of speech

The key difference between speech production and speech intelligibility measures is that in the former the assessment will usually include scoring the linguistic content of the output; while in the latter case, the focus is on the clarity or pronunciation of the productions, and this is usually scored by one judge or a panel of judges. However, as will be seen in some of the studies described in this review, there is some confusion between the use of terms, and studies do not always distinguish between the two outcomes.

Speech production and age at implantation

The imitative nature of the IMSPAC test means that findings concerning correlation between speech perception and age at implantation will most likely be replicated for speech production in the investigation of Boothroyd and Eran (1994). Those implanted at an earlier age derived greater sensory benefit from their implants – no details specifically regarding speech production are provided in their report. Tye-Murray et al. (1995a) investigated the ability to produce the speech features of nasality, voicing, duration, frication and place of articulation in three different perceptual conditions in 23 young cochlear-implanted children. They concluded that information received from cochlear implants might influence young cochlear-implanted children's speaking behaviours after an average of 34 months of experience, but results are equally characterized by the large numbers of errors made by the children. Tye-Murray et al. (1995b), in their sample of 28 cochlear-implanted children, concluded that while older-implanted subjects achieved higher scores prior to implantation, this performance gap was closed two years post implantation.

Vermeulen et al (1999) used the Reynell scale to consider the rate of spoken language development after implantation. Allen and Dyar (1997) focused on a sample of pre-verbal deaf children who were implanted; they found that three years after implantation all children in their sample were able to be reliant on spoken language communication. Molina et al. (1999) investigated the speech production of eight implanted 2-year-olds, noting that post implantation the children increased use of spoken language, while the use of sign language steadily decreased – these were children placed in a mainstream kindergarten with logopedic support. McDonald Connor et al. (2000) concluded from their findings on 147 cochlear-implanted children that implantation during preschool years resulted in higher gains relative to implantation during primary school years – in fact, the younger the child at implantation, the better the spoken language outcomes. This was particularly true for their measures of consonant production and vocabulary development. There were also contradictory findings for the combination of age at implantation and placement, with oral subjects implanted below the age of 5 demonstrating an advantage in consonant production, and total communication subjects implanted below age 5 demonstrating an advantage in vocabulary development.

Speech production and age at onset of deafness

Gantz et al. (1994) report overall greater rates of improvement for prelingual implanted children relative to post-lingual implanted children, although they offer few detailed findings in relation to speech production (as opposed to speech perception). The sample is distorted, with 54 prelingually deafened cochlear-implanted children (of whom 44 are congenitally deaf) being properly described, in contrast with only five postlingually deafened cochlear-implanted children for whom no descriptive demographic detail is offered. Uziel et al. (1995) report on a population of deaf children implanted at Montpellier, and observed that phoneme detection was achieved by all subjects 3 months post implantation, with a mean group score of 85%; a ceiling effect was evident at one year post implantation. The prelingually deaf children tended to outperform the congenitally deaf children by 6–18 months post implantation, an effect possibly due to brief auditory experience prior to the onset of deafness.

Speech production and long-term findings

Tye-Murray et al. (1995b) report that after two years of cochlear implant experience the younger children performed mostly level with children who were older; for those children using sign language communication prior to implantation, the use did not discontinue, so that across the population there was an increase in simultaneous communication. Although the paper claims to focus on 'prolonged' implant experience, it is not made entirely clear how this is to be interpreted. As a criterion of inclusion, the children had worn their implants for at least two years. Waltzman et al. (1997) report five-year over-time findings for a research sample that dropped from 48 children at implantation to just three children at the five-year interval. They report a mean growth of 48 months for expressive vocabulary, but their reporting provides insufficient detail to interpret that finding meaningfully.

Speech production and comparisons with other aided populations

Boothroyd and Eran (1994) assessed performance on IMSPAC (imitative test of the perception of phonologically significant speech pattern contrasts) to evaluate the predictive power of this test for eventual sentence production; they failed to achieve a clear result, but did find a correlation between IMSPAC scores and assessments of equivalent hearing loss as an effect of age at implantation. Geers and Moog (1994) set up a triadic comparison in the ongoing CID programme of research, comparing cochlear-implanted subjects with hearing aid and tactile vocoder users. They report that cochlear-implanted subjects significantly outperformed those in other groups by three years post implantation. In a comparison of cochlear-implanted children with two groups of hearing-aided children in the CID programme, Geers (1997) reported equivalent speech production scores for the cochlear-implanted children and the 90–100 dB hearing aid users. Although there was no statistical difference, Spencer et al. (1998) found that children with cochlear implant experience produced significantly more English-inflected morphemes than did a comparison group of hearing-aided children. Molina et al. (1999) reported a tentative correlation between psychomotricity, bucco-facial ability, auditory perception and discrimination and speech articulation in eight implanted subjects. Tomblin et al. (1999) report superior story retell scores for cochlear-implanted children compared with scores for hearing-aided children, but the result was not statistically significant across the 29 children. Blamey et al. (2001) concluded that children showed a wide scatter about the average speech production score of 40% of words correctly produced in spontaneous conversations, with no significant upward trend with age and no real difference between cochlear-implanted and hearing-aided children.

Speech production and educational placement

McDonald Connor et al. (2000) observed over-time improvement of consonant-production accuracy and expressive and receptive vocabulary, regardless of oral or total communication programme, in a study involving no fewer than 147 cochlear-implanted children. Diller et al. (2001) claim that development of hearing and speech skills correlates with how well the hearing device has been adapted and the quality of education received, as well as with the actual language spoken by the family.

Speech production and other factors

One reason to differentiate between congenitally deaf implanted children and deafened implanted children is the effect that prior experience of audition – no matter how brief – might have on children's ability to adapt to, and make the most of, their cochlear implant. Gantz et al. (1994) compared prelingually implanted children with congenital implanted children and noted encouraging findings for speech production in the prelingual cohort, but overall, experiencing 'a brief exposure to acoustic input does not appear to be a significant advantage for the group with prelingually acquired deafness' (p.5). Dawson et al. (1995) report on a pre- and postoperative interval speech articulation test on 12 late-implanted subjects (average age at implantation 9 years, range 8–19 years) and observed significant improvement. Allen and Dyar (1997) report in very general terms on a profiling exercise three years following implantation. Perrin et al. (1999) compared cochlear-implanted children with matched hearing control children on a story retell task; they concluded that cochlear-implanted children took longer to retell the story, but they could not find any systematic differences in the output. Tait et al. (2000) report that three-year postoperative data on telephone use and speech-production ability were not significantly associated with pre-implant (communicative behaviour) measures.

Reviewed material on speech production

Allen SE, Dyar D (1997)
Blamey PJ, Sarant JZ, Paatsch LE, Barry JG, Bow CP, Wales RJ, Wright M, Psarros C, Rattigan K, Tooher R (2001)
Boothroyd A, Eran O (1994)
Dawson PW, Blamey SJ, Dettman LC et al. (1995)
Diller G, Graser P, Schmalbrock C (2001)
Gantz BJ, Tyler RS, Woodworth GG, Tye-Murray N, Fryauf-Bertschy H (1994)
Geers AE (1997)
Geers A, Moog J (1994)
McDonald Connor C, Hieber S, Arts HA, Zwolan TA (2000)
Molina M, Huarte A, Cervera-Paz FI, Manrique M, Gracia-Tapia R (1999)
Perrin E, Berger-Vachon C, Topouzkhanian A, Truy E, Morgon A (1999)
Spencer LJ, Tye-Murray N, Tomblin JB (1998)
Tait DM, Lutman ME, Robinson K (2000)

Tomblin JB, Spencer L, Flock S, Tyler R, Gantz B (1999)
Tye-Murray N, Spencer L, Gilbert-Bedia E (1995a)
Tye-Murray N, Spencer L, Woodworth GG (1995b)
Uziel AS, Reuillard-Artieres F, Sillon M et al. (1995)
Vermeulen A, Hoekstra C, Brokx J, van den Broek P (1999)
Waltzman SB, Cohen NL, Gomolin RH, Green J, Shapiro W, Brackett D, Zara C (1997)

Speech intelligibility

A key feature of the measure of speech intelligibility, which measures the extent to which utterances are understood, is the use of judges. Here, too, different options are used. Most studies opt for the use of multiple judges, often paired with a measure of inter-rater reliability, or at the least a method of randomizing speech production sample distribution among judges. In cases where only a single judge is used, this is usually a trained professional in a cochlear implant rehabilitation team. Some studies include a scheme for scoring the quality of spoken language.

Speech intelligibility and long-term findings

Tye-Murray et al. (1995) report disappointing speech intelligibility outcomes, in terms of 10 listeners' ratings and their correct story identification, in research on 28 implanted children aged between 31 and 170 months at implantation. Mondain et al. (1997) observed steady improvement in speech intelligibility over time in 64 French-speaking implanted children, but found no correlation between speech-intelligibility and speech-perception scores over time. Allen et al. (1998) used the speech intelligibility rating scale (SIR) with a population of 84 children (all below 7 years at implantation) and found 'some intelligible connected speech' for 85% after four years. Improvements were significant over the first years, but not significant 4–5 years post implantation.

Speech intelligibility and comparisons with other aided populations

McConkey Robbins et al. (1995) compared speech intelligibility of 61 cochlear-implanted children with that of two groups of hearing aid users. After 3.5 years the speech intelligibility of cochlear implant users was generally between that of 'gold' (90–100 dB) hearing aid users and 'silver' (101–110 dB) hearing aid users, as scored by experienced listeners.

Speech intelligibility and mode or placement measures

Osberger et al. (1994) report that greater improvement in speech intelligibility over time is associated with placement, but the reporting is not based on significant numbers or statistical evaluation. Miyamoto et al. (1999) found that only the main effect of communication mode was significantly correlated with their measure of speech intelligibility for 33 children. Archbold et al. (2000) found that cochlear-implanted children using oral communication remained one standard category above cochlear-implanted children using total communication on the SIR. Tobey et al. (2000) found that children with 4–6 years' experience of their cochlear implant in oral education had better speech intelligibility outcomes than did children with similar implant experience in a total communication setting, but the oral cohort received double the amount of speech therapy. Finally, Lachs et al. (2001) observed that children who received more benefit from audiovisual presentation also produced more intelligible speech, and they suggest a close link between speech perception and production and a common underlying linguistic basis for audiovisual enhancement effects. Implanted children in oral education outperformed those in total communication settings. On average, naive adult listeners could correctly identify 17.13% of the words produced by the implanted children on an elicited sentence-production task.

Speech intelligibility and other factors

Tye-Murray et al. (1996) observed no significant relationship between implant on- and implant off-scores on a story retell activity, in research on 20 subjects; one single trained listener assessed the output. Chin et al. (2001) compared sub-lexical speech performance with sentence-level speech performance and found that perception and production of overall consonant and vowel contrasts correlate positively and significantly with sentence intelligibility; but they noted that at finer levels of analysis the pattern of correlation is weak.

Reviewed material on speech intelligibility

Allen C, Nikolopoulos T, O'Donoghue GM (1998)
Archbold SM, Nikolopoulos TP, Tait M, O'Donoghue GM, Lutman ME, Gregory S (2000)
Chin SB, Finnegan KR, Chung BA (2001)
Lachs L, Pisoni DB, Kirk KI (2001)
McConkey Robbins MS, Kirk KI, Osberger MJ et al. (1995)
Miyamoto RT, Kirk KI, Svirsky MA, Sehgal ST (1999)
Mondain M, Sillon M, Vieu A, Tobey E, Uziel A (1997)

Osberger MJ, McConkey Robbins AM, Todd SL, Riley AI, Miyamoto R (1994)
Tobey EA, Geers AE, Douek BM, Perrin J, Skellet R, Brenner C, Toretta G (2000)
Tye-Murray N, Spencer L, Gilbert-Bedia E (1996)
Tye-Murray N, Spencer L, Woodworth GG (1995)

The development of language and communication

Most studies in this category focus on spoken language development rather than the development of sign language or of communication in general. In addition, many studies in the research listed below use the term 'language development' to refer to the acquisition of spoken language. Usually, the term refers simply to the measures of speech perception and speech production combined into a single overall measure of (spoken) 'language development'. Studies of children's narrative or story-telling ability are also included here. In some instances, the term 'language development' is used to refer to results of a specific test, such as the Reynell Developmental Language Scale, which can be problematic and is discussed in more detail in Chapter 4. Sign language is the focus of very few studies, and the use of sign language by the children is rarely assessed and often not recorded.

Spoken language development outcomes

Most studies of spoken language development report progress, but at a slower rate than that for hearing children. For example, Blamey et al. (2001) concluded that language development progress for 47 cochlear-implanted children and matched hearing-aided children was steady, but slower than for hearing children. Brinton (2001) used a standardized spoken language development test, measuring only the early development of spoken language structures including grammar, vocabulary and syntax in monitoring intelligibility and auditory performance (PLS-3), to test 12 implanted children, and observed steady improvement over time. Moog and Geers (1999) reported that all but one of the 22 cochlear-implanted children in their study scored within two standard deviations of hearing children of the same age, and four of the cochlear-implanted subjects scored within 80% of their hearing peers on reading. Allen and Dyar (1997) concluded, using a generalized profile, that it takes 18 months for implanted children to achieve 'functional language status'. The work of Tait and Lutman (1994, 1997, 2000) also supports this finding. However, the main emphasis of Tait and Lutman's work is the establishment and validation of an assessment of early pre-verbal communication to provide a means of assessing the role of early communication as a predictor of later language development.

Some studies do report development at a rate similar to that of hearing children. Miyamoto et al. (1997) found, for 23 cochlear-implanted children aged between 1.5 and 8 years, their spoken language developed at a rate roughly equivalent to that of hearing children, noting that a rate of half that of hearing children is commonly reported in the literature for non-implanted deaf children

A series of studies by McConkey Robbins and colleagues (1995, 1997, 1999), based on the Reynell, suggest that children with cochlear implants show improvement greater than that due to maturation alone. In their study in 2000, they reported faster rates of improvement at 6 months compared to the 12-month postoperative interval, and suggest this may be attributable to an 'equilibration period'.

Crosson and Geers (2000) found that the narrative ability of cochlear-implanted children, whether in oral or total communication programmes, was different from that of a hearing control group. The cochlear implant appeared to have a positive effect on narrative ability, although this function was not found to be statistically significant. In a follow-up study published one year later (Crosson and Geers, 2001), they comment that the syntax of deaf and hearing groups is different, with the deaf children using fewer temporal conjunctions. Moreover, they found that narrative ability is a good predictor of reading skill.

Szagun (2001) tested differing theories of language acquisition triggers and patterning on a sample of 22 cochlear-implanted children. She concluded that language development continues to be delayed relative to that of hearing peers. However, since some cochlear-implanted children did acquire language at a comparable developmental rate, the evidence overall points towards a 'sensitive period' model of language acquisition which does not draw on the notion of a 'trigger age'.

Reviewed material on spoken language development

Allen SE, Dyar D (1997)
Blamey PJ, Sarant JZ, Paatsch LE, Barry JG, Bow CP, Wales RJ, Wright M, Psarros C, Rattigan K, Tooher R (2001)
Brinton J (2001)
Coerts JA, Mills AE (1995)
Crosson J, Geers A (2000)
Crosson J, Geers A (2001)
Cullington H, Hodges AV, Butts SL, Dolan-Ash S, Balkany TJ (2000)
Inscoe J (1999)
Lutman ME, Tait DM (1995)
McConkey Robbins AM, Bollard PM, Green J (1999)
McConkey Robbins AM, Green J, Bollard P (2000)
McConkey Robbins AM, Osberger MJ, Miyamoto RT, Kessler KS (1995)
McConkey Robbins AM, Svirsky M, Kirk KI (1997)

Miyamoto RT, Kirk KI, Svirsky MA, Sehgal ST (1999)
Miyamoto RT, Svirsky MA, Robbins AM (1997)
Moog JS, Geers AE (1999)
Szagun G (2001)
Tait DM, Lutman ME (1994)
Tait DM, Lutman ME (1997)
Tait DM, Lutman ME, Robinson K (2000)
Wang HL, Toe D (1998)

Sign language outcomes

This review did not identify any studies that examined the development of
sign language following implantation; rather studies considered whether
or not children who sign continue to do so after they have been implanted. The small number of studies identified (3) indicates that this was the
case. Tye-Murray et al. (1995) suggest that over a two-year period, most
of the 28 children studied continue to rely heavily on a combination of
speech and signing. Preisler et al. (1997) present data for 19 young
cochlear-implanted deaf children in Swedish sign-bilingual education.
They suggest that 16 of the implanted children continue to use sign language as their primary mode of communication three years after
implantation. However, these results come from studies where the focus is
sign language. Other studies that focus on spoken language development
suggest more variability in the use of sign language after implantation.

Reviewed material on sign language

Coerts JA, Mills AE (1995)
Preisler G, Ahlstrom M, Tvingstedt AL (1997)
Tye-Murray N, Spencer L, Woodworth GG (1995)

Educational placement and communication approach

In recent years, there has been a worldwide trend towards the inclusion
of all children with any disability into mainstream schools, and this has
been reflected in the educational provision for deaf children. Although the
terminology used in different countries may differ, the usual choices for
placement of deaf children are: schools for the deaf; special classes in
mainstream schools, often called units or resource bases; or placement in
a mainstream school with varying degrees of specialist support. Studies of
deaf children with cochlear implants have looked at the placement of
these children and endeavoured to identify trends in comparison to those
without cochlear implants.

For deaf children, the communication approach in education is identified in terms of the language or mode used. Three main categories may be identified: oral/aural methods without the use of sign; the use of sign language and the spoken language of the community (a sign bilingual approach); and total communication, where spoken language is used, supported by varying degrees of sign language. The difficulty for researchers is not only to classify the method being used with, and by, the child (as there is a wide range of styles in practice), but also to assess the extent to which the communication used in the classroom actually reflects the child's preferred language.

Educational placement outcomes

The implicit assumption of many of the studies is that mainstream placement is a measure of success of implantation, and Nevins and Chute (1995) reported that all but two of 16 implanted children performed outstandingly in their mainstream setting. Age at implantation, duration of deafness and length of cochlear implant experience have all been found to be significant predictors of placement (Archbold et al. 1998; Francis et al. 1999).

The research suggests that children with implants experience placements similar to severely, rather than profoundly, deaf pupils. Archbold et al. (2002) found that 42 profoundly deaf cochlear-implanted preschoolers shared their placement characteristics with severely deaf children of the same age. Fortnum et al. (2002) reached a similar conclusion in a UK study that included 757 cochlear-implanted children.

Some studies also report a change in placement following implantation. Daya et al. (2000) report that of 30 cochlear-implanted children in non-mainstream settings, nine moved to mainstream schools some time after implantation. Archbold et al (2000) raise questions as to the implications of such moves.

Communication approach outcomes

Some studies report no difference in outcomes for oral and total communication settings. For example, McDonald Connor et al. (2000) found no difference in speech perception or production performance in 147 implanted children, and McConkey Robbins et al. (1997) report roughly equivalent outcomes for 23 cochlear-implanted children.

Where a difference is reported, it is in favour of oral settings. Osberger et al. (1998) observed that 19 cochlear-implanted children in oral settings were significantly outperforming 11 cochlear-implanted children in total communication settings. Miyamoto et al. (1999) found significant effects of communication mode in results in speech-perception and speech-production assessments, and on the Reynell Developmental Language Scale (RDLS). Cullington et al. (2000) found that oral subjects demonstrated significantly less spoken language delay than did total communication subjects, based on speech-perception scores only; speech-production scores were not significantly correlated with communication mode. Geers et al. (2000) studied 31 cochlear-implanted children and concluded that those enrolled in programmes reliant on spoken language were better able to derive auditory benefit from their cochlear implant than those in settings that included the use of sign, although the oral and signing groups had different levels of support. Geers et al. (2002) report on a study that included 136 8- to 9-year-olds, and concluded following elaborate multivariate analysis that an oral approach is an important option for children with cochlear implants.

Reviewed material on educational placement and communication approach

Archbold SM, Nikolopoulos T, Lutman ME, O'Donoghue GM (2002)
Archbold SM, Nikolopoulos TP, O'Donoghue GM, Lutman ME (1998)
Archbold SM, Nikolopoulos TP, Tait M, O'Donoghue GM, Lutman ME, Gregory S (2000)
Cullington H, Hodges AV, Butts SL, Dolan-Ash S, Balkany TJ (2000)
Daya H, Ashley A, Gysin C, Papsin BC (2000)
Fortnum HM, Marshall DH, Bamford JM, Summerfield AQ (2002)
Francis HW, Koch ME, Wyatt JR, Niparko JK (1999)
Geers AE (2004)
Geers A, Brenner C, Nicholas J, Uchanski R, Tye-Murray N, Tobey E (2002)
Geers A, Nicholas J, Tye-Murray N, Uchanski R, Brenner C, Davidson L, Torretta G (2000)
McConkey Robbins AM, Svirsky M, Kirk KI (1997)
McDonald Connor C, Hieber S, Arts HA, Zwolan TA (2000)
Miyamoto RT, Kirk KI, Svirsky MA, Sehgal ST (1999)
Nevins ME, Chute PM (1995)
Osberger MJ, Fisher L, Zimmerman-Phillips S, Geier L, Barker MJ (1998)

Psychological and social outcomes

Despite their clear significance, psychological and social outcomes are an under-reported element of cochlear implant outcome research, an issue that is discussed in Chapter 4.

Psycho-social outcomes

Positive social and psychological outcomes are reported by Knutson et al. (2000), who observed no evidence of negative psychological consequences of cochlear implantation for the 24 cochlear-implanted children aged between 2 and 13 years in their study. Filipo et al.'s (1999) analysis of post-implant findings showed a reduction of stereotype elements, more dynamic modes of figurative expression, quite good relationships within their own social environment, and gradual, positive integration both at home and at school among cochlear-implanted children researched. Bosco et al. (1999), in a paper that is more a discussion paper than a research report, suggest positive psycho-social outcomes for a group of adolescents in terms of communication and social interaction.

Knutson et al. (1997a) sought to investigate suggestions – apparently deriving from within the deaf community – that those parents seeking an implant for their child are in some socio-psychological way different from those parents who do not. They concluded that children with hearing impairments and their families who were seeking cochlear implants are not significantly different from children with hearing impairments whose parents were not seeking a cochlear implant. Spencer et al. (1997) report that cochlear implantation improves reading, comparing users and matched non-implanted deaf adolescents, and Wald and Knutson (2000) report that both groups were most inclined towards a bicultural (deaf/hearing) identity. No differences between the two groups were found for measures on social competence; moreover, implanted adolescents were largely in agreement with non-implanted peers on beliefs about deafness and deaf culture.

Reviewed material on psycho-social outcomes

Bosco E, D'Agosta L, Ballantyne D (1999)
Filipo R, Bosco E, Barchetta C, Mancini P (1999)
Knutson JF, Boyd RC, Goldman M, Sullivan PM (1997a)
Knutson JF, Boyd RC, Reid JB, Mayne T, Fetrow R (1997b)
Knutson JF, Wald RL, Ehlers SL, Tyler RS (2000)
Spencer L, Tomblin JB, Gantz BJ (1997)
Wald RL, Knutson JF (2000)

Parents' perspectives

These studies break down into two distinct types. In one group, the parents are invited to communicate their own views on process or outcome. This feedback can be taken at face value, or it can be re-interpreted – as, for example, in calculations of parental stress, or in research using discourse analysis to capture underlying patterns of significance to responses. The second group of studies includes those in which parents are considered 'gate-keepers' to information that may otherwise be difficult to obtain; for example parents may be asked for information on their implanted child's peer friendship patterns. A further difference is the methodology employed. Parents will usually either be sent a questionnaire or be interviewed. Either method can use open or closed responses, leading towards either qualitative or quantitative types of analysis.

A number of studies report parents' satisfaction with the outcomes of implantation. Archbold et al. (2002) report an open-ended, written questionnaire study that included parents of 30 children with cochlear implants. Parents reported positive changes in behaviour and communication. Kluwin and Stewart (2000) suggest that from parents' perspective, language and speech rather than improved social skills or social contact are the primary benefits of the implant. Studies have also considered whether parents' initial expectations were realistic. Beadle et al. (2000) report for parents of 17 implanted children that they were pleased with the outcomes; no particular stress was noted, and prior expectations were found to be reasonably matched with outcomes. Kelsay and Tyler (1996) report that parents have 'realistic expectations' of cochlear implant outcome and parents also report steady improvements over time.

Bat-Chava and Deignan (2001) found that parents reported positive outcomes for their cochlear-implanted children in terms of communication and other factors, but also felt that their sons and daughters would continue to benefit from interaction with deaf peers, since despite the potential for improved relationships with hearing peers, communication obstacles will continue to limit free association.

Other studies report on parental stress. Purdy et al. (1995) report high stress levels among parents of cochlear-implanted children in a study in New Zealand, and Incesulu et al. (2004) suggest that cochlear implantation is a stressful process for families, although their results are not straightforward.

Reviewed material on parents' perspectives

Archbold SM, Lutman ME, Gregory S, O'Neill C, Nikolopoulos TP (2002)
Bat-Chava Y, Deignan E (2001)
Beadle EA, Shores A, Wood EJ (2000)
Incesulu A, Vural M, Erkam U (2003)
Kelsay DMR, Tyler RS (1996)
Kluwin TN, Stewart DA (2000)
Osberger MJ, Geier L, Zimmerman-Phillips S, Barker MJ (1997)
Purdy SC, Chard LL, Moran CA, Hodgson SA (1995)

Cognitive outcome measures

These measures are represented by a mixture of studies looking at various aspects of cognition, often alongside other variables. Some of the studies examine an outcome that demands more specialized input and assessment tools, such as work on memory skills or temporal sequencing.

Preisler et al. (1997) concluded from their qualitative study into a sample of cochlear-implanted preschool children in Sweden that teachers tended to overestimate implanted children's spoken language skills, while at the same time tending to underestimate children's cognitive ability. Spencer et al. (1997) investigated reading skills, and Crosson and Geers (2001) identified narrative ability as an important predictor of reading comprehension ability, in particular over and above IQ and syntactic competence.

Quittner et al. (1994) tested cochlear-implanted deaf children, non-implanted deaf children and hearing children on a visual speeded selective response task, and concluded that the results show evidence for developmental dependencies between sensory modalities – in this case between vision and hearing. Smith et al. (1998) continued the work by Quittner et al. (1994). This investigation was more clearly targeted, used a larger sample, and allowed the authors to elaborate a multicomponent model of development and task performance, following from their findings that sensitivity to environmental sounds is related to the beginning of developmental changes in the control of visual attention.

Cleary et al. (2001) concluded that deaf children (irrespective of input modality and with no distinctions between implanted and non-implanted children) have atypical working memories, characterized by differences in memory span observed between hearing and deaf cohorts. Pisoni and Geers (2000) looked specifically at correlations between digit span (working memory) and speech-perception and intelligibility measures. They identified working memory as a systematic source of variation in performance on these measures.

Reviewed material on cognitive outcomes

Cleary M, Pisoni DB, Geers AE (2001)
Crosson J, Geers A (2001)
Pisoni D, Geers A (2000)
Preisler G, Ahlstrom M, Tvingstedt AL (1997)
Quittner AL, Smith LB, Osberger MJ, Mitchell TV et al. (1994)
Smith LB, Quittner AL, Osberger MJ, Miyamoto RT (1998)
Spencer L, Tomblin JB, Gantz BJ (1997)

Economic evaluation outcomes[1]

A small number of economic evaluations have been undertaken with reference to the paediatric population of cochlear implant users. The consensus among these papers is that cochlear implantation is cost-effective compared to other healthcare interventions. The magnitude of cost-effectiveness varied most in sensitivity analyses which adjusted length of device use and outcome. However, these papers have been based on assumptions and data from a limited number of centres of excellence and countries (USA, UK, Australia and Germany). Of particular concern is the reliance upon assumptions concerning outcome – only two studies used empirical values elicited in their own study (Bichey et al. 2002; Cheng et al. 2000). The type of economic evaluation undertaken has been mainly cost–utility analysis, where outcome is measured in terms of quality-adjusted life-years (Bichey et al. 2002; Carter and Hailey 1999; Cheng et al. 2000; Hutton et al. 1995; Lea and Hailey 1995; O'Neill et al. 2000, 2001; Summerfield et al. 1997).

Since utility does not measure all the appropriate outcomes from paediatric cochlear implantation (that is, it focuses on health-related quality of life outcomes only), a number of authors have attempted to perform cost-benefit analyses (Francis et al. 1999; Summerfield and Marshall 1999; Schulze-Gattermann et al. 2002). However, since these studies incorporate only the costs avoided (i.e. educational cost savings), they would be most appropriately termed cost-minimization or cost analyses. The results from these studies cannot be used to make resource allocation decisions as they only consider financial resources and, as such, interventions would only be funded if they were cost saving without regard to the outcomes of the intervention in question. To attach monetary values to the outcomes of the intervention in cost-benefit analysis, studies need to perform techniques, such as contingent valuation, to measure the willingness of individuals in society to pay for paediatric cochlear implantation. All studies have been classified according to authors' published reports, for example where authors state education costs as indirect costs, even where this classification may be technically incorrect. Some of these issues will be picked up on in the observation sections.

By 2002 no published study had reported results from cost-effectiveness analysis. The main reason for this lies in the fact that authors were addressing the allocative efficiency issue of whether or not paediatric cochlear implantation offered value for money compared to other healthcare interventions. However, this focus has meant that technical efficiency

---

[1] Terms used in health economics are described in the Glossary of Health Economic Terms.

issues, that is how resources can be better deployed within cochlear implantation in order to improve outcomes, have been overlooked.

Reviewed material on economic evaluation outcomes

Bichey BG, Hoversland JM, Whynne MK, Miyamoto RT (2002)
Carter R, Hailey D (1999)
Cheng AK, Rubin HR, Powe NR, Mellon NK, Francis HW, Niparko JK (2000)
Francis HW, Koch ME, Wyatt R, Niparko JK (1999)
Hutton J, Politti C, Seeger T (1995)
Lea RA, Hailey DM (1995)
O'Neill C, Archbold S, O'Donoghue GM, McAllister DA, Nikolopoulos TP (2001)
O'Neill C, O'Donoghue GM, Archbold S, Normand C (2000)
Schulze-Gattermann H, Illg A, Schoenermark M, Lenarz T, Lesinski-Schiedat A (2002)
Summerfield AQ, Marshall DH (1999)
Summerfield AQ, Marshall DH, Archbold SM (1997)

Other outcome measures

In addition to the categories discussed so far, a number of other outcomes of paediatric cochlear implantation have been investigated. What characterizes these outcomes is that, in comparison with those covered earlier, they have been given less attention to the date of the search – the modest number of studies focused on the outcomes reported in them is indeed the only reason why these studies are grouped together here. This is not at all to suggest that these are outcomes that are less important. In some instances, they concern an outcome, such as cultural identity, that is extremely difficult to measure or interpret. They may focus on a group that is not often considered, such as children with additional disabilities. Also included here is another literature review, a meta-analysis using published texts to form a secondary analysis sample population (Cheng et al. 1999).

Archbold et al. (1998) surveyed 273 teachers of deaf children; they report that teachers of deaf children see working with cochlear-implanted deaf children as a positive professional experience, with most of them supporting the practice of cochlear implantation in deaf children. Easterbrooks and Mordica (2000) investigated teachers' ratings of the functional communication with cochlear-implanted children; they report two correlations between teachers' ratings and address (of the child), and teachers' ratings and known aetiology, concluding merely that this topic needs further investigation.

Koch et al. (1997) investigated the cost implications of cochlear implantation on educational resources and concluded that the cochlear implant has favourable financial effects on the system, but their assessment is hampered by an overly simplistic model of deaf education provision.

Rose et al. (1996) surveyed US schools and reported the often-quoted finding that 47% of those implanted were no longer using their implant; the findings are heavily contested, in particular by cochlear implant centres' local figures.

With the interesting exception of telephone use, 80% of parents reported 'at least some' benefit of their child's cochlear implant in 20 categories of assessment, an assessment made by Chmiel et al. (2000) following the circulation of a closed-question questionnaire to 21 parents. Significantly, the questionnaire also included 11 responses by the cochlear implantees themselves. The question format was derived from that used by Kelsay and Tyler (1996).

Gfeller et al. (1998) investigated music activities and appreciation in a sample of cochlear-implanted children. They found that music activities are common, especially in mainstream primary education, although generally few accommodations are made for cochlear-implanted pupils.

Reviewed material on other outcomes

Archbold S, Robinson K, Hartley D (1998)
Cheng AK, Grant GD, Niparko JK (1999)
Chmiel R, Sutton L, Jenkins H (2000)
Easterbrooks SR, Mordica JA (2000)
Gfeller K, Witt SA, Spencer LJ, Stordahl J, Tomblin B (1998)
Harrigan S, Nikolopoulos TP (2002)
Koch ME, Wyatt JR, Francis HW, Niparko JK (1997)
Lesinski A, Hartrampf R, Dahm MC, Bertram B, Lenarz T (1995)
Paganga S, Tucker E, Harrigan S, Lutman M (2001)
Rose DE, Vernon M, Pool AF (1996)

Chapter 3

The research reviews

This chapter contains the research reviews listed in alphabetical order.

Allen C, Nikolopoulos T, O'Donoghue GM (1998) Speech intelligibility in children following cochlear implantation. American Journal of Otology 19: 742–746.

Population size
   84
Population comments
   11 at 5 years
Demographics
   Age at onset: ≤ 3 years (mean 6 months, range 0–34 months)
   Age at CI: 7 years (mean 52 months, range 21–84 months)
   Duration of deafness: mean 46 months, range 2–81 months
   Up to five years' cochlear implant use
Selection criteria
   Consecutive implantation at one centre (Nottingham)
Dependent variables
   Speech intelligibility (speech intelligibility rating scale, SIR) at yearly intervals for five years
Independent variables
   Age at onset
   Aetiology
   Socio-economic status range (no detail)
   Educational needs range (no detail)
   Communication mode (no detail)
Method
   Mann-Whitney U-test
Results
   Speech intelligibility ratings increased significantly across all children each year for four years (years 4–5 did not). 'Intelligible speech' was achieved three years after CI. At four years 85% had some intelligible connected speech. At five years, median intelligibility was category 4 (speech is intelligible to a listener who has little experience of a deaf person's speech).
Conclusions
   Congenital and prelingually deaf children gradually develop intelligible speech that does not plateau five years after implantation.
Observations
   The SIR test administration obtained a high inter-observer reliability (0.9). The highest and lowest performances are detailed in the article, accompanied by background information. Some language delay in three children was put down to illness in intervening periods, and language delay in two children to gradual device failure leading to reimplantation.

Allen SE, Dyar D (1997) Profiling linguistic outcomes in young deaf children after cochlear implantation. American Journal of Otology 18: s127–s128.

Population size
47
Demographics
Age: 'preverbal'
Age at CI: range 2.7–8.6 years (mean 4.2 years)
Selection criteria
No selection criteria or sampling method given. Most likely the sample was selected from one cochlear implant centre (Nottingham)
Dependent variables
Descriptive purpose only
Independent variables
Communication (pragmatics)
Receptive skills
Expressive skills
Voice
Speech skills
Profile of Actual Linguistic Skills profile
Method
General profiling
Results
All 'preverbal' children were able to rely on speech as a primary means of communication three years post implantation. The majority of children had achieved 'transitional linguistic competences' (PALS category) by the end of year 1.
Conclusions
It takes at least 18 months or longer for preverbal cochlear-implanted children to attain functional language status.
Observations
The research was not aimed at measuring outcomes; instead it aimed to introduce PALS as a profiling tool. Even so, there is limited descriptive information on the sample. In particular, home situation, ethnicity, socio-economic status, additional needs and educational placement might be expected to impact on the results quoted.

Allum JH, Greisiger R, Straubhaar S, Carpenter MG (2000) Auditory perception and speech identification in children with cochlear implants tested with the EARS protocol. British Journal of Audiology 34(5): 293–303.

Population size
71
Demographics
Aetiology: unknown (51), meningitis (14) progressive (2)
CI device: Med-El C40+ (21), Nucleus Mini 22 (35), Mini 24 (15)
Speech processing strategy: CIS (Med-El), SPEAK replaced with ACE for Mini 24 (Nucleus)
Age at CI: range 1:7–14:6 years, average 6:9 years (Med-El), range 1:9–14:0 years, average 6:7 years (Nucleus)
CI experience: average 14 months
PTA: 1–8 kHz > 100 dB HL
Programme: auditory rehabilitation programme (= oral placement)
Selection criteria
None detailed

Dependent variables

EARS (LiP, MTP, MAIS, MUSS) in mother tongue – German, French, Italian or Spanish

Independent variables

Age at implantation

CI experience

Method

Ad-hoc statistical evidence using repeated measures ANOVA (significance levels identified with Bonferroni (adjusted) t-test)

Results

Preoperative scores on LiP and MAIS were significantly greater for over-7-year-olds relative to below 7 ($p < 0.01$) (p.295). Those aged below 3 scored significantly lower on LiP at 1-month ($p < 0.10$), 3-month ($p < 0.05$) and 12-month ($p < 0.01$) post-implant intervals (p.295).

Individual scores show that all children made improvements over time with a significant interaction between age and time ($p < 0.0001$) (p.296). This followed an initial drop in outcome significant only for the over-7-year-olds ($p < 0.1$).

With preoperative scores used as baseline (as opposed to the first postoperative scores), improvements were significantly greater at 6 months for the under-7-year-olds compared to over-7-year-olds ($p < 0.05$), with first significant improvements for under-3-year-olds at 12 months. Although results revealed faster improvement rates after 6 months, at 18 and 24 months postimplantation there were still significant differences in LiP scores between age groups (p.296).

MTP scores were significantly influenced by time for the over-7-year-olds ($p < 0.0006$) (p.298); an average plateau value of 0.8 was reached at 24 months (p.299). These results were largely replicated for MAIS scores ($n = 55$).

Conclusions

'... all children except the very young with meningitis showed significant improvements by 1–3 months' (p.300).

'... those over 7 years of age having higher preoperative performance are highly susceptible to an adaptation effect of repeated "new" auditory stimulation and therefore to performing more poorly immediately after first fitting of the cochlear implant speech processor' (p.300).

'... very young children (those aged 3 years and younger), deafened as a result of meningitis, appear to improve very little in the first 6 months, but thereafter improve rapidly. Thus, the most important factors influencing post-operative performance appear to be duration of cochlear implant experience and prior auditory experience as a result of advanced (over 7 years) age. Other factors, such as aetiology, play a secondary role' (p.300).

Observations

A Swiss study looking at two critical factors, age of the child at implantation and the amount of experience with the CI. Speech perception measures (derived from the EARS protocol) are recorded as dependent variables in a population of 71 children divided into three groups: those implanted above aged 7, those below aged 7, and those aged 3 or below (deafened by meningitis) at the time of implantation. The central hypothesis of this study is that duration of stimulation with a cochlear implant correlates with maturation of the audiology cortex once stimulation is provided; the question is whether performance improvements vary between age groups. The authors report that an earlier study has shown that 15 years of auditory input are required for cortically evoked potentials to develop normal adult latencies, while delays in access merely delay the maturation process (p.294). Such evidence might appear to contraindicate the notion of a 'critical age' for language development (and is contrary to the evidence on vocabulary acquisition) as a pure audiological measure of that development, so that '... time exposed to sound is a more significant variable than the onset or duration of deafness (Kiefer et al. 1996; Miyamoto et al. 1995; Tye-Murray et al. 1995)...' (p.294).

This study therefore concerns the ability of children with cochlear implants to 'catch up' with (near) normal auditory development patterns. The period of analysis is very limited – there are only two years' worth of data post implantation – but the population size is significant.

All children showed improvements after 6–12 months, with the rate of improvement differing between age groups. The eldest children showed greater pre-implant performance that dropped following cochlear implantation and recovered over 1–3 months, to demonstrate improvements at later test intervals. Children under age 7 approached performance levels of the older children after 12 months' cochlear implant experience. Under-3-year-olds made little progress over the first 6 months but approached test levels of under-7-year-olds by 18 months.

Archbold SM, Lutman ME, Gregory S, O'Neill C, Nikolopoulos TP (2002) Parents and their deaf child: their perceptions three years after cochlear implantation. Deafness and Education International 4(1): 12–40.

Population size
  30
Population comments
  Parents of 30 children with cochlear implants
Demographics
  'All social strata ... educated in a wide range of schools' (p.14)
  Age at onset: at birth (9), acquired (21)
  Age at CI: range 30–131 months (mean 50 months)
  Gender: boys (16), girls (14)
  The sample may not be representative of those now receiving implants, since deafness
    threshold criteria have been widened (p.14)
Selection criteria
  First 30 children implanted at Nottingham to fulfil the following criteria: born deaf, or
  deafened under age 3
Dependent variables
  Not applicable
Independent variables
  Child functioning
  Parental implications
  Family implications
  Process of implantation
  Educational liaison
  Most useful influences on progress
  Intrusiveness of intervention and rehabilitation
  Future needs
  Advice to other parents
  Open-ended written response questionnaire sent to parents three years post implantation
Method
  Randomized reporting of written responses according to themes addressed in open-
  ended written questionnaire
Results
  Widespread comments pertaining to increased self-confidence, easier communication,
  positive changes in spoken language development, improved behaviour and greater
  independence are reported (p.19). A majority of the parents commented on links between
  the cochlear implant and educational placement and achievement (p.21).

  An issue emerging across themes is improved potential for social interaction, at
  school, at home, with peers and with the wider family.

  The operation, and the first few months following it, are reported to be the most
  challenging to families (p.26–27).

One of the strongest issues to emerge from the parents was the perceived need for long-term educational liaison between implant centre and school (n = 29, :31).

Conclusions

'Three issues particular to this group emerged from the scripts:

(1) the change in confidence and communication abilities [...]

(2) their reliance on the functioning of the technology and on the expertise of the cochlear implant centre [...]

(3) the necessity for close liaison between implant centre and educational services' (p.38).

Observations

This is a recent study reporting on the parents' views of 30 children with cochlear implants. The study aimed to explore the perceptions of parents without limiting them to prescribed issues (p.14), with a view to deriving a closed questionnaire that can be used in future quantitative assessments of the impact of paediatric cochlear implantation on families and their children.

The scripts reported are rich in detail on personal considerations and beliefs, and demonstrate the strength of a qualitative approach. Themes covered are relatively wide-ranging, starting at child behaviour and communicative ability prior to cochlear implantation, via the operation itself, to the impacts of the implant on family and school life for both parents and child.

Given the clear focus on spoken language acquisition following cochlear implantation, more information on the parents' child communication strategies prior to cochlear implantation, and the nature of the advice given to them as parents by specialists and educational services, would have been welcome. This would have given a better understanding of any 'change in approach' taken with the child, and in particular to what extent the post-implantation effects on, for example, behaviour and communication might derive from more focused and 'expert' input by the implant team and its resources. But it must be recognized that this concerns children who would have been very young prior to cochlear implantation.

What emerges from the scripts is a more general recognition of a logic of common sense among the parents, taking stock of the current state of interaction between deafness, the community, resources and policy making. For example, in making the case for putting their deaf child through a serious operation, it is reported that:

'We felt this gave him a CHOICE for his future using both or either British Sign Language or spoken language' (p.23).

'... in order to make the best of himself in a hearing world, for whether we like it or not, that is what it is' (p.23).

Archbold SM, Nikolopoulos T, Lutman ME, O'Donoghue GM (2002) The educational settings of profoundly deaf children with cochlear implants compared with age-matched peers with hearing aids: implications for management. International Journal of Audiology 41(3): 157–161.

Population size

42

Population comments

Profoundly deaf three years post CI, comparison groups of 635 severely deaf and 511 profoundly deaf age-matched children

Demographics

Age at CI: 5 years (mean 3.3 years, range 1.8–4.8 years)

CI use: ≥ 3 years (age range 4.8–7.8 years)

Socio-economic status range (details not given)

Educational backgrounds (details not given)

Aetiology: meningitis (25), congenital (14), other (3)
Communication mode: 24 oral, 18 total communication
CI device: Nucleus multichannel

Selection criteria

Age-matched
All CIs received implants before beginning school (<5 years)
UK selection
No exclusions

Dependent variables

Placement: school for the deaf, unit or special class in mainstream, and full-time mainstream

Independent variables

CI

Method

Comparison of placement with groups listed in BATOD (British Association of Teachers of the Deaf) survey. Chi-square analysis

Results

Three years after implantation 38% (16) of the cochlear-implanted children attended mainstream, 57% (24) were in a special class attached to mainstream, 5% (2) were in deaf schools. Of the non-cochlear-implanted profoundly deaf children these figures are 12% (63), 55% (239), 33% (167); in the severely deaf group the figures are 38% (239), 51% (326) 11% (70).

The difference with the profoundly deaf children was significant ($p = 0.00001$), while the difference with the severely deaf group was not.

Conclusions

The population of profoundly deaf children implanted before school share placement characteristics with severely deaf children of the same age in the UK.

Observations

This study arose from an interest in the current emphasis on mainstreaming and inclusion in current education provision in the UK, and the impact this might have on children with cochlear implants.

The focus in this study on preschool cochlear-implanted children probably removed the likelihood of the child's educational settings remaining fixed regardless of progress with the implant system, due to funding issues or local inflexibility in the educational system, so that this particular measure provides information for future comparisons.

Factors such as socio-economic status, geographic location, LEA budgets, other disabilities and ethnicity, may all influence placement, suggesting that a more detailed study over larger numbers remains necessary.

Despite these provisos, it will be clear that the focus on spoken language skills in cochlear implantation intervention, cochlear implantation rehabilitation and inclusionary policies will mean that children with cochlear implants are more likely to attend mainstream schools than children with hearing aids with the same degree of deafness.

Archbold SM, Nikolopoulos TP, O'Donoghue GM, Lutman ME (1998) Educational placement of deaf children following cochlear implantation. British Journal of Audiology 32: 295–300.

Population size

48

Population comments

In addition, a group of 121 pre-implantation placements, of which 47 were classified as preschool prior to implantation.

Demographics

Placement prior to CI (121): preschool (47), school for the deaf (27, 37%), units (35, 47%), mainstream (12, 16%).

Geography: national distribution

Socio-economic status: varied

Age at onset: acquired (61, 49 result of meningitis), range 6–79 months, average 19 months; born deaf (60)

Age at CI: average 44 months, range 21–203 months

Deafness: > 95 dB HL

CI device: Nucleus 22 multichannel

Speech processor: latest type

Rehabilitation: wide variation involving local teachers and cochlear implant teachers

Subgroup (n = 48)

Age at onset: acquired (30), range 0–79 months, average 16:4 months; congenital (18)

Age at CI: most common 51 months, average 65:8 months

Placement: oral (20), total communication (28)

Selection criteria

First 121 consecutively implanted children, Nottingham; no exclusions reported

Dependent variables

Placement: preschool, school for the deaf, unit or resource base (mainstream) and full-time mainstream

Independent variables

Age at CI

Duration of deafness

Prior placement

Preschool placement

Method

Chi-square analysis, one-way analysis of variance (ANOVA) between duration of deafness and placement; Mann-Whitney U-test to compare age at implantation between placement groups at two-year interval

Results

Age at implantation and duration of deafness found to be significant predictors of placement two years after CI. The duration of deafness of children in schools for the deaf, or units, was double that of those in mainstream education. Fifty-three percent of children who were in preschool at the time of implantation were found to be in mainstream schools two years after CI, while the respective percentage of children who were already in educational placements at the time of implantation was 6% (statistically significant difference) (p.295).

Of the 17 children in preschool prior to implantation, eight were in mainstream two years after CI. Two were in schools for the deaf, while five were in units. Compared with the early placements of those in education prior to implantation, this represents a shift from deaf school placements towards mainstream placement that is significant ($p = 0.001$) (p.297).

Age at implantation was statistically significantly lower in children in a mainstream setting compared with those in a unit ($p = 0.002$) and compared with those in a school for the deaf ($p = 0.004$), suggesting a correlation between experience of the cochlear implant and placement (p.297). Discriminant analysis confirmed that children with shorter duration of deafness are more likely to be found in mainstream schools ($p = 0.004$) (p.297).

Conclusions

Children implanted earlier were more likely to go to mainstream schools than the profoundly deaf children in the UK (p.295).

Age at implantation and duration of deafness are predictors of educational placement two years after implantation (p.298).

Placement overall is stable, with little change across individuals (p.298); this may have causes prior to cochlear implantation itself, including funding arrangements.

'… if mainstream education is considered a desirable goal, these results argue for early implantation, where possible prior to an educational placement decision' (p.298)

Observations

The authors report that since the mid-1970s, more and more deaf children have been placed in mainstream schools full time in the UK (with varying levels of support, p.295), indicating a trend that predates paediatric cochlear implantation and which has been supported by government policies over that time, initially using the term 'integration' and more recently the term 'inclusion'. Nevertheless, it is reported that profoundly deaf children in the UK are often placed in schools for the deaf; in this study 37% of school pupils were in this provision prior to cochlear implantation (p.296). This study aimed to measure the effect of cochlear implantation in this group of deaf pupils on placement.

The authors report a link between both age at implantation and duration of deafness and placement, with shorter durations and earlier ages at implantation presenting a positive correlation with mainstream education. The authors also note a reluctance to move children between provision once in a school setting.

Archbold SM, Nikolopoulos TP, Tait M, O'Donoghue GM, Lutman ME, Gregory S (2000) Approach to communication, speech perception and intelligibility after paediatric cochlear implantation. British Journal of Audiology 34(4): 257-264.

Population size
46
Population comments
Decreasing to 20 at the five-year test interval
Demographics
Onset of deafness: before age 3 years
Age at CI: before age 7 years, range 30-82 months, average 53 months
CI device: Nucleus 22
Socio-economic status: full range (details not given)
Educational settings: preschool, mainstream, units, schools for the deaf
Communication mode: all variations in UK represented
Aetiology: congenital (19), acquired (27)
Hearing loss: < 60 dB across speech frequency range (aided)
Selection criteria
Consecutively implanted (unselected) population of the Nottingham Cochlear Implant Centre. No child lost to follow-up
Dependent variables
Speech perception and intelligibility tests:
closed-set speech perception: Iowa
open-set speech perception: CDT
speech perception rating: CAP
speech production rating: SIR
Independent variables
Communication mode
Method
Student's t-test used for statistical comparison for normally distributed continuous measures; Mann-Whitney U-test for other comparisons
Results
All statistical comparisons were significant at the $p < 0.05$ level in favour of children using oral communication at the assessment intervals (p.260). The Iowa test results are

affected by clear floor and ceiling effects, but within these, scores reveal differences between oral and total communication groups (p.261).

The CDT remains a demanding task for total communication users at all intervals; after five years of implantation, the median score of the oral group was 61 words per minute, significantly better than the total communication group ($p < 0.05$) (p.261).

On the CAP test, the overall population's median score remained constant from three years following implantation, with the level of the oral group one category level above that of the total communication group (6 versus 5) (p.261).

At the follow-up intervals of the SIR, the median SIR of the oral group was one category higher than that of the total communication group right up to the five-year interval, ending at category 4 (intelligibie to a listener with little experience) versus category 3 (intelligible to an experienced listener) (p.261).

The dataset was corrected for movement among pupils from total communication to oral environments, but this recomputation demonstrated no levels of significance (p.261).

Conclusions

'... on measures of speech perception and intelligibility obtained three, four and five years after implantation, children using oral communication outperformed those using signed communication' (p.263).

'Of the 46 children, 30 began using signed communication. Ten of these changed to oral communication in the first three years' (p.262). Note that four children moved from oral communication to total communication (p.262). 'We need to consider whether these children transfer from signed to oral communication on the basis of developing spoken language, or whether they move on the expectation of it; whether the change was the cause, or result, of developing spoken language skills' (p.262).

'The finding that those who changed communication approach do as well as those using an oral approach consistently could be taken to support the view that early (pre-implant) signing is not a disadvantage to developing later oral skills' (p.263).

Observations

The aim of this study was to explore the relationship between approach to communication, speech perception and speech intelligibility after cochlear implantation of young children with profound early deafness. A prospective speech perception and speech intelligibility assessment was undertaken on a consecutive group of implanted children.

It is generally accepted that a major aim of cochlear implantation in young children is to promote the development of spoken language; the expectation is that children will either develop only spoken language, or develop spoken language as part of a bilingual system (p.257). The authors comment that there is little evidence to support greater effectiveness of any one approach in terms of educational or linguistic outcomes (p.258).

The authors report that in relation to communication mode and outcomes of paediatric implantation, the research is divided, both in terms of outcome placement (e.g. oral or total communication) and in terms of the amount of support that is derived from signing after implantation (p.258). One difficulty in such research is the sheer amount of intervening variables typically involved but not measured, the small samples often available and the comparatively short follow-ups reported.

This study also investigates the correlation between communication approach and spoken language outcome measures for up to five years post implantation for children deafened before age 3 years or born deaf. All received cochlear implants before the age of 7. The population size decreased over the time intervals from 46 at the three-year to 26 at four- and 20 at the five-year test interval. Communication modes covered oral and those using a signing approach (total communication).

Results suggest that those in oral environments achieved significantly higher spoken language outcome scores than did those in total communication environments ($p < 0.05$). However,

'... it remains to be explored whether children use oral communication after cochlear implantation because they are doing well, or whether they do well because they are using oral communication' (p.257).

In their attempt to correct for placement mobility among children in the study, the authors note that four children transferred from using oral to use of total communication during the test period; all these children had known additional learning difficulties that would affect speech perception and intelligibility (p.262). Although the significance of this is downplayed in the report with reference to the lack of statistical power of these children to affect the overall results, it is interesting that an approach using sign is considered more appropriate for children with learning needs, despite the benefits of a cochlear implant.

Archbold S, Robinson K, Hartley D (1998) UK teachers of the deaf – working with children with cochlear implants. Deafness and Education 22(2): 24–30.

Population size
497

Population comments
Teachers of deaf children working with cochlear-implanted children

Demographics
273 teachers of the deaf, working with 497 children with CI (= 83% of 600 CIs in 1998)

Selection criteria
Questionnaire sent to BATOD members. Return rate 23% (non-targeted)
182 (67%) of respondents had experience of working with CI; 111 (41%) experience of working with more than one CI

Dependent variables
Not relevant

Independent variables
Not relevant.

Method
Open- and closed-question survey. Likert scale closed questions reported in percentages

Results
Eighty-five percent of teachers said working with cochlear-implanted children was a positive experience. Teachers foresaw expansion of cochlear implantation among the population. Around 50% of teachers estimated that cochlear-implanted children require more educational support than hearing aid users; ±25% estimated less support required. About 50% believed support needs would decrease over time.

The response suggests that about 50% (154/309) believed that the majority of cochlear-implanted children would be placed in mainstream schools, in special classes/units attached to mainstream (135/309, 44%) or in deaf schools (20/309, 6%). In response to which provision would be most favourable, 204 responded [see comments]. Forty-five percent considered mainstream favourable, 22% units or resource bases, 1% (n = 3) 'signing school for the deaf' was favourable.

For communication mode, the predominant response quoted favours flexibility of sorts. Twenty-three percent report oral/aural as most effective, 14% total communication, 2% BSL.

A number of support functions were rated by the teachers as affecting child progress, including management and device efficiency. Age at implantation and rehabilitation were also rated.

Conclusions
Archbold et al. conclude that most of the respondents support the practice of cochlear implantation for young deaf children, and see it as a positive professional experience. Although figures are quoted as representative against the total number of cochlear implants, the numbers quoted are confusing to interpret [see comments]. In summary, however, the authors amply demonstrate that:

'... given the rapidly growing numbers of children with implants, it is apparent that Teachers of the Deaf are increasingly taking on the role of long-term management of implant systems on a daily basis and appear to be willing to do so' (p.29).

Observations

The paper considers attitude measurement among teachers of deaf children towards cochlear implantation on the basis of a blanket distribution of closed-response questionnaires to all BATOD (British Association of Teachers of the Deaf) members. The questionnaire targeted teachers' experience of working with cochlear-implanted children, their views about educational implications, and the quality of liaison between implant centres and local teachers (p.25).

Different population sizes are quoted for the responses, and not all questions seem to be fully reported; this leads to confusion in the interpretation of findings (see further below). Although the total number of returns is quoted as 273, the question re future placement quotes '154/309, 50%', i.e. a population of 309.

With respect to the conclusion, the article quotes highly favourable views of CI, but this does not necessarily seem to follow from the responses reported here, although support may of course exist elsewhere in the dataset. Regardless of an interpretation of findings, however, given the variation in the responses quoted and the confusion in interpreting them, it is quite probable that the views of teachers merely confirm pre-existing issues concerning placement, communication mode, support requirements and 'ideal type' situations, allied to the need for 'flexibility'. To that extent there is no compelling evidence presented here that respondents have been able to base their responses on actual relevant experience of cochlear implantation rather than on commonplace and widespread views on what constitutes appropriate pedagogy. An assessment of this distinction would benefit from a more targeted investigation, and much more detailed reporting.

Bat-Chava Y, Deignan E (2001) Peer relationships of children with cochlear implants. Journal of Deaf Studies and Deaf Education 6(3): 186–199.

Population size
25
Population comments
Parents of cochlear-implanted children
Demographics
Demographics tabled with SD (p.189). Means:
Age: 97 months (range 59–127 months)
HL PTA: 109 dB (range 100-120 dB)
Age at diagnosis: 13 months (range 0–30 months)
Age at CI: 43 months (range 20–78 months)
CI experience: 55 months (range 19–91 months)
Gender: male 40%, female 60%
Aetiology: acquired 48%, congenital 52%

The sample differs from national US population in that the vast majority (92%) used oral communication. Nationally, 61% of cochlear-implanted children use total communication (versus 31% oral only; details from Gallaudet Research Institute).

Overall, the parents interviewed were well educated, with 63% of fathers and 58% of mothers having completed college or graduate school. Eighty-three percent of family incomes exceeded $40,000.

Selection criteria
'Recruited from clientele of the communication department in a large hearing rehabilitation organization in the NorthEast United States' (p.188)
Client list sample relying on 'institutional memory'
Between ages 6 and 10, CI experience at least two years

Dependent variables
Not relevant
Independent variables
Not relevant
Method
Face-to-face interviews with parents, including Achenbach's Child Behavior Checklist (CBCL) for ages 4–18

Ordinal scales derived from coding responses into categories. Inter-rater discrepancies resolved by discussion (initial inter-rater agreement ranged from 88 to 100%)
Results
Peer relationships

Sixty-eight percent ($n = 17$) of parents reported improvement in peer relationships. Forty percent ($n = 10$) reported increase in degree of 'attachment' to peers. While seven reported improvements only, 14 reported both improvements and limitations, four limitations only.

Oral communication

Both improvements and limitations were reported. Chi-square analysis showed significant association between peer relationship improvements and oral communication ability ($p = 0.011$). Eighty-one percent ($n = 17$) reported improvements in oral communication. 72% ($n=18$) reported one or more limitations due to continuing difficulties in oral communication skills (correlation with early diagnosis). Acceptance by peers, familiarity with other children, residual lags in speech and hearing (e.g. poor articulation) and group communication versus one-to-one communication were dominant subthemes.

Personality

Thirty-three percent ($n = 7/21$) reported changes in personality following CI; increased extrovert behaviour was a dominant theme.

Participation in sports

Twenty-eight percent ($n = 7$) reported difficulties in athletic activities attributable to the CI. Potential for physical damage and insufficient hearing were dominant themes.

Relationships with other deaf children

Twenty-four percent ($n = 6$) reported relationships with other deaf children (unprompted), suggesting that these were important for their child. All of these children derived originally from self-contained programmes for deaf children.
Conclusions
Results show that the implant has the potential to improve deaf children's relationships with hearing peers. Nonetheless, children with implants still face communication obstacles, which impede their social relationships with hearing peers. Even satisfied parents reported continuing difficulties, mostly concerning communication problems; interaction with deaf peers may be helpful in attempts to overcome some or all of these.

The authors refer to Rose, Vernon and Pool (1996) in suggesting that continuing problems may explain high levels of non-use of CI. They also report Hoden-Pitt's (1997) analysis; using the GRI's Annual Survey, he reported 50% discontinued use of implant in adolescence.

Possible research limitations are suggested by the authors themselves: first, parents not satisfied with cochlear implantation might be reluctant to report; and second, other data sources currently unavailable are limiting the generalizability of the findings.
Observations
Previous research on children with cochlear implants has focused mostly on their speech perception and production. With the growing numbers of children who use implants, the authors note that it is important to assess other aspects of these children's functioning. This article offers a qualitative and quantitative analysis of interviews with 25 parents who described their 5- to 10.5-year-old children's communication skills and peer relationships before they had the implant and afterwards. The authors quote, incidentally, that by the end of 2000 about 8000 children were implanted in the US (p.186).

The authors focus here on the social development of children with cochlear implants specifically because the literature on this is thin on the ground, while they suggest that most of the extant research has focused on speech perception and production – an observation that is supported by the reviews in this volume. The authors also discuss literature reporting non-use of cochlear implants against the relative 'success' of the results reported here. They suggest that on the one hand, the reported literature largely concerns populations implanted at later ages than reported on here, and on the other hand, that the results reflect different 'stake-holders'. Self-reporting for non-use (by electing to switch off) might be low when compared with the willingness to report relative parental satisfaction, so that the returns might be skewed towards the latter.

Given the small numbers involved, there is a danger of over-interpreting the outcomes of the research reported here. Not only is the sample small, the research used a 'standard', closed form of questioning.

However, in particular, the fact that all parents (without exception) continued to report problems should not be played down – as the authors propose – for the same reason as stated earlier: the threshold for reporting negative experience is likely to be higher than for positive experience. Moreover, in the absence of any other real evidence either way, such problems are logically as likely to become cumulative as they are likely to diminish over time, not least because, as the authors equally suggest, social relationships become more important as children get older.

Baumgartner WD, Pok SM, Egelierler B, Franz P, Gstöttner W, Hamzavi J (2002) The role of age in pediatric cochlear implantation. International Journal of Pediatric Otorhinolaryngology 62(3): 223–228.

Population size

33

Demographics

CI experience: ≥ 36 months

Communication mode: German as primary language

Aetiology: 79% congenital deafness; 9% meningitis; 9% other.

Age at CI: ≤ 3 years (15), > 3 years (18), range 0.9–9 years (mean 4.0 years)

Prior achievement: 8 achieved non-zero scores on LISP before CI

Selection criteria

All children participated in individually tailored intensive audiological rehabilitation programmes after receiving their implants. None had congenital malformations of the inner ear or other handicaps. Computed tomography (CT) and magnetic resonance imaging (MRI) were performed on all children to exclude malformation and auditory nerve aplasia.

Dependent variables

EARS (Evaluation of Auditory Responses to Speech) test battery at 1-, 3-, 6-, 12-, 18-, 24- and 36-month intervals following implantation. Open-set tests were performed as early as 12 months after implantation.

Independent variables

Age at CI

Method

Linear regression analysis (not detailed) based on group outcome scores

Results

The average of all tests in the EARS test battery showed significant improvements. Starting at 3 months after the first fitting, the mean overall scores of the early implanted children were observed to be higher than the scores of those implanted later. At 12, 18 and 24 months after first fitting, this difference was significant ($p < 0.021$, $p < 0.047$, $p < 0.034$). Children who were implanted under the age of 3 achieved higher levels of speech perception performance.

Conclusions

It was observed that a minimum of 18–24 months of implant experience was necessary for the children to achieve adequate speech perception.

To shorten the process of central maturation of the auditory system, it is desirable to implant the children as young as possible. Early intervention seems to be the ideal strategy in enabling prelingually deaf children to derive maximum benefit from cochlear implantation.

Nevertheless, the later-implanted children were able to slightly reduce the gap between their speech perception scores and those of the children implanted at a younger age at the last test interval of three years following implantation.

Observations

This is an article specifically concerned with age at implantation. The sample was subdivided into a population implanted below age 3 and one implanted at age 3 or more. This does impose an artificial effect within the population to the extent that the eldest implanted child was 9 years of age and therefore not in a comparable language situation, especially in terms of prior experience and achievement. But equally, and on a more methodological level, this study is a follow-up to that reported in Gstöttner et al. (2000), which was hampered by small numbers and ceiling effects in the EARS test at three years' cochlear implant experience.

Individual variation in outcome of cochlear implantation is reported in the introduction, but not treated or discussed as part of the results reported here. The authors do precede their discussion of results with the comment that, ideally, each child should be reported on separately (p.228), but that is not the case here.

The demonstrated outperformance by children implanted at a younger age is consistent with other such research (e.g. the Fryauf-Bertschy/Tyler series based on a population described in Fryauf-Bertschy 1997). Since the findings present a straightforward single point in time analysis, very little can be said about them. Even so, it is difficult to factor out the likely intervening factor of normal language development (or maturation) in this type of research; the most methodical approach might be to include language development measures in a control group of hearing children matched for age, and factor that element out.

Beadle EA, Shores A, Wood EJ (2000) Parental perceptions of the impact upon the family of cochlear implantation in children. Annals of Otology, Rhinology and Laryngology 185: s111–s114.

Population size

17

Population comments

Sets of parents of implanted children

Demographics

None detailed

Selection criteria

None detailed

Dependent variables

Questionnaire responses

Independent variables

Quality-of-life measures

Method

Chi-square of single linear correlations

Results

With respect to parental expectations, the validity of the retrospective measure was shown to be weak, with only seven statements showing a positive correlation with pre-implant expectation responses (p.112). Results are suggested to indicate that parental expectations were not inappropriately increased; expectations were predictably lower for children who were relatively young or old at the time of implantation.

Responses showed higher ratings for finding schoolwork easier and for progress in reading (p.112).

The stress results provide a comment that siblings of children with cochlear implants have some difficulty in coping (p.113).

The different mean ratings of support grouped by formal (rehabilitation) and informal (family) showed a difference that was statistically significant ($p < 0.001$). No further analysis or explanation is offered (p.113).

Conclusions
'Overall, the parents who participated in the study seemed pleased with their implant-recipient children's progress. Some children with implants learn to communicate orally with great proficiency; those who achieve less success in learning to talk still benefit from the ability to perceive environmental sounds, which they would lack without the device. [...] This study has indicated that social support may decrease stress and ameliorate the quality of life in such families' (p.114).

Observations
The overall aim of the study was to assess parents' perspectives on outcome of paediatric implantation, and early on in the report reference is made to the aim of the intervention itself. The description of quality of life was not clear and all embracing: '...a multidimensional concept that involves physical aspects, psychological adjustment, and social well-being' (p.111).

It is later noted that the quality of life of an implanted child is also affected by that of the whole family (p.112).

A number of quality-of-life aspects worthy of investigation are listed, including benefits from the implants, assessments of the impact of stress factors over time and the benefits when correlated to wider social support (p.112). This study focused on increasing knowledge about the stress factors and coping factors involved in the implant process, as reported by parents, using a rating scale in relation to 74 statements in four sections: parental expectations prior to implantation, parental views on the realization of outcomes, parental views on wider social support and items relating to quality of life (p.112).

Unfortunately the research does not detail any demographic details of either the parents or of the children, so that any interpretation becomes difficult.

The results are summarily given, and are occasionally not significant – for example where it is reported that negative correlation coefficients suggest a link between stress and quality of life (p.113) – while the conclusion is apparently based on data not reported in the study, since little evidence for it is located in the report. The authors conclude that social support may decrease stress and ameliorate the quality of life in families with a cochlear-implanted child, which would suggest the need for a longitudinal approach to this issue.

Bichey BG, Hoversland JM, Whynne MK, Miyamoto RT (2002) Changes in quality of life and the cost-utility associated with cochlear implantation in patients with large vestibular aqueduct syndrome. Otology and Neurotology 23: 323–327.

Population size
20 patients with large vestibular aqueduct syndrome (10 with a cochlear implant and 10 without)

Population comments
Small sample size

Demographics
Current age: median 44.3 years for the cochlear-implanted (range: 9.9–75.6 years) and median 22.5 years for those with hearing aids (range: 8.6–65.1 years)

Age at onset: median 25 years in implanted population (range: 5.0–69.0 years) and 7 years in hearing aided (range: 5.0–59.0 years)
Age at CI: not reported
Duration of deafness: not reported
Life expectancy: 76 years (assumed)
Setting: Indiana University School of Medicine Department of Otolaryngology and Neck Surgery, USA

Method

Economic evaluation type: cost-utility analysis
Study perspective: health payer
Comparator intervention: hearing aids
Source of effectiveness data: primary research – patients
Direct costs: charges – including preoperative assessment, surgical fees, anaesthesia, hospitalization, implant device, postoperative therapy/implant training, audiological assessment and communication assessment
Indirect costs: not included
Discount rate for costs and benefits: 5%
Outcome measure: Health Utilities Index (HUI) (version used unclear)
Currency and price year: US$, price year unreported
Sensitivity analysis: the gain in the HUI score was changed to 0.15 (sensitivity 1 – decreasing the hearing portion of the proxy score by one level) and 0.05 (sensitivity 2 – decreasing the hearing portion of the proxy score by two levels) to examine the impact on cost-utility

Results

In the base case, cochlear implantation resulted in a utility gain of 0.20 (SD = 0.13, with 95% CI = 0.12, 0.28). The undiscounted cost per QALY was $6,426, while the discounted cost per QALY was $12,774. In sensitivity analysis 1, the gain in utility was changed to 0.15 and resulted in an undiscounted cost per QALY of $8,970 and a discounted cost per QALY of $17,832. In sensitivity 2, where the gain in the utility fell to 0.05, the respective costs per QALY were $27,120 and $53,913.

Conclusions

'Some clinicians initially doubted any clinical benefit of cochlear implantation in patients ... with LVAS.... The results indicate an improvement in quality of life associated with postlingually deafened implant recipients. When compared with other disease states, favorable cost-utility figures were also noted for this group of patients' (p.327).

Observations

An interesting study, because it looks at the cost-utility within a clearly defined patient subpopulation experiencing large vestibular aqueduct syndrome.

Blamey PJ, Sarant JZ, Paatsch LE, Barry JG, Bow CP, Wales RJ, Wright M, Psarros C, Rattigan K, Tooher R (2001) Relationships among speech perception, production, language, hearing loss, and age in children with impaired hearing. Journal of Speech, Language and Hearing Research 44(2): 264–285.

Population size

47

Population comments

Hearing aided group of 40

Demographics

CI

PTA (unaided): mean 106 dB HL (SD = 11), range 77–125 dB HL
Onset of deafness: mean 0.3 years (SD = 0.7), range 0–3.4 years

Age at CI: mean 3.5 years (SD = 1.5), range 1.2–8.2 years
Age at evaluation: mean 7.7 years (SD = 2.0), range 4.3–13.0 years
Duration of deafness: mean 3.2 years (SD = 1.5), range 0.5–8.2 years
Auditory experience: mean 4.2 years (SD = 2.0), range 09–9.2 years

HA

PTA (unaided): mean 78 dB HL (SD = 1.7), range 40–103 dB HL
Onset of deafness: mean 0.4 years (SD = 1.1), range 0–4.6 years
Age at evaluation: mean 9.0 years (SD = 2.4), range 4.5–13.5 years
Auditory experience: mean 8.5 years (SD = 2.5), range 0.6–13.5 years

Selection criteria

Enlisted from four schools in Melbourne and from the Children's Cochlear Implant Centre
in Sydney
Attending primary school (ages 4–12 years)
Bilateral PTA of at least 40 dB HL
Cochlear implant or hearing aid or both
English at home as their first language
Enrolled in an educational programme using spoken language without signing
   supplement
Experienced onset of deafness before age 5 years

Dependent variables

Speech perception

Consonant–Nucleus–Consonant (CNC) monosyllabic word test; Bench–Kowal–Bamford
   (BKB) sentence test

Language measures

Peabody Picture Vocabulary Test (PPVT-R and -III); the Clinical Evaluation of Language
Fundamentals (CELF)

Speech production

Transcription of conversations with Computer Aided Speech And Language Analysis
(CASALA)

Independent variables

PTA
Age

Method

Linear regression with computation of variance for selected variables. Authors point out
that this assumes a constant difference between variables; however, this is an artificial
byproduct of the assumption of linearity. Moreover, variables may not have a truly
additive effect (p.269)

Results

Little difference in the level of performance and trends was found for the two groups of
children, so the perceptual effect of the implant is equivalent, on average, to an
improvement of about 28dB in hearing thresholds. The children's scores were widely
dispersed around the mean speech production score of 40% of words correctly produced
in spontaneous conversations, with no significant upward trend with age. After allowing
for differences in language, speech perception scores in the auditory test condition
showed a slight downward trend over time, which is consistent with the known biological
effects of hearing loss on the auditory periphery and brainstem (p.264).

   'It is clear [from the results] that the perception scores are more strongly
   related to lexical knowledge than chronological age, suggesting that the rate of
   lexical development and the rate of change of speech-perception scores over
   time in individuals are likely to be correlated' (p.276).

So that, therefore,

   'Rather than inferring a cause-and-effect relationship between language scores,
   speech production scores, and speech perception scores in either direction, we

suggest that the three scores are significantly correlated because they all depend on three underlying variables: hearing, language, and speech production abilities. The underlying variables may be weighted differently for different test measures. [Moreover] The trends and levels of performance in the language and speech production tests were not strongly dependent on residual hearing level' (p.278).

'On average, the analyses [...] account for 60% of the variance, which is a significant improvement over previous studies. The remaining variance is partly due to random variation arising from test–retest and inter-transcriber variability [averaging 21%]. This leaves an average of 19% of the total variance arising from systematic factors other than those considered in this study' (p.280).

'The rate of improvement for the children in the CI group preoperatively is slightly higher than the rates of improvement previously reported for other groups of children in the preoperative period. The average rate of vocabulary improvement postimplantation seems to be lower for the children in this study than the average rates previously reported' (p.281).

Conclusions

The model suggests that most of the children in the study will reach a level of over 90% sentence recognition in the auditory-visual condition when their language becomes equivalent to that of a normally hearing 7-year-old, but they will enter secondary school at age 12 with an average language delay of about four or five years, unless they receive concentrated and effective language training (p.264).

'The results show that the language performance of children with either a hearing aid or a cochlear implant improved at a rate that was steady, but slower than for children with normal hearing. There was wide variation in rate of language acquisition within the two groups, but individual rates were not correlated with hearing thresholds in either group, nor were speech production scores highly correlated with hearing thresholds. If individual children follow the group trends, the average language delay will be about four or five years by the time the children enter secondary school at about age 12 years' (p.283).

And finally, there is a strong need for language-based habilitation to enable these children to understand material that will be presented to them in secondary school.

Observations

The statistical analysis in this report is detailed and responsive, and a clear account of statistical effects is given at each point along the line: a good model to follow. The authors evaluated speech perception, speech production and language skills for 47 children with profound hearing loss and cochlear implants, and 40 children with severe hearing loss and hearing aids over a three-year period. The authors set up a clear set of hypotheses, and add:

'... our expectation was that severely hearing-impaired children using hearing aids and profoundly deaf children using implants would perform similarly on a range of measures. It is already apparent that these groups of children are enrolled in the same types of habilitation and educational programs in Australia' (p.266).

Since placement was a constant in this research (all were placed in auditory oral settings), this article seems to suggest that the language improvements measured for both a cochlear-implanted group and a severely deaf hearing-aided group across a number of English language tests were almost entirely due to 'normal' language development progress. In other words, although hearing loss impacts significantly on the rate of development, hearing (and hearing aids) contributes relatively little to performance.

Blamey et al. elaborate significantly on the notion of equivalent hearing loss throughout their assessments, but in particular at the point where they give a clear and concise summary:

'... it can be said that an average cochlear implant user with a hearing loss of 106 dB HL performs like an average hearing aid user with a hearing loss of about 78 db HL. Svirsky and Meyer (1999) found that the average phoneme and word perception scores of children using the Clarion cochlear implant were slightly below those of children with hearing loss between 90 and 100 dB HL using hearing aids. Boothroyd and Eran (1994) found that the performance of 18 children using the Nucleus cochlear implant with the MPEAK speech processing strategy was equivalent to average performance of children with hearing aids and a hearing loss of 88 dB HL (range from 74 to 113 dB HL for individual children). The improvement of implant users relative to hearing aid users in the current data may result from the improvement in implant speech processing strategies and hardware since the data of Boothroyd and Eran (1994) were collected [...], or from the greater auditory experience of the present group (4.2 years compared with 3.3 years for Boothroyd and Eran or 18 months for Svirsky and Meyer)' (p.278).

A strong relationship was observed between speech-perception scores and language skills, suggesting a relationship between lexical knowledge and speech-perception measures. By contrast,

'There is no significant effect of onset age, indicating that hearing is unchanged before the onset of the hearing loss. A slight negative effect with increasing device experience does not reach statistical significance for most of the perception measures' (p.282).

Boothroyd A (1997) Auditory capacity of hearing-impaired children using hearing aids and cochlear implants: Issues of efficacy and assessment. Scandinavian Audiology Supplement 26(46): s17–s25.

Population size
50
Population comments
Control group of 96 hearing aid wearers
Demographics
CI device: Nucleus (MSP)
Age: range 3.5–15.4 years (mean 8.8 years)
Age at onset: range birth–11.2 years (mean 1.4 years)
CI use: range 0.9–5.3 years (mean 2.6 years)
Communication mode: oral (31), total communication (19)
HA users are roughly matched to the CI children.
Selection criteria
None indicated. Groups were tested in various clinics and schools around the US
Dependent variables
IMSPAC scores
Independent variables
Current age
Age at onset
Age at CI
Duration of profound deafness
CI use
Communication mode
Minority status
Aetiology

Method

Multiple regression analysis

Results

Composite audio-only IMSPAC scores ranged from under 10% to over 80% in both groups. The mean score for the children with implants was 45%, while that for the aided children was 37% (p.20).

[For the hearing aid group] performance was unrelated to age, communication mode, age at onset of deafness, minority status and aetiology (p.20).

[For the cochlear implant group] two variables explained significant amounts of variance – communication mode (13%) and duration of implant use (7%) (p.20).

There was significant improvement in test scores over time, in the months following implantation. Growth rates varied considerably between individuals; superiority of auditory-visual over auditory only performance was present at all times (p.21).

Conclusions

Results supported the conclusion that the IMSPAC test (an auditory-only measure) is insensitive to linguistic and cognitive status. For cochlear implant users, results showed significant effects of communicative mode (despite the above) and duration of use, while auditory capacity increased over time.

The data showed a distribution of auditory capacity in paediatric users of the Nucleus implant (with the MSP processor) that was similar to that of hearing aid users with hearing losses in the range 90–99 dB (p.24).

Observations

This article further builds on evidence collected in support of an imitative test of phonetic contrast perception (IMSPAC) as a measure of inherent auditory capacity, describing data obtained from paediatric hearing aid and cochlear implant users. It is reported that the primary predictor of IMSPAC performance for aided children is degree of hearing loss, with little or no influence of age and communication mode.

Applying the test to young cochlear implant users, they observed that their IMSPAC scores suggested that communication mode and experience of cochlear implant use are primary predictors of auditory performance (p.17).

IMSPAC requires imitation of non-language sounds (all within phonological range of language). IMSPAC tests are conducted in two administrations: auditory-visual and auditory only. The results are digitized and scored by four listeners.

Results also indicate that IMSPAC is a suitable test to measure auditory capacity in young cochlear implant users (see Boothroyd and Eran 1994 for an earlier report on this).

Equivalent hearing loss

Results from the cochlear implant group compared post hoc to an earlier hearing aid group confirm the notion of equivalent hearing loss, in that they showed a distribution of auditory capacity in paediatric users of the Nucleus implant (MSP processor) similar to that of hearing aid users with hearing losses in the range of 90–99 dB.

The hearing aid data suggest that the IMSPAC test is effective in measuring auditory sensory capacity without confounding by linguistic status. If this is true, the implant data must be interpreted as evidence of the development of auditory perceptual skills during the post-implant period.

Boothroyd A, Eran O (1994) Auditory speech perception capacity of child implant users expressed as equivalent hearing loss. Volta Review 96(5): 151–168.

Population size

18

Population comments

+76 HA users

Demographics

CI

Age: range 4.5–14.9 years (mean 9.3 years)

Age at onset: range 0–3.5 years (mean 1.3 years)

Age at CI: range 2.3–11.8 years (mean 6.0 years)

Pre-implant average. threshold: range 110 to > 120 dB HL (mean > 118 dB HL)

Onset to implant: range 0.6–10.3 years (mean 4.7 years)

CI use: range 1.5–5.3 years (mean 3.3 years)

Gender: male (11), female (7)

Ethnic minority: yes (3), no (15)

Communication mode: oral (18), total communication (0)

Aetiology: meningitis (10), unknown (5), high fever (2), Mondini dysplasia (1)

HA

Age: range 5.3–14.6 years (mean 4.5 years)

Age at onset: range 0–4 years (mean 0.5 years)

Age aided: range 0.2–5.5 years (mean 1.9 years)

Average threshold across three frequencies: range 82-117 dB HL (mean 99 dB HL)

Gender: male (37), female (39)

Ethnic minority: yes (14), no (62)

Communication mode: oral (45), total communication (31)

Selection criteria

Not detailed

Dependent variables

IMSPAC (imitative test of the perception of phonologically significant speech pattern contrasts)

The test is claimed to reduce the potential effects of lexical and higher levels of language knowledge

Independent variables

Age

Hearing loss

Communication mode

Method

Linear regression analysis and stepwise multiple regression analysis based on a model provided by the HA group around IMSPAC scores

Results

The IMSPAC score at which an average cochlear implant user would equal the score of an average hearing aid user (calculated through a linear regression function and referred to as 'equivalent hearing loss') averaged 88 dB for the 18 implant users, with a range of 74 to 113 dB (p.159).

'As might be expected, implantation at an earlier age led to greater sensory benefit from the implant (i.e. a higher IMSPAC score and a lower equivalent hearing loss). The effect is not marked, however. The typical equivalent hearing loss rises by only 10 dB (from 85 dB EHL to 95 dB EHL) as age at implantation increases from 4 to 10 years. [...] Duration of implant use was not a significant predictor of IMSPAC score or equivalent hearing loss' (p.160).

'The predictive value of the auditory IMSPAC score in terms of eventual performance at the sentence level has not been determined. Using a related test with normally hearing adults listening to filtered speech, however, it has been shown that a 60% composite contrast perception score is sufficient for 80% recognition of words in sentences of known topic (Boothroyd 1991). With this level of function, it should be possible to sustain an unstructured conversation over the telephone. Approximately half of the 18 implant users studied here scored 60% or better on IMSPAC' (p.162).

Conclusions

'The results provide support for the conclusion that a multichannel implant can provide many otherwise very profoundly deaf children with auditory speech perception capacity similar to that of severely deaf children who wear hearing aids' (p.151).

'Although this level of performance is by no means guaranteed, the high proportion of such children in the present sample is very encouraging and further confirms the cochlear implant as a viable option for the sensory management of profoundly hearing-impaired children' (p.165).

Observations

The authors set out to assess, for each implant user, the unaided threshold at which test scores of a typical hearing aid user would equal that of the implant user – the expression that results is that of 'equivalent hearing loss', presented as unaided HL level. The advantage of this expression is that it enables different outcome measures to be reduced into a single common metric (p.152). This article is one of the earliest in the dataset to undertake this type of description. The disadvantage is, of course, that it does reduce a wide variety of experiences to a simple point on an audiological metric scale, to a degree of hearing loss.

For a much more recent and large-scale project reporting in a similar fashion, see Blamey et al. (2001) and Svirsky and Meyer (1999). For a further detailed assessment of IMSPAC, see Boothroyd (1997).

The IMSPAC test allows for both auditory/visual and auditory only conditions. The test uses non-words, which means the test is, theoretically speaking, language independent and therefore appropriate for a wider age group at the bottom end of the scale. However, for those with existing or developing language skills, the test might introduce a level of confusion in attempts to map the non-words to one's existing vocabulary. There is no mention of the test having been normed across different populations.

As an additional related finding, communication programme (oral/total communication) did not affect outcome to any degree of significance among the hearing aid group (all children in the cochlear implant group were in oral settings). This finding contrasts with that of, for example, Miyamoto et al. (1999), who do note a correlation between language development and communication mode.

Bosco E, D'Agosta L, Ballantyne D (1999) 'Small group' rehabilitation in adolescent cochlear implant users: learning experiences. International Journal of Pediatric Otorhinolaryngology 47(2): 187–190.

Population size
6
Demographics
CI device: Clarion
No details
Selection criteria
Non-selection from the ENT Clinic of Rome University 'La Sapienza'
Age sample
Dependent variables
Not appropriate
Independent variables
Not appropriate
Method
Discussion
Results
Outcomes are a range of improved psycho-social outcomes, in addition to constant use of the implant (p.190). Participants tended to spend more time on homework, develop more

natural peer relations, have more natural language interaction ability/confidence, and have improved skill of argument and debate.

Conclusions

'The most significant learning experiences after 18 months of treatment were the socialization of experience, the socialization of individual learning processes, the direct relationship between adolescents, practice discussion of topics of common interest, emphasizing of personal opinions and beliefs, experiencing collective 'products', the reinforcement of interpersonal relationships and the emphasizing of individual initiatives both at home and at school' (p.187).

Observations

This text is more a discussion paper than a research report. It is included because it focuses on adolescents, and is one of the few published papers to do so. It is linked to D'Agosta L, Bosco E, Cordier A (1999) 'Small group' rehabilitation in adolescent cochlear implant users: Aims, methods and results. International Journal of Pediatric Otorhinolaryngology 47(2): 191–194.

The project appears to form part of an action research programme, in that the aims of the research spell out improvements in the communication and interactions with their peers of those enrolled in the programme:

'Experience with group sessions is central in that it enables us to lay grounds for what has been defined as non-egocentric communication. Conditions for this mode are: semantic flexibility, flexibility in the reference scheme, meta-linguistic awareness, role-taking, ability to do verbal recoding for another person and emotional availability. In our opinion it is particularly useful to work on this aspect in deaf teenagers because they are usually brought up along very rigid lines with methods which do not take into due consideration the tendency of many deaf children at this age to consider given words as necessarily linked to a specific object' (p.188).

The authors do not discuss their findings in any detail, or contextualize their project with reference to other research on outcomes.

Brinton J (2001) Measuring language development in deaf children with cochlear implants. International Journal of Language and Communication Disorders 36: s121–s125.

Population size

12

Population comments

12 at 6 months post implantation, dropping to 4 at the five-year interval.

Demographics

No demographics detailed

Selection criteria

No selection criteria detailed: 'All children under 11 years of age were included in this study (p.123)

Dependent variables

Preschool Language Scales-3 at one-year intervals from 6 months to five years post implantation

Independent variables

CI experience

Method

Graphs

Results

All graphs show steady improvement over time. There is no further detail provided, and no analysis or comparison attempted.

Conclusions

'The use of the PLS-3 has been shown to be sensitive to change over time in both comprehension and expressive communication in children following fitting with a cochlear implant. Without a control group it is however impossible to state that the fitting of the cochlear implant caused the score improvements' (pp. 124–5).

'... early indications are that the implanted children are following the pattern of hearing children acquiring language' (p.125).

Observations

The authors note that there is a need for a test that assesses a wide range of language abilities and which is also sensitive to change. To this end they selected the Preschool Language Scales-3 (PLS-3), which has been standardized on a British population and was chosen to be part of a test battery at The South of England Cochlear Implant Centre (SOECIC). The test is suitable for ages 0–7 years; it concerns the precursors of language, the early development of spoken language structures, including grammar, vocabulary and syntax in monitoring intelligibility and auditory performance, namely speech perception and speech production (p.122).

Only spoken language was used in administering the assessment: 'The test was administered orally and only oral responses were credited [...] a record was kept of children who responded to the test instructions given in a manual mode and responses that were manual. The results given [however,] represent aural/oral test results' (p.123).

The population is small, dropping from just 12 at the 6-month post-implantation interval to only 4 at five years post implantation. Moreover, 'some' (p.123) children were already aged between 8 and 10 years, and were between four and six years post implantation, so that for them the test might no longer have been an appropriate assessment tool – as that age range is beyond the range for which the test is standardized. Therefore no standardized scores were available for these children, while no standardized scores exist at all for a deaf population (p.123). Consequently only over-time improvements are usefully reported.

Carter R, Hailey D (1999) Economic evaluation of the cochlear implant. International Journal of Technology Assessment in Health Care 15(3): 520–530.

Population size

Based on a hypothetical cohort of 40 children using published data and expert opinion

Demographics

Current age: not reported
Age at onset: not reported
Age at CI: not reported
Duration of deafness: not reported
Life expectancy: 10-, 15- and 20-year time period covered

Setting

Australia

Method

Economic evaluation type: cost-utility analysis
Study perspective: societal (partial)
Comparator intervention: no intervention
Source of effectiveness data: assumed
Direct costs: assessment costs, surgery, device, tuning and rehabilitation session costs included
Indirect costs: changes in education costs
Discount rate for costs and benefits: 5%
Outcome measure: assumed based on the HRQOL-15D
Currency and price year: AUS$, 1994

Sensitivity analysis: undertaken – variables changed included the discount rate (7.5% and 10%), device cost (increased from $18,220 to $22,500), electrical maintenance (increased from $400 to $800 per year), upgrade cost (increased from $4,378 to $6,000 per five years), rehabilitation increased (from 145 hours to 200 hours year 1, from 2 hours to 100 hours in year 2, and from 3 hours in year 3+ to 100 hours in year 3 and 75 hours in year 4), and decreased in mainstream schooling (from 65% to 50%)

Results

Implantation is assumed to improve the hearing disability by 0.04 to 0.05 while the functional consequences improve HRQL by 0.13 to 0.32. Thus total HRQL for children was assumed to improve by 0.17 to 0.37. The cost per QALY estimates based on this gain ranged from AUS$5,940 to $13,020 (in 2001/2 prices – £2,945 to £6,455 or US$4,241 to $9,295) for 10 years, AUS$5,070 to $11,100 (in 2001/2 prices – £2,513 to £5,503 or US$3,619 to $7,924) for 15 years and AUS$1,580 to $3,465 (in 2001/2 prices – £783 to £1718 or US$1,128 to $2,474) for 20 years. Results are not particularly sensitive to the assumptions made, although sensitivity analysis did show that cost per QALY (base case for 15 years $7,480 – middle value) estimates did vary according to the rates of long-term rehabilitation (cost per QALY AUS$16,125 (in 2001/2 prices – £7,994 or US$11,511)) and proportion of implantees attending normal schools (cost per QALY AUS$13,680 (in 2001/2 prices – £6,782 or US$9,766)) assumed. Regardless of the changes made in sensitivity analysis, the cost per QALY estimated for CI still suggested good value for money.

Conclusions

'The results of this study reflect the further development of cochlear implantation and give a strong indication that it is an effective technology that is acceptable value for money in Australia' (p.525).

Observations

This study builds on the analysis reported in Lea (1995). The study relies on a lot of assumptions, for example that the educational benefits are not felt until 18 months post implantation or that there is a 5% complication rate in the first year.

Cheng AK, Grant GD, Niparko JK (1999) Meta-analysis of pediatric cochlear implantation literature. Annals of Otology, Rhinology and Laryngology 108(4/2): 124–128.

Population size

Although the authors detail overall numbers included in their original collection of articles, they do not provide such a population description for the final selection of articles – therefore the overall numbers involved are not known

Selection criteria

Medline range of published research 1966–1999; n = 6 articles
Unpublished results with at least one-year follow-up from clinical trial data submitted to the US FDA submitted by Cochlear and Advanced Bionics Corporations

Dependent variables

Speech reception: scored synthesis of 22 different tests

Independent variables

Age at cochlear implant
Aetiology or age at onset

Method

Published test results were rescaled into ordinal categories. Comparison between published and non-published results of outcomes carried out with the non-parametric Wilcoxon test statistic

Results

There is concordance between the two datasets, with the exception of higher scores on oldest age group (> 6 years). There was found to be no plateau of benefit over time, with higher scores for congenitally implanted children after two to three years of implant use.

Conclusions

Open-set speech understanding was observed in over 50% of implanted children within two years of implantation.

Earlier implantation associated with higher outcomes.

No plateau in speech perception increase observed over time.

Performance differences between congenital and acquired causes diminish over time.

A comparison of published/unpublished results indicates no publication bias.

Observations

This article is unlike all others included in this review, in that it uses secondary sources for its dataset (meta-analysis). The report analyses a number of published reports for their reporting on the effect of age at implantation, the cause of deafness and the age at onset of deafness in relation to speech perception benefits in children with cochlear implants. Results were rescored into an ordinal classification to allow for comparisons between different datasets. The authors suggest that since they did not observe any differences between results reported in published and unpublished literature, there is no publication bias in the literature. The populations of the reports analysed are only described (to some extent) *before* making the final selection of papers, which means that the meta-analytical rescoring is hard to interpret. Moreover, the rescoring of results across the literature weakens the statistical significance of the original results, with ordinal score reinterpretation creating a single band of outcome that is lacking in detail. It is also worth noting in this respect that the literature reported results on 22 different speech perception tests alone (p.125).

To allow for more in-depth comparative analyses, the authors recommend that future articles either report, or make available, a full range of individual patient data, including age at implantation, cause/age at onset of deafness, and speech perception scores on a yearly basis (p.127).

Cheng AK, Rubin HR, Powe NR, Mellon NK, Francis HW, Niparko JK (2000) Cost-utility analysis of the cochlear implant in children. Journal of the American Medical Association 284: 850–856.

Population size

Parents of 78 profoundly deaf children using a cochlear implant

Demographics

Current age: mean age 7.5 years (SD = 4.5 years)

Age at onset: 93% prelingually deafened under the age of 3 years, 3% prelingually deafened between the ages of 3 and 5 years, and 4% postlingually deafened over the age of 5 years

Age at CI: mean 5.7 years (SD = 4.2 years)

Duration of deafness: mean 4.5 years (SD = 3.6 years)

Life expectancy: average life expectancy of 78 years so implant use for a further 73 years (90 to 40 years used in the sensitivity analysis)

Setting

The Listening Center at Johns Hopkins, Baltimore, USA

Method

Economic evaluation type: cost-utility analysis

Study perspective: societal

Comparator intervention: no intervention

Source of effectiveness data: primary data – parents

Direct costs: Charges – hospital charges, including device, surgery, processor upgrade

costs, patient-borne costs, e.g. cost of warranty, loss or damage insurance and batteries
Indirect costs: time off work, travel expenses, changes in education costs and future earnings (assumed)
Discount rate for costs and benefits: 3% (range 0–5% in sensitivity analysis)
Outcome measure: visual analogue scale (VAS), Time Trade Off (TTO) and Health Utilities Index – mark III (HUI-III)
Currency and price year: US$, 1999
Sensitivity analysis: the ranges on a number of variables were tested, including the gain in health utility (0.39 to 0.10), direct medical costs, time off work (0–8 hours per visit), salary of parent taking time off work (US$0-100,000), travel distance (5 to 200 miles), additional children mainstreamed (70 to 30%), gain in future earnings (US$0 to $148 198) and special living equipment (US$0 to $38 374).

Results
The authors found that cochlear implants for children are cost-effective regardless of which outcome measure is used (HUI $5,197 per QALY, VAS $7,500 per QALY or TTO $9,209 per QALY) (in 2001/2 prices – £3,937 or US$5,919 for the HUI, £5,671 or US$8,542 for the VAS and £6,976 or US$10,489 for the TTO). The gain in utility measured on the three instruments differed (HUI = 0.39, VAS = 0.27 and TTO = 0.22) and was found to be the most significant determinant of the magnitude of the cost per QALY in sensitivity analysis. The utility gain was varied from 0.39 to 0.10 (best to worst case) to give a range of $5,196 to $20,278 (in 2001/2 prices – £3,936 to £15,361 or US$5,918 to $23,096) as possible cost-per-QALY ratios.

Conclusions
'This analysis suggests that the cochlear implant is highly cost-effective in children, with a net expected saving of $53,198 over a child's lifetime. Considering only direct medical costs yields cost-utility ratios of $9,029 per QALY using the TTO, $7,500 per QALY using the VAS and $5,197 per QALY using the HUI' (p.854).

Observations
No justifications are given for the assumptions and ranges of values used in this analysis. It is not clear why only direct medical costs were used in the cost-per-QALY calculations when the authors had also measured other costs, for example travel, parental time off work, special equipment. What is particularly interesting in this study is that the gain in utility varies depending on which instrument is used to measure it. This may be explained by the instruments purporting to measure the same thing when they are actually measuring or valuing the same health states differently. The implication of this finding for economic studies requires that economists justify their choice of instrument in terms of the intervention/question stated. Clearly the choice of instrument is likely to determine the magnitude of the cost per QALY estimated and if the choice is not justified, one may suspect it was chosen in order to show the desired outcome.

Chin SB, Finnegan KR, Chung BA (2001) Relationships among types of speech intelligibility in pediatric users of cochlear implants. Journal of Communication Disorders 34(3): 187–205.

Population size
20

Demographics
Age at onset: range 0–2.4 years, mean 0.18 years (SD = 0.56)
Age at implantation: range 1.4–5.3 years, mean 3.42 years (SD = 1.15)
Age: range 4.8–7.8 years, mean 6.8 years (SD = 1.1)
CI experience: range 2.1–5.0 years, mean 3.4 years (SD = 0.8)
Detailed individually in Table 1 (p.192)

Selection criteria
Children followed at the Indiana University School of Medicine; age at onset 3 years; age at implantation <6 years; use of SPEAK or CIS; CI experience ≥ 2 years
Dependent variables
Speech intelligibility, as an overall function of:
• speech perception: Minimal Pairs Test (MP1)
• speech production: Minimal Pairs Test (MP2)
• speech intelligibility: MP2 scored by judges
• sentence elicitation using the BIT, scored by judges.

Sixty adult listeners served as judges; their ages ranged from 18 to 40 years and they had no experience with hearing impaired speech (p.192)
Independent variables
Speech intelligibility
Method
Arcsine transformed percentage scores (scatterplots with regression lines) modelled through descriptive statistics followed by correlational analyses (p.195)
Results
Table 5 (p.197) presents scores from the three tasks as aggregate means; Table 6 (p.198) shows correlations of sentence intelligibility scores (BIT) with MP1 and MP2 feature classes, showing significant correlations of two of the three consonant feature classes and both vowel feature classes with MP1, while two of three consonant feature classes but none of the two vowel feature classes correlated with MP2 (p.198).

Results indicate a general trend, demonstrating intercorrelations among perception of contrasts (MP1), the production of contrasts (MP2) and productive sentence intelligibility (BIT), and 'that especially, the perception and production of overall consonant and vowel contrasts both correlate positively and significantly with sentence intelligibility' (p.199).

Results are not consistent with findings that perception of place of articulation tends to lag behind perception of manner of articulation and sometimes behind perception of voicing (p.199).
Conclusions
Although the three types of intelligibility are related at a gross level, relationships are more tenuous at finer levels of analysis, suggesting that the separate skills may need to be addressed separately in remediation.

'Most perception and production feature classes correlated significantly with sentence intelligibility, but there were no significant correlations between individual perception feature classes and their corresponding production feature classes' (p.201).

So that, in summary, improvement in one is insufficient to countenance expectation of improvement in another – speech perception and production skills do not predict improvements in speech intelligibility per se (p.201).
Observations
The authors quote a definition of intelligibility as the degree to which the speaker's intended message is recovered by the listener (p.188), which, as they suggest, is neutral with respect to perception, transmission and production. This assessment precisely characterizes a linear, signal-based description that has been criticized in linguistics as ignoring agency or individual language user characteristics and the crucial role of interpretation or variation in 'reading' in any communicative act. The study aimed to assess the relative value of different types of closed- and open-set speech intelligibility tests in an assessment of: (a) the relationship between the perception of contrasts and the production of contrasts; and (b) their relationship to another measure of speech intelligibility, a sentence elicitation task (BIT) judged by listeners.

The authors locate the clinical implications of cochlear implantation in the area of speech-language pathology, but suggest that the management of speech intelligibility is a tractable problem (pp.190–1), thereby stressing the role of remediation and specific management of phonological development postimplantation.

Chmiel R, Sutton L, Jenkins H (2000) Quality of life in children with cochlear implants. Annals of Otology, Rhinology and Laryngology 185: s103–s105.

Population size

21

Population comments

Concerns families (group A) of cochlear implanted children, and a subset of 11 children (group B) responding personally

Demographics

Group A

Age: range 3–20 years

Gender: girls (10), boys (11)

CI device: Nucleus

Mode of communication: auditory-oral (16), total communication (4), cued speech (1)

Group B

Age: range 6–20 years

Gender: girls (8), boys (3)

CI use: mean 4.78 years, range 0:6–9:9 years

Selection criteria

Voluntary participation; all recipients targeted; no details on returns

Dependent variables

Parents and children with cochlear implants closed-question forced answer (Lickert scale) survey. Questions derived from Kelsay and Tyler (1996). Ratings negative to positive on scales from 1–5

Independent variables

Not applicable

Method

Rating scales of quality-of-life measures

Results

Eighty percent of parents reported at least some benefit in each of the 20 areas addressed, with the exception of telephone use (65%). A mean rating of 3.82 was calculated by averaging across all of the specific areas represented, suggesting 'quite a bit' (p.104) of benefit.

Mean problem scores ranged from 1.30 to 3.52, with the highest score (3.52) given for parents' concern about potential damage to the internal device, followed by limitations in sports and unrealistic expectations by others (p.104).

The responses of parents and children were largely in agreement, although children self-reported less benefit for speech production skill (p.105).

Conclusions

Parents and children report substantial quality-of-life benefits and few problems with cochlear implants. Parents' and children's reports were largely similar, although children reported slightly more problems.

The quality-of-life questionnaire is a valuable tool in the clinical assessment of the benefits of cochlear implantation (p.105).

Observations

The authors report that few studies have focused on quality-of-life measures following paediatric cochlear implantation. One reported exception is the study by Kelsay and Tyler (1996), which used an open-ended questionnaire to query parents. Chmiel et al. comment that this approach does not allow for quantification of the degree of benefit or the magnitude of problems reported (p.103).

Moreover, this study is unique in that it questioned cochlear implant recipients as well as their parents; this concerns a subset of 11 children out of the total response population of 38 families (p.104).

The results are largely in agreement with those reported in Kelsay and Tyler. The benefits are shown to be quantitatively greater than are the problems reported.

The advantages of a closed-question format are less clearly demonstrated, although it is easier to administer to larger populations; the response categories, and especially aggregating the responses, limit the conclusions that can be drawn.

Cleary M, Pisoni DB, Geers AE (2001) Some measures of verbal and spatial working memory in eight- and nine-year-old hearing-impaired children with cochlear implants. Ear and Hearing 22(5): 395–411.

Population size
44

Demographics
Age: range 8.1–9.10 years (mean 8.10 years)
Age at onset: range 0.0–3.0 years (mean 0.4 years)
Duration of deafness: range 0.3–5.0 years (mean 3.0 years)
CI experience: range 4.3–6.9 years (mean 5.5 years)
Gender: males (25), females (19)
CI device: Nucleus 22 (active electrodes range 6–20, mean 17)
Educational programme: range of oral and total communication
Control group of age-matched hearing children

Selection criteria
CI experience > 4 years
Recruited as part of ongoing CID study at summer camps, selected for characteristics
One child failed to complete the memory game task

Dependent variables
Working memory task requiring memory for sequences of either visual-spatial cues or visual-spatial cues paired with auditory signals (new design); WISC Digit Span task of the Wechsler Intelligence Scale

Independent variables
CI/hearing

Method
2×3 and 2×2 mixed factorial repeated measures analyses of variance for independent measures

Results
'The cochlear implant group obtained shorter span scores on average than the normal-hearing group, regardless of presentation format. The normal-hearing children also demonstrated a larger "redundancy gain" than children in the cochlear implant group – that is, the normal-hearing group displayed better memory for auditory-plus-lights sequences than for the lights-only sequences. Although the children with cochlear implants did not use the auditory signals as effectively as normal-hearing children when visual-spatial cues were also available, their performance on the modified memory task using only auditory cues showed that some of the children were capable of encoding auditory-only sequences at a level comparable with normal-hearing children' (p.395).

'Exposure to an oral-only language environment was not found to be associated with higher memory span scores when the memory game task included visual-spatial signals' (experiment 1, p.404).

'We found that experienced school-age users of cochlear implants did not integrate a semantic redundancy present in a memory span task across the auditory and visual sensory modalities as effectively as age-matched normal-hearing children. This finding suggests that fundamentally different sensory encoding and/or rehearsal processes may be operating in these two populations. Although the cochlear implant is now providing the cochlear implant children with access to sound and spoken language, their atypical early sensory and perceptual experiences are still evident in how they perceive and encode sensory information even after more than four years of experience with a cochlear implant' (pp.407–8).

'CI children relied primarily on visual-spatial encoding of the target sequence to perform the task. These results were obtained despite the fact that many of these cochlear implant children did well on the auditory WISC digit span task and on the auditory-only presentation condition of the memory game' (p.409).

Conclusions

'The finding of smaller redundancy gains from the addition of auditory cues to visual-spatial sequences in the cochlear implant group as compared with the normal-hearing group demonstrates differences in encoding or rehearsal strategies between these two groups of children. Differences in memory span between the two groups even on a visual-spatial memory task suggests that atypical working memory development irrespective of input modality may be present in this clinical population' (p.395).

Observations

The purpose of this study was to examine working memory for sequences of auditory and visual stimuli in prelingually deafened paediatric cochlear implant users with at least four years of device experience. The research arose, in part at least, from the authors' impression that:

'Increasingly, clinicians are beginning to see pediatric cochlear implant users that have reached ceiling levels of performance on the traditional standardized measures of speech perception and spoken word recognition that are typically used with this population – and yet these children are still clearly having problems with reading and other more advanced language skills that are based on listening, phonological encoding, and other metalinguistic abilities' (p.409).

The research concerns a group of 44 8- to 9-year-olds with relatively significant experience (average 5.5 years) of cochlear implants. The research is also of interest since it addresses working memory and cognitive tasks, and because of the comparison that is set up with hearing children. This report forms part of a cluster of projects (see also Crosson and Geers 2001).

The authors hold that early sensory experience predetermines the later strategies used in working memory. Deafness therefore has modal effects on the stimuli used in recall:

'Literature published between the 1950s and 1970s suggested that hearing-impaired children in general were less adept overall than normal-hearing children in their working memory for some types of visual (but verbally codeable) sequences because these children lacked effective verbal strategies for rehearsal [...]. In the 1980s and 1990s, however, the focus of research shifted to showing that manually signed equivalents to verbal strategies could be adopted to analogous benefit, although the comparable efficiency of these manual strategies, and the frequency of their use by signing individuals came under debate' (p.396).

The task set to the children is described as 'the presentation of a sequence of sounds in conjunction with a sequence of colored lights located behind a series of four large translucent buttons mounted on a response box modelled after the popular Milton Bradley electronic game Simon. The task requires the child to immediately reproduce the target sequence by pressing on the appropriate buttons in the proper order thereby causing the synchronized sounds to be heard again as the buttons are pressed. The difficulty of the task is adjusted by increasing the list length of the sequence to be reproduced when the child is doing well, and shortening it after an error is made' (pp.398–9).

The results relate to Preislers et al.'s (1997) assessment that cochlear-implanted children are still deaf, since the authors conclude that 'the encoding strategies and working memory mechanisms of pediatric cochlear implant users seem to differ measurably from those of normal-hearing children' (p.409).

In summary, the authors suggest that much of the results reported here can be explained by a different sensory focus resulting from deviant sensory experience in early life.

Coerts J, Mills A (1995) Spontaneous language development of young children with a cochlear implant. Annals of Otology, Rhinology and Laryngology 166: s385–s387.

Population size

6

Population comments

Subsample of a research project involving 20 children with cochlear implants

Demographics

Age at onset: range 2.2–3.0 years

Duration of deafness: range 1.5–3.11 years

Age at CI: range 4.5–6.6 years

Method of communication: oral (4), total communication (2)

Selection criteria

None detailed

Dependent variables

Analysis of linguistic pattern in recordings of spontaneous language of the children 6, 12 and 18 months post implantation. Covers mean length of utterance (MLU) and mean length of five longest utterances (MLUL) for both spoken Dutch and Sign Language of the Netherlands

Independent variables

Pre-implantation performance

Age at implantation

Duration of deafness

Chronological age

Communication mode

Method

Percentage reporting per child. The small number of children precludes statistical reporting

Results

The oral children had a clear preference for spoken Dutch (p.385), but all children produced all three types of utterance (spoken Dutch, SLN and simultaneous Dutch/SLN).

All six children demonstrated development in the morphology-syntax of their spoken language over the study period, although starting point and rates of improvement varied. Important variables appeared to be language environment and age at onset of deafness. The TC children produced better results in spoken Dutch than the oral subjects in the 18-month follow-up period; neither duration of deafness nor age explained this (p.386).

There was little development in SLN over the period of study for any of the children (p.386).

Conclusions

'If age at onset of deafness is relevant, it appears to interact with the factor of language environment. Children who become deaf early appear to profit most from a language environment in which signs are used (TC) in order to learn Dutch' (p.386).

Observations

Although the sample includes only six children, the research is included in the review because the measures used are not commonplace but may have relevance elsewhere, because it presents evidence from a different locale (the Netherlands) where there may be differences in approach to the process of cochlear implantation, and because the researchers pay attention to modally independent (overall) language development, which is rare in the available research.

Because of the small number of children involved in the study, the findings are tentative – the authors note that the findings need to be checked against the full research population of 20 children. More importantly, the follow-up period is limited to 18 months post implantation, so that the outcomes may not reflect a stable over-time pattern. Nevertheless, the methodology is of interest because it addresses spontaneous language interaction:

> 'The rationale for using spontaneous language is based on the assumption that it reflects the functional language of the deaf child and hence is of real relevance, instead of only leading to better test results' (p.385).

Cowan RS, DelDot J, Barker EJ, Sarant JZ, Pegg P, Dettman S, Galvin KL, Rance G, Hollow R, Dowell RC, Pyman B, Gibson WP, Clark GM (1997) Speech perception results for children with implants with different levels of preoperative residual hearing. American Journal of Otology 18(6 Suppl): s125–s126.

Population size
117

Demographics
CI device: Nucleus 22
No demographics detailed; grouped in four categories of preoperative aided residual hearing

Selection criteria
The first 117 children to undergo implantation in the Melbourne and Sydney Cochlear Implant Clinics

Dependent variables
'Standard speech perception tests scores' review; not detailed

Independent variables
Preoperative aided residual hearing

Method
Category percentages; no statistical analysis, presumably due to low numbers in some categories

Results
'The results showed that children in the higher categories of aided preoperative residual hearing showed significant scores on open-set word and sentence perception tests using the implant alone. For children in lower categories of residual hearing, results were variable within the groups. More than 90% of children with implants with aided residual hearing thresholds in the speech range above 1 kHz achieved open-set understanding of words and sentences' (p.s125).

Conclusions
'... children with severe to profound hearing impairments should be considered for cochlear implantation' (p.s125).

Observations
The project reported arose because of findings in paediatric cochlear implantation, suggesting the possibility that cochlear implantation might be appropriate for severely or severely-to-profoundly deaf children and thus they should be considered for implantation. Therefore the retrospective study design considered a cohort of implanted children subsampled by categories of preoperative residual hearing, evaluated in terms of postoperative speech perception benefits.

The results of this study produced some clear findings leading to an unambiguous conclusion. However, the results are not unproblematic.

First, the research concerns post hoc analysis on a dataset that included a range of variable statistics on each child. To cancel out the intervening variables, the authors recode outcomes into a limited and reduced range of a seven-step scale of auditory benefits, which may or may not suit any particular individual's characteristics; in any case the statistical power is therefore reduced. Second, children were assigned into a speech perception benefit category by a 'clinician familiar with the children's results' (p.s126). The original source of the outcomes used in this recoding (i.e. the speech perception tests originally administered) is not detailed.

Third, although the total number of children (117) is relatively high, the numbers in the subsampled groups are more modest; since the final table is based on percentages, care is needed in interpreting the results. As the authors suggest:

> 'These preliminary data should be confirmed in a larger patient group, and the effects of particular factors, such as preoperative aided residual hearing, etiology, length of deafness before implant, and education setting, should be assessed...' (p.s126).

And finally, the fact that overall clear benefit is derived by the group (however they may vary internally in terms of aided residual hearing) might actually reflect effective and appropriate selection by the implant programme teams. In other words, although these children vary minimally in hearing loss, it does not necessarily follow that this improved score-effect will behave as a simple linear variable with reference to a group of children with severe hearing loss.

For comparison, see Blamey et al. (2001), who conclude that there is no reason to believe that the criteria should be relaxed.

Crosson J, Geers A (2000) Structural analysis of narratives produced by young cochlear implant users. Annals of Otology, Rhinology and Laryngology 109(12)s185: 118-119.

Population size
43
Population comments
Control group of 28 hearing children from private schools matched for age
Demographics
Age: range 8–9:11 years (mean 9:1 years)
Age at onset: prelingual (not detailed)
IQ: normal nonverbal distribution
Communication mode: oral, simultaneous communication (not detailed)
Selection criteria
CID programme students; no selection criteria detailed, apart from normal distribution IQ
Dependent variables
Narrative ability; elicited narratives coded with the use of a modified version of the high-point analysis, including orientations, complicating actions, evaluations, and resolutions (p.118)
Independent variables
Communication mode
Improved speech perception results
Method
F-test linear correlation measure of significance .
Results
Narrative structures

> 'The average proportional use of each narrative structure type exhibited by the NH [normally hearing] 8- and 9-year olds was about 30% complicating actions, 30% evaluations, 20% orientations, and 20% resolutions. The two deaf samples

differed from this pattern in the following ways: (1) the SC [simultaneous communication] group used significantly more orientations [...] and (2) both the SC and oral groups used significantly fewer resolutions...' (p.118).

The levels of significance are reported as $p < 0.01$ and $p < 0.05$ respectively.

Conjunction analysis

The SC group was found to use significantly fewer causal conjunctions than the NH group ($p < 0.01$). Oral children produced significantly more causal conjunctions in their narratives. The NH group used significantly more conjunctions in their narratives than the oral and SC groups ($p < 0.01$) (pp.118–19).

Those children who received more benefit from their cochlear implants used fewer orientations and more evaluations and were more likely to use conjunctions to link semantic relations in their narratives (p.119).

Conclusions

'The narratives of deaf children from both oral and SC groups differed substantially from those of NH children. To the extent that the cochlear implant improved speech perception, it appeared to have a positive impact on narrative production' (p.119).

Findings underscore the importance of measuring beyond the sentence level in the assessment of children with cochlear implants (p.119).

Observations

The study arises out of a suggested link between narrative skill and predicted later academic achievement (p.118). The suggestion here is that better narrative production may lead to earlier entry into mainstream education. It is hypothesized that children with improved speech perception resulting from implantation and children who depended on oral communication would produce narratives more closely approximating those of their hearing peers (p.118).

The results are less conclusive: while the authors find correlations between speech perception and narrative structuring skills, the narrative structures produced by both oral and simultaneous communication children differed significantly from those of hearing children.

As the authors suggest, measures of language skills are a useful addition to sentence and subsentence level tests, and may provide better predictors for later academic achievement in so far as this is linked to spoken language ability.

Crosson J, Geers A (2001) Analysis of narrative ability in children with cochlear implants. Ear and Hearing 22(5): 381–394.

Population size

87

Demographics

Age: range 8.0–9.9 years (mean 9.0 years)

Age at onset: range 0–36 months (mean 5.6 months)

Age at CI: range 2.0–5.0 years (mean 3.5 years)

CI experience: range 4.0–6.9 years (mean 5.5 years)

Wechsler performance IQ: range 80–136 (mean 103.9)

CI device: Nucleus 22

Educational programmes: full range

Comparison group of age-matched hearing children

Selection criteria

Summer research camp cohort (US/Canada)

Normal nonverbal intelligence;

Monolingual English-speaking family

Dependent variables

Narrative productions were prompted from an eight-picture sequence story. The stories were transcribed and a scoring system for narrative ability was developed based on the use of complete narrative structure, conjunctions linking semantic relations, and referents that served to identify and distinguish characters in the narrative. The child's preferred mode of communication was used in the process. Results reflected the independent contribution of discourse level language skills, as measured by the narrative ability score, as well as sentence level language skills in predicting reading test scores

PIAT-R (reading test); TACL-R (receptive language); WIPI (closed set speech perception test)

Independent variables

Age
IQ
Speech perception
'Language'
Reading test scores
Comparison with hearing children's scores

Method

Use a modified version of High Point Analysis (Labov and Waletsky 1967) to code the structural components of narratives

Narrative ability test correlated significantly with all other tests in multiple regression analysis, and was thus accepted as a valid measure. Narrative ability accounted to 11% added variance in reading scores (total 52%)

ANOVA (analysis of variance) of speech perceptions scores and narrative ability for three groups: normal hearing, CI with good speech reception ($n = 44$), CI with bad speech perception ($n = 43$); division based on WIPI median score of 43% correct

Results

Within the sample of hearing-impaired children, narrative ability scores correlated significantly with speech perception, language syntax and reading test scores. A multiple regression analysis was conducted to predict reading comprehension scores from four predictor variables (age, IQ, language syntax and narrative ability). Results reflected the independent contribution of discourse-level language skills, as measured by the narrative ability score, as well as sentence-level language skills in predicting reading test scores.

Deaf children who received above-average speech-perception scores with a cochlear implant (i.e. scored above 48% on the Word Intelligibility by Picture Identification speech-perception test) told narratives that were similar in structure and use of referents to those of age mates with normal hearing.

Below-average [CI] speech perceivers exhibited significantly poorer use of narrative structure and cohesive devices than either hearing age mates or children who achieved above-average speech perception with a cochlear implant.

Conclusions

Narrative ability is an important predictor of reading comprehension ability in deaf children above and beyond IQ and syntactic competence. Children who receive a cochlear implant under 5 years of age and obtain above-average speech-perception benefit from the device construct narratives that are similar in structure and cohesion to those of their hearing age mates by age 8 to 9.

Above-average speech perceivers still did not achieve the level of narrative ability of hearing age mates, while the syntax used by the deaf and hearing groups was noticeably different (p.391). The deaf children used very few temporal conjunctions (p.392).

Observations

The aims of this study were to develop a scoring system to assess narrative ability in children, to evaluate the impact of auditory speech perception with a cochlear implant on narrative ability and, finally, to evaluate the importance of narrative ability to reading comprehension in deaf children. The objectives covered developing an appropriate scoring system to measure narrative ability in paediatric cochlear implant users, to correlate narrative ability with speech-perception outcome, and to investigate the relationship between narrative ability and reading ability. The method uses a picture-sequence to elicit talk in the children. This project forms part of a cluster of projects based on the CID summer-camp population: (for earlier work in this area see Crosson and Geers 2000, but see also Cleary et al. 2001). As with the other element of this research, the interest in the results arises in part from the targeted age-group of children (8–9 years) with some considerable experience of cochlear implants.

> 'A narrative ability score was developed based on use of narrative structure, use of conjunctions, and use of referents that served to identify and distinguish characters in the narrative' (p.384).

The findings of this project are relatively straightforward:

- overall narrative ability (English structure) continues to lag behind that of hearing peers (no details of gap)
- cochlear implant, in so far as it improves speech perception, improves narrative ability
- not all cochlear implant results lead to improved narrative ability
- some narrative structure differences remain between deaf and hearing; one notably relates to temporal conjunctions, where deaf children use spatial framing rather than temporal ordering of events.

These outcomes appear to confirm the outcome reported in another part of the study concerning working memory: despite cochlear implantation deaf children are deaf (Cleary et al. 2001; Preisler et al. 1997) in the sense that they have narrative abilities 'properly' their own. In addition, from the very fact that outcome score on WIPI (used to divide the cochlear implant group) ranged from 0 to 92, it is clear that at least some implanted children in the group had very minimal speech perception skills after four years' experience.

This research, together with the Crosson and Geers (2000) study, makes a welcome contribution to a little-researched area of outcome in paediatric cochlear implantation.

Cullington H, Hodges AV, Butts SL, Dolan-Ash S, Balkany TJ (2000) Comparison of language ability in children with cochlear implants placed in oral and total communication educational settings. Annals of Otology, Rhinology and Laryngology 185: s121–s123.

Population size
24

Demographics
Detailed in table per communication group
Age: range 76–197 months
Age at onset: prelingual except one deafened at 19 months (no details)
Aetiology: range not reported
CI use: range 15–80 months
Age at CI: range 31–135 months
CI device: Nucleus (22), Clarion (2)
Gender: boys (11), girls (13)
Communication mode: oral (12), total communication mode (12)
Total communication group has a much longer experience of cochlear implant

Selection criteria
Miami Ear Institute study children. No selection criteria detailed

Dependent variables
Speech perception
  PPVT-III
  EVT
Speech production
  TACL-R
  GAEL
Independent variables
  Communication mode
Method
  Parameters were examined with F-test; comparable variances analysed with two-tailed t-test; all other assessments were analysed with the Mann-Whitney U-test
Results
  'The oral children demonstrated significantly less language delay than the total communication children on the EVT test. Although they also performed better on the PPVT-III, TACL-R and GAEL, these differences were not statistically significant' (p.122).

  '... the oral children are better at demonstrating their vocabulary knowledge in an open expressive format rather than a receptive format' (p.122).

  There were too few children in the study to attempt a direct comparative quantitative analysis between oral and total communication children. The latter finding reported above is therefore based on comparisons with normed (hearing) populations.
Conclusions
  The authors suggest that oral children performed 'significantly better', but on the EVT speech-perception test only. Other differences were not statistically significant. It is anyway possible that early indicators of language ability affect the selection of educational mode (p.122).
Observations
  As a reason for conducting the study, the authors comment that most previous research has demonstrated that children with cochlear implants in oral settings attain comparatively better speech-perception outcomes than do cochlear-implanted children in total communication settings (p.121). The authors employ a narrow focus in their approach because they perceive that linguistic development is the targeted outcome of paediatric implantation, although they comment that speech-perception scores do not reflect linguistic development well.

  They test 24 children (12 each in oral and total communication setting) using the PPVT-III, EVT, TACL-R and GAEL tests, but without explaining why such formal clinical measures present a better overall measure of linguistic development in any way (p.121).

  Test administration was performed in the communication mode preferred by the child, although in practice this meant that the non-spoken language assessment was undertaken by two audiologists who had taken college-level courses in American Sign Language. The authors suggest that the results indicate that cochlear-implanted children in oral settings attain higher language skills than their peers in total communication settings (p.122). Yet relative to the lack of statistically significant correlation (p.122) on three out of four measures, the conclusion seems rather over-interpreted. The measures furthermore concern spoken-language targets exclusively using tests normed on spoken-language children, while the communication with children in total communication settings does not focus on spoken language in auditory mode exclusively; hence this type of assessment does not reflect a cross-modal assessment of the linguistic development more typical of those in total communication settings.

  Furthermore, as the authors note, 'It is possible that early indicators of language ability affected the selection of education mode' (p.122) independent of cochlear implantation and its effects on language development.

Davids L, Brenner C, Geers A (2000) Predicting speech perception benefit from loudness growth measures and other map characteristics of the Nucleus 22 implant. Annals of Otology, Rhinology and Laryngology 109(12)s185: 56–58.

Population size
46
Demographics
Age: 8- to 9-year olds
Age at CI: < 5 years of age
CI use: range 3.98–6.94 years (average 5.5 years)
Encoding: MPEAK, 36 moved to SPEAK
Active electrodes: 20 or more (24), 14–19 (20), 7 (2)
Selection criteria
None detailed
Dependent variables
Speech perception (WIPI)
Independent variables
Loudness growth measures
Method
Linear correlation
Results
'The greater the ability to perceive differences between loudness categories and the smaller the variability in judgments, the higher the child's speech perception score' (p.58).
Conclusions
'... the better the growth of loudness across the intensity scale and the greater the frequency and dynamic range available, the better the perception of speech (p.58).
Observations
This research is principally of relevance because it demonstrates that the better the working of the device is matched with user's needs, the higher the auditory benefit will be. It is worth noting that despite the considerable average experience of cochlear implants among the sample (5.5 years), the WIPI scores still ranged from 0 to 92% (p.58).

Dawson PW, Blamey SJ, Dettman LC et al. (1995) A clinical report on speech production of cochlear implant users. Ear and Hearing 16: 551–561.

Population size
12
Population comments
Two groups of 10 and 11 administered different tests, out of which a group of nine were administered both tests
Demographics
Listed in table on individual basis
Age: range 8–20 years
Age at onset: range congenital to age 4 years progressive
Aetiology: meningitis (4), Usher's (4), Mondini malformation (1), unknown (3)
Duration of deafness: range 5:10–19:9 years
Age at CI: range 8–19:9 years
PTA: range 103–125 dB HL
Gender: male (6) female (6)
CI use: range (across tests) 0:70–4:5 years

Selection criteria
Implanted at age 8 years or over

Dependent variables
McGarr's procedure: read aloud 36 sentences. Scored by listeners familiar with deaf speech articulation:

Test of Articulation Competence (TAC). Scored by listeners familiar with the individual children

Not every child did both tests, and the time of test administration varied widely between children. Tests were taken preoperatively and postoperatively

Independent variables
Speech articulation

Speech intelligibility

Method
'The t-test for dependent samples was used with a one-tailed criterion to test the directional hypothesis that the group mean postoperative performance would be significantly greater than the group mean preoperative performance' (p.555)

The chi-square analysis was used for individual scores in preference to a linear regression or correlation analysis because the trends are not necessarily linear and values not necessarily normally distributed

Results
Speech intelligibility

'Mean group performance (for total scores) of 11 patients on the latest postoperative assessment was significantly higher than the performance on the preoperative assessment ($p < 0.01$)...' (p.555).

Error bars show considerable variation in performance among patients. Preoperatively scores ranged from 0 to 36%, postoperatively from 19 to 81%, although the majority of patients scored below 50%.

Speech articulation

Results suggest a significant increase over time in the overall accuracy of articulation ($p < 0.05$), and again error bars reveal substantial variability in individual performance (pp.555–6).

'With the exception of nasals and affricates, there were significant gains in accuracy for each of the consonant categories. Significant increases in accuracy also occurred in each of the three word positions. Consonants produced at the front of the mouth were significantly more accurate than those produced further back in the mouth, regardless of implant status (pre- versus postoperative) or position in the word ($p < 0.001$ for a two-tailed chi-square test). Affricates were, by far, the group of consonants that were produced the least accurately' (p.556).

Across individuals, performance appeared to plateau at about 13 months postimplantation, with five out of 10 children showing significant improvements over time (p.557).

Conclusions
Sentence intelligibility prior to implantation is reported to be similar to that of previous studies, ranging between 18 and 26% sentence intelligibility for American and British profoundly deaf speakers (p.557).

'The group average postoperative scores for low and high context sentences were remarkably similar to those [reported elsewhere] for experienced listeners judging a group of 20 congenitally hearing-impaired children with a mean pure tone average of 98.6 dB HL' (p.557).

'Despite the significant group results not all individual patients improved. Fifty-five percent of the patients demonstrated a significant improvement over time in speech intelligibility' (p.558).

'Fifty percent of the patients in this study demonstrated significant
improvement over time for the total score on the articulation test' (p.558).

Observations

In this study, the authors investigated the speech articulation and speech intelligibility of
later-implanted children (ranging from age 8–20 years). Although the study is exemplary
in its demographic and methodological detail and description, it is also characterized by a
few uncontrolled factors. First, the number of participants is relatively low (12 children).
Moreover, not all children took both tests, and they took them at different time intervals.
Findings require conservative interpretation in light of the wide age distribution and the
fact that experience of implantation and time of testing varied greatly between them.
Nevertheless, detailed attention to individual performance and statistical analysis
sensitive to the variations involved have allowed the authors to report some notable
findings.

The authors comment that poor speech intelligibility is commonly reported for
profoundly deaf children, and that it appears to be influenced by the amount of residual
hearing. Restoration of hearing via cochlear implantation appears to have a positive
influence on speech intelligibility in some children using multichannel implants, with
reports predictably and typically reporting higher scores for experienced listeners than
naive listeners (p.551).

Since past research, according to the authors, has reported depressed outcomes in
profoundly deaf children after late childhood, the current study selected children aged 8
and over (including two prelinguistically deafened adults) to investigate the effects of
cochlear implantation (p.552).

The results suggest overall group improvements that are significant relative to
preoperative scores, but it also reports wide individual distribution of scores, with only
roughly 50% making measurable improvements over the variable period reported.
Moreover, one child did not have sufficient reading skill to complete the speech
intelligibility measure (p.554).

The wide distribution of age produced some observations to be noted, such as the fact
that:

'... four of the patients in this study were over the age of 17 years at
implantation and three of these showed significant improvement on the
sentence intelligibility test and one significantly improved on the articulation
test. These results show clearly that it is not impossible for older deaf
adolescents and adults to improve their speech production skills' (p.559).

There was no clear-cut relationship between gains in speech production and speech
perception performance on a sound-alone word-recognition task, so it is likely that other
factors (such as the use mentioned of tactile and visual cues and speech therapy in the
educational setting) were also important in influencing outcome scores (p.559).

Neither was there a clear-cut relationship between duration of implant use and speech
production changes following implantation: 'For both articulation and intelligibility
measures the patients with the greatest duration of implant use did not consistently
show the greatest gains in production. Furthermore, preoperative performance in
articulation and intelligibility did not appear to be related to changes in production
postimplantation' (p.559).

For a more reliable assessment it will be critical to replicate this research with much
larger population sizes, possibly grouped for age and experience with their cochlear
implant. Nevertheless,

'... data are in accord with previous studies detailing increased speech
production performance with implant use in younger groups of children.
Improvements cannot be attributed unambiguously to implant use since no
control group was used in this clinical work' (p.560).

Dawson PW, McKay CM, Busby PA, Grayden DB, Clark GM (2000) Electrode
discrimination and speech perception in young children using cochlear implants. Ear
and Hearing 21(6): 597–607.

Population size
17

Demographics
Age: range 4.5–10.8 years
CI device: Nucleus 22
Processing strategy: Spectra (16), MPeak (1)
Onset of deafness: range congenital to 2.3 years
Communication mode: total communication (10), oral/aural (7)
Age at CI: range 1.9–5.7 years
CI experience: 1.5–7 years

Selection criteria
Not detailed, but likely to correspond with those published in Dawson et al. (1998):
volunteers residing in metropolitan Melbourne, age-selected

Dependent variables
Adaptation of play audiometry procedure used to assess electrode discrimination; also
assessed on a speech feature discrimination test, a closed-set word recognition test and
a nonverbal intelligence task

Independent variables
Electrode discrimination
Age
Mode of communication

Method
Correlations, and multiple regression analysis

Results
Sixty-five percent of children demonstrated ability to discriminate adjacent electrodes in
mid- and apical regions of the cochlea, whilst the remaining children needed electrode
separations of between two and nine electrodes for successful discrimination. In a
forward stepwise regression analysis, electrode discrimination ability was found to be the
strongest factor in accounting for variance in the speech perception scores. Child
variables such as duration of deafness, nonverbal intelligence and implant experience did
not significantly account for further variance in the speech-perception scores for this
group of children.

Communication mode was the only independent variable to account for a significant
portion of the variance (24%) in the electrode discrimination task. Those children in the
aural/oral educational setting had better electrode discrimination performance on
average than those children in the total communication settings.

As in the study by Busby and Clark (2000), some children in the present investigation
had much poorer electrode discrimination. Both studies found that lower closed-set
speech perception scores were significantly associated with poorer electrode
discrimination in the apical region of the cochlea. In contrast to Busby and Clark's
findings, this study also observed a significant correlation between speech perception
scores and electrode discrimination in the mid-region of the cochlea.

Conclusions
As an overall summary of findings, electrode discrimination ability was the strongest
factor in predicting performance on speech-perception measures in a group of children
using cochlear implants.

Observations
In terms of aims and objectives this research proceeds from that published by Dawson et
al. (1998), which suffered a number of weaknesses largely addressed here. The aim was

to determine the efficacy of a child-appropriate procedure to assess electrode discrimination ability in young children using cochlear implants and to investigate the relationship of electrode discrimination ability and speech perception performance in children implanted at a young age.

There appears to be some consensus in the literature that electrode discrimination ability is a factor that accounts significantly for some of the variance in speech perception ability for postlinguistically deafened adults and for early deafened older children, teenagers and young adults.

In contrast to previous studies, the factors of duration of deafness, age at implantation, onset of profound loss and implant experience did not account for significant variance in the speech perception scores in this investigation. This could be at least partly explained by the fact that all the children were implanted at a relatively young age (≤ 6 years) and had a short duration of profound deafness relative to that for children in previous studies. Furthermore, the majority of the children were congenitally deafened and all were deafened before 2.5 years of age. There is another possible interpretation of the findings. This study used speech feature discrimination and closed-set word recognition tasks, which are influenced less by the child's linguistic skills than open-set speech perception tasks. It is likely that linguistic skills are strongly influenced by factors such as duration of implant experience. Finally it should be remembered that the sample size for this study was relatively small.

In all, it appears that technology is heavily implicated in the variation of outcomes across populations researched, introducing factors that are difficult to normalize; in part, therefore, variation in individual performance must be attributable to technological factors such as electrode discrimination.

Dawson PW, Nott PE, Clark GM, Cowan RS (1998) A modification of play audiometry to assess speech discrimination ability in severe-profoundly deaf 2- to 4-year-old children. Ear and Hearing 19(5): 371–384.

Population size
12

Population comments
Also included 30 hearing and 36 hearing aid users

Demographics
Age-grouped as 2-, 3- and 4-year-olds
Age: 3 years (1), 4 years (11)
CI device: Nucleus 22
Age at CI: range 1.8–3.10 years
CI experience: range 10 months–3.3 years
Aetiology: range, many unknown
Active electrodes: ≥ 12
Educational placement: integrated (7), segregated (5)
Mode of communication: oral (9), total communication (3)

Selection criteria
Volunteers residing in metropolitan Melbourne. Age-selected

Dependent variables
Non-meaningful speech contrasts, consisting of repeated CV syllables, one acting as a 'background stimulus', the other as a 'change' stimulus. Eight speech contrasts selected.
Play audiology assessment in six trials per child

Independent variables
Comparison between cochlear-implanted children, hearing aid users, and hearing children

Method
Percentage scores. 2-way ANOVA using age as independent measure

Results

More than 82% of the 3- and 4-year-old hearing and hearing-impaired children were able to complete the testing for the eight speech sound contrasts within three 20-minute sessions. Fifty percent of the 2-year-old hearing and hearing-impaired children were able to condition and complete the task. All the hearing children who completed the task successfully discriminated all speech sound contrasts. On average, hearing-impaired children took a greater number of sessions than hearing children to complete the task.

For hearing aid users, contrast type rather than age influenced the discrimination performance of those children using hearing aids who completed the task. Hearing loss (PTA) accounted for a significant amount of the variance in individual scores, especially for the speech contrasts requiring use of finer spectral cues.

For the cochlear-implanted group (n = 10), the average performance was similar to that of the hearing aid users for the three easier contrasts: /ba/b^/, /ba/ba[drarr]/, /ba/bi/. For the other contrasts, average performance was approximately midway between the performance of the severely deaf hearing aid users and the performance of the profoundly deaf hearing aid users. Removing atypical children, four of the remaining six implant users passed all eight contrasts, performing similarly to the mild to moderate hearing aid users.

Conclusions

The new SFT is a modification of existing procedures used, and appeared to be a reasonably efficient and reliable test for the majority of 3- and 4-year-old severe-profoundly deaf children tested and for about 50% of 2-year-old children tested. Performance on the task was influenced by PTA hearing loss but not by age at testing for the particular speech contrasts tested. The procedure has the potential to be used as a clinical and research tool in the assessment of very young, severe-profoundly deaf children using hearing aids or cochlear implants.

Observations

This report is of a fairly technical nature, with considerable detail on test procedures and test–retest reliability; for those less familiar with the technical linguistic detail, the research is more readily accessible in the 2000 publication.

The aim of the research was to develop an assessment procedure that was independent of language and speech-production ability, to test speech feature discrimination in severe-profoundly deaf children aged between 2 and 4 years. To this end, the test uses non-meaningful utterances. Respondents were expected to respond to changes in a speech stimulus presented in a repeated fashion through a speaker (i.e. auditory condition only testing).

Outcomes were affected by low numbers and atypical users of cochlear implants (including cognitive delay, health problems, device problems and infrequent use). Correction for atypical instances leaves only six children, who scored equivalent to moderate hearing loss hearing aid users – and in this respect the results confirm other assessments.

Daya H, Ashley A, Gysin C, Papsin BC (2000) Changes in educational placement and speech perception ability after cochlear implantation in children. Journal of Otolaryngology 29(4): 224–228.

Population size

83

Demographics

Ethnicity: 18 children were from multilingual homes 'with only some members of the family speaking English' (p.226)

No demographic details provided

Selection criteria

Attending the Cochlear Implant programme at The Hospital for Sick Children (Toronto, Canada) between 1990 and 1998

Included if PB-K test scores at least 6 months post-CI available

No selection criteria detailed

Dependent variables

PB-K test scores pre-CI and at 6-month intervals after CI

Parent questionnaire

Independent variables

PB-K pre- and post-CI

Placement post-CI

Method

Plain percentage scores; chi-square calculation of significance between selected factors

Results

Of the children who were in non-mainstream school programmes at implantation (n = 30), 50% moved towards mainstream with nine (30%) reaching mainstream placement. Of the children who were preschool at implantation (n = 34), 24 (70%) were placed or planned to be placed in mainstream after implantation. The rate of improvement in speech perception ability was significantly higher in those children who moved toward or remained in mainstream than those who stayed at the same non-mainstream educational placement or moved away from mainstream. Children from a multilingual background were able to achieve similar educational placements and similar rates of progress of speech perception outcome as the only English-speaking children. The 'move towards' mainstream was, however, not found to be significant (p.226), although there was a significant positive correlation between mainstream and speech perception skills (p > 0.05; p.226).

Of the 80 sent questionnaires, 61 were returned. Of the preschool group, 82% of parents desired mainstream schooling for their child.

Conclusions

Children with cochlear implants have increased educational opportunities, with those children in mainstream and those who have moved towards mainstream demonstrating improved progress in speech perception ability.

Observations

The purpose of this study was to evaluate the effect and relationship of paediatric cochlear implantation on educational placement and speech perception ability and to determine the effect of a multilingual background on educational placement and speech perception ability after cochlear implantation.

The study concerns a retrospective chart review, followed by a one-off questionnaire sent to parents of cochlear-implanted children. The authors suggest that until the advent of cochlear implants educational opportunities were restricted for profoundly deaf children, while mainstream education was attended typically only by children with moderate hearing loss (< 70 dB). The authors express their hope that cochlear implantation will widen the educational opportunities for profoundly deaf children (p.225). In this study, they correlate changes in speech perception ability with post-implant changes in placement. In addition, parents are questioned about the educational opportunities of their implanted child.

It is particularly illuminating to compare these results with those of McDonald et al. (2000), who note no differences in total communication/oral placements. The finding in this study that children from non-English-only backgrounds make similar progress suggests that the clear correlation between placement and increased speech perception scores following cochlear implantation may be misunderstood. It may be because inclusion/mainstreaming is adopted by education authorities and parents independently of cochlear implantation outcomes.

Or, as the authors recognize:

'It remains speculation whether these children were only able to remain in less supervised educational settings because of their speech perception ability or whether this improved because of their educational setting' (p.227).

Unfortunately, there is no clearly detailed assessment of multilingual backgrounds and outcomes reported, so that this element must be discounted.

Contradictory findings may also partly be explained by the fact that numbers are low for the chi-square test of significance, and may have been affected by extreme individual scores.

Diller G, Graser P, Schmalbrock C (2001) Early natural auditory-verbal education of children with profound hearing impairments in the Federal Republic of Germany: results of a 4 year study. International Journal of Pediatric Otorhinolaryngology 60(3): 219–226.

Population size

103

Population comments

CI: 4 (year 1), 33 (year 2), 49 (= 50.8%, year 3) of study

Demographics

Age at CI: 'who were fitted with hearing aids or CI until 24 months old'

Age at onset: 88% congenital, 12% postnatal

Parents' HL status: 81.6% had no hearing impairments

Ethnicity: 18.4% (n = 19) were from ethnic minority background (did not use German to communicate)

Age at start of survey: range 0–23 years (average 15.2 years)

Selection criteria

Contacted schools with natural aural-verbal programmes nationwide; 41 agreed to take part in four-year study

No other handicaps

Dependent variables

Denver development scales

Senso-motoric developmental scale

Vademecum

Munich functional development test

Independent variables

Age at diagnosis

Age at aid provision (including CI)

Degree of use ('acceptance')

Type of aid: hearing aid or CI

Educational programme

Family language

Comparison with hearing population

Method

Measure scores. Interval measures compared with age-matched hearing peers. Chi-square (Spearman coefficient) used to correlate independent variables

Results

In 1997, fewer than 40% of the children reached hearing language development levels comparable to hearing children. At the end of the study, development of about a half of the children was such that their progress and speed in hearing and language learning was comparable to that of hearing children. More children (63%) with cochlear implants had typical language development than hearing aid users (35%). Typical rates of speech development were related to whether the cochlear implant or hearing aid was worn. The development of hearing and speech skills correlated with how well the hearing device had been used, the quality of education received, as well as with the actual language spoken by the family. Statistical evidence of an additional factor emerged, namely, which type of hearing device was worn, in other words, whether a cochlear implant or hearing aid was used.

Conclusions

When the best conditions currently available are actually present, then children with profound hearing impairments (about half according to this current study) are as capable of developing hearing and language skills as hearing children – perhaps with a slight time lapse, and certainly with a large amount of effort on the part of the children themselves – yet in principle, along the same natural path as with their own native language, and of very similar quality.

Observations

This is a wide-ranging study, and consists mainly of broad statistical assessments. By means of background to their study, the authors note that early education of children with hearing impairments has been carried out in Germany for the past 40 years using a variety of different educational concepts. One of these concepts, they go on to note, is the natural auditory-verbal approach, which by supporting the use of hearing even among children with profound hearing impairments makes the claim of being capable of initiating the children's development of natural auditory-verbal skills, which are subsequently comparable to those of children with hearing.

The authors' focus is the auditory-verbal approach and this influences the assessments they use. 'During the course of this study, the measures involved in a hearing-oriented system of early education were comprehensively examined' (p.219).

During the course of the study the selected children were tested three times (once per year), while teaching professionals practising the auditory-aural approach were sent questionnaires at each of these test intervals. The study focuses on approach, not on cochlear implants; therefore the cochlear implant responses are a subset of the total response set, and are treated as such:

> 'The early education system must urgently be improved by the introduction of screening for newborn infants. As far as devices are concerned, the cochlear implant (CI) will very soon be standard equipment for infants with profound hearing impairments. Within institutional facilities, there is a broad consensus that the goal of these measures consists of the development of speech communication skills in children' (p.219).

The authors report that during the phase when data were compiled, a tendency towards using cochlear implants and a corresponding progressive reduction in relevance of the use of hearing aids became apparent for children with profound hearing impairments (p.220).

> 'Only 46.0% of parents and 58.1% of the professionals provided education that was consistent in a natural auditory-verbal way' (p.222).

This assessment involved a range of assessments. However, the sample is not representative as the authors themselves indicate:

> 'It can be conspicuous that families in which the parents were involved in a comprehensive natural auditory-verbal program, were characterised as having a secure social standing, a non-working mother with experience in raising children, a father who played an active role in the child's education and a consistent and constant attitude towards the education programme' (p.225).

Dorman MF, Loizou PC, Kemp LL, Kirk KI (2000) Word recognition by children listening to speech processed into a small number of channels: data from normal-hearing children and children with cochlear implants. Ear and Hearing 21(6): 590–596.

Population size

56

Population comments

Control group of 36 matched hearing children

Demographics
Age: range 3.5–5.7 years
CI device: Nucleus 22
Age at CI: 43 'late-implanted' (mean 5.4 years), 13 'early implanted' (mean 3.3 years)
Age at onset: mean 0.2 years
Age at onset: 82%/92% congenital
CI experience: mean 4.5 years/3.1 years
Active electrodes: mean 17

Selection criteria
Recruited from on-campus preschools at Arizona State (no demographics reported)

Dependent variables
MLNT adapted to the CHILDES assessments of age-appropriate child vocabulary

Independent variables
Number of channels of output (6 and 12)

Method
In the first experiment, the words from the Multisyllabic Lexical Neighborhood Test (MLNT) were processed into 6 to 20 channels and output as the sum of sine waves at the centre frequency of the analysis bands. The signals were presented to hearing adults and children for identification. In the second experiment, the wideband recordings of the MLNT words were presented to early-implanted and late-implanted children who used the Nucleus 22 cochlear implant

Results
Hearing children needed more channels of stimulation than adults to recognize words. Ten channels allowed 99% correct word recognition for adults; 12 channels allowed 92% correct word recognition for children. The average level of intelligibility for both early- and late-implanted children was equivalent to that found for hearing adults listening to four to six channels of stimulation. The best intelligibility for implanted children was equivalent to that found for hearing adults listening to six channels of stimulation. The distribution of scores for early- and late-implanted children differed. Nineteen percent of the late-implanted children achieved scores below that allowed by a six-channel processor. None of the early-implanted children fell into this category.

Conclusions
The average implanted child must deal with a signal that is significantly degraded. This is likely to prolong the period of language acquisition. The period could be significantly shortened if implants were able to deliver at least eight functional channels of stimulation. Twelve functional channels of stimulation would provide signals near the intelligibility of wideband signals in quiet.

Observations
This research takes an interesting approach in the comparison between deaf and hearing children by equalizing them: the hearing children were presented with auditory input (MLNT words) in an impoverished fashion, which approaches the quality of sound afforded by cochlear implants. The sound was compressed into a range between six and 20 channels, and this provided the test conditions for listening by the hearing children. The results were then compared to the auditory recognition performance of the children with multichannel cochlear implants.

As an approach, this provides information on the number of channels that present a normative threshold for sufficient (in the light of the test taken) auditory discrimination.

The performance deficit of children versus adults reported in the article may be explained by lexical access and/or by nonlinguistic task-related factors. The study demonstrates that children need more auditory input for age-appropriate speech reception than do adults. Early-implanted children are slightly closer to hearing performance than are later-implanted children.

Easterbrooks SR, Mordica JA (2000) Teachers' ratings of functional communication in students with cochlear implants. American Annals of the Deaf 145(1): 54–59.

Population size
51
Population comments
Concerns teachers of deaf cochlear-implanted children
Demographics
Limited demographic data
Gender: male (28), female (23)
Age: range 4.25–21.67 years
Address: rural (21), non-rural (30)
Selection criteria
CI experience at least two years, 'large metropolitan area'
Dependent variables
Teacher's ratings of CI 'functionality' into one of three categories:
• does not use
• uses for environmental awareness
• uses as primary means of communication
Independent variables
Placement
Address (rural/non-rural)
Aetiology
Home use of American Sign Language
Method
Percentage scores; chi-square analysis of correlation
Results
Correlations with aetiology ('known' or 'unknown'), rural address, home use of ASL and school placement were found to be significant at $p < 0.01$.
Conclusions
The authors suggest that the teacher's role in implant use warrants more attention.
Observations
This study examined factors associated with teachers' ratings of functional communication skills of students with cochlear implants. Deaf students living in and around a metropolitan area were surveyed to locate 51 with cochlear implants, while teachers rated each student's functional use of the implant, given three defined ratings. Additional information regarding sex, communication option, placement, home language, rural or non-rural address, aetiology and presence or absence of an additional disability was also gathered.

This report is constructed out of a subsample of a larger study (not detailed here) that comprised 284 students in total. This study reports on the 51 (18%) who had cochlear implants. The authors suggest that it is incumbent on teachers to have 'a clear picture of when an implant is most successful' (p.54) since implants are becoming more widespread. The authors claim to have undertaken this add-on study to assess whether teachers' ratings of benefits were associated with any 'risk factors' (p.54) for functional communication among other potential candidates for a cochlear implant – no further clarification is given. A more detailed account of the overall, larger study would have been helpful to assist readers in placing the current study into a more clearly defined theoretical framework.

The authors recognize that teacher opinion might have affected the findings, as might teacher bias, listed as a separate 'possible limitation' of the research (p.57). Yet at the same time the authors conclude that 'numeric measures of specific speech or language skills, while important, mean nothing if the teacher is not satisfied that he or she may use the auditory channel as a channel for instruction' (p.57). An important suggestion is that the validity of some longitudinal studies based around cochlear implant centres or rehabilitation networks might be affected by a process of 'self-selection', through which better performing students remain in the programmes while others drop out, thereby artificially increasing the average outcomes over time (p.57).

As a contribution to the available literature this article serves to raise one or two questions in what is already a very complex set of issues (for perhaps another example of this kind, see Bennet and Lynas 2001).

Eilers RE, Cobo-Lewis AB, Vergara KC, Oller D et al. (1996) A longitudinal evaluation of the speech perception capabilities of children using multichannel tactile vocoders. Journal of Speech and Hearing Research 39(3): 518–533.

Population size
28
Population comments
In the comparative element the population of Osberger et al. (1991) is being used
Demographics
Population of 30 children with tactile vocoders (TVs) and hearing aids
Comparison populations of 13 TVs (Robbins et al. 1992) and 28 CIs (Osberger et al. (1991)
CI (as reported in Eilers et al.)
CI device: Nucleus 22
Age at CI: range 2–14 years, mean 7.4 years
CI use: range 0.5–3.5 years, mean 21 months
Selection criteria
The TV children were enrolled in a full-day educational programme that uses the CHATS (Cochlear Implant, Hearing Aid, Auditory and Tactile Skills) curriculum at the University of Miami Tactual Speech Project
Dependent variables
6-month intervals over two-year period
Test battery of vocabulary development, speech perception and speech production ranged at four test levels. Battery includes:
• MTSP
• ESPT
• SCIPS
• change/no change
• maximal pairs test
• PSI
• minimal pairs
• NU-CHIPS
• contextual word
• common phrases
• familiar word
• PB-K word lists
Independent variables
CI group and other TV group test battery outcome scores
Method
Pearson coefficients for correlating independent in-group variables (auditory, auditory+tactile, and auditory+tactile+visual test administrations), converted to z-score metrics group inter-group comparisons
Results
Detail is provided only on progress with tactile vocoders over time and under different test conditions. The variables test condition and time were both found to be significantly

correlated with outcome. For comparisons with the cochlear-implanted population, scores from both reports were converted to z-scores, with regression reliability (R) ranging from .96 to .98 between the four outcome levels:

> 'The high reliability of the regression equations suggest that the conversion of Robbins' and Osberger's data to z-scores, measured on the present study's scale, can be done with confidence. The procedure allows direct comparison across studies' (p.525).

On level 1 scores:

> 'The mean for the Osberger, Miyamoto et al. dataset falls less than one-third of a standard deviation above the TA [tactile+auditory] condition mean. The pooled and transformed CI child scores are, therefore, quite similar to the TA scores in the present study, whereas the Robbins et al. Tactaid 7 data fit our T [tactile only] condition data quite well' (pp.525–6).

The findings are replicated across the four conditions (pp.527, 528, 530). For example, at level 3:

> 'the tactile data represented in [the table] are striking in their similarity to the mean cochlear implant data from Osberger, Miyamoto et al. (1991). Children's performance at a mean duration of 21 months post-implant without the benefit of lipreading is indistinguishable from children's performance with tactile aids plus hearing aids. Similarly, performance of both groups is indistinguishable when lipreading is available to both. In these comparison data, the effects of lipreading are substantially larger than any differences in performance that can be attributed to implants, tactile aids, or hearing aids' (p.529).

Conclusions

Overall, performance of cochlear-implanted children at 1.7 years post-implant was similar to that of tactually and auditorily aided children at similar time post-fit.

Observations

Although this article reports on children using a combination of tactile vocoders and hearing aids, it is of particular interest since it compares the results directly with matched-population data from an earlier cochlear implant project with a matched set of data, also published earlier, of deaf children using vocoders (incidentally, neither of the two secondary source data studies are reported here). Although this approach will mean that cochlear implant results have since been improved for various technical, rehabilitation and group-size reasons, the same might well be true for those using tactile vocoders. Nevertheless, the observation that must be made is that a developmental time gap of five years exists between the tactile vocoder cohort reported here and the post hoc inclusion of Osberger's group of children with cochlear implants, reported in 1991. At least in terms of cochlear implant development, this means that an earlier generation of speech-processing strategies in particular, and even perhaps single-channel technology, may affect the interpretation of results.

The two reports used in the comparison are: Osberger MJ, Miyamoto RT, Zimmerman-Phillips S, Kemink JL, Stroer BS, Firszt JB, Novak MA (1991) Independent evaluation of the speech perception abilities of children with the Nucleus 22-channel cochlear implant system. Ear and Hearing 12(4): s66–s80; Robbins AM, Todd SL, Osberger MJ (1992) Speech performance of paediatric multichannel tactile aid or cochlear implant users. Paper presented at the Second International Conference on Tactile Aids, Hearing Aids and Cochlear Implants, Stockholm, Sweden.

In these comparison data, the effects of lipreading are substantially larger than any differences in performance that can be attributed to implants, tactile aids or hearing aids (p.529). This suggests a more modest (but effective) effect of negation of hearing loss itself for cochlear implants. In fact, the authors note the precise 'fit' of the outcomes between the groups reported as raising questions on choice and decision:

'Comparisons with the literature showed similarities between performance of children using cochlear implants versus children of similar age and hearing impairment using tactile aids plus hearing aids. Both implanted children and users of tactile aids plus hearing aids showed similar levels of open-set word recognition, pattern recognition, and closed-set word recognition on a common battery of tests' (p.530).

The authors also note that there is large individual variation in outcome, but this is noted for both groups:

'the patterns across time of individual children using tactile aids look similar to those observed for children using cochlear implants (i.e. individual children differ markedly in their rate and degree of success with perceptual tasks using the aids...)' (p.530)

so that even in this respect the two groups perform in a similar fashion:

'performance of children using cochlear implants for an average of 21 months from the Osberger, Miyamoto et al. (1991) study seems quite similar to TA performance of children using tactile aids over an equivalent period of time' (p.530).

In fact, the authors note that the initial hearing status across the studies is so similar that a number of children in the present study have gone on to receive implants. The performance levels of these children on levels 1 to 4 tasks remain similar to their matched controls who still use tactile aids and hearing aids (Eilers et al. 1995). In the light of such findings, the authors move to consider that tactile vocoders present a possible alternative to cochlear implants, suggesting that medical criteria may become decisive.

'Given the similarities found between performance of a small group of children using cochlear implants in one study in the literature and performance of children using tactile aids in the present study, can we feel comfortable suggesting use of tactile devices instead of surgical intervention? The question is obviously complex and difficult. For children for whom surgery is medically contraindicated or financially out of reach, we can feel confident about the value of multichannel tactile aids used in a suitable training environment' (p.531).

Finally, it is worth noting that the educational environment of the children in the active sample includes not only spoken language but also sign language, because CHATS uses an early-signing environment to move to speech later in the curriculum:

'As academic children are introduced, spoken language becomes a more and more prominent part of the routine' (p.520).

See Geers and Moog (1994) and Geers and Brenner (1994) for similar types of comparison of cochlear-implanted children and children using tactile vocoders, obtaining contrasting findings.

Filipo R, Bosco E, Barchetta C, Mancini P (1999) Cochlear implantation in deaf children and adolescents: effects on family schooling and personal well-being. International Journal of Pediatric Otorhinolaryngology 49s1: s183–s187.

Population size

12

Demographics

Age: 6 adolescents (range 12–18 years), 6 children (range 4–9 years)
Gender: 4 males, 2 females in each group
CI device: all adults Clarion, 2 Med-Els in children group

Selection criteria

Selected from Rome implant centre out of a total of 30 children with implants
Sampling procedure or selection process not detailed

Dependent variables

Battery of psycho-social tests, including projective personality tests, self-assessment scales, interviews with parents and teachers, and hetero-assessment scales concerning emotional instability, pro-social behaviour and physical and verbal aggressiveness
Measures were taken pre-CI and repeatedly post-CI

Independent variables

Not applicable

Method

Test result interpretations, normed against a control group of hearing children of comparable age (not detailed). The authors provide general data only, making reference to the lack of homogeneity as a characteristic of the control group

Results

The analysis of post-implant findings shows a reduction of stereotype elements, more dynamic modes of figurative expression, quite good relationships within their own social environment and gradual, positive integration both at home and at school.

Results

'seem to indicate a greater discrepancy between how implanted children evaluate their behaviour and how in turn this is assessed by adults, in comparison to the tendency in the hearing group. However one variable that should be taken into consideration is the fact that these profoundly deaf children inevitably had fewer speech skills even though all the items used were previously illustrated to them and accurately explained' (s186).

Following implantation, more integrated behaviour includes children telling lies, answering when called, asking why, being able to wait and being more attentive, while adolescents answer when called, take part in discussions, are interested in what happens around them (home, school), want explanations, greater respect for rules, play around with peers, offer solutions and are more constant.

In drawings, richer detail and more dynamic modes of expression were observed; some graphic elements indicating lack of order and difficulty in interpersonal relationships; this

'last mentioned finding can be considered a positive factor since it indicates a greater awareness of personal limits and confirms that the child is beginning to take note of various new aspects of reality' (s185).

Greatest discrepancy between deaf cochlear-implanted children and hearing controls was between self-evaluation and perceptions of adults. Both children and adolescents considered themselves more inadequate and vulnerable in comparison (under-esteem).

Conclusions

Cochlear implantation would seem to cause no psychological disruption. Our sample group shows an improvement in their modes of expression – more consistent with the mental and effective age – and a greater awareness of personal limits, together with the ability to judge the appropriateness of their own behaviour.

Observations

The study is motivated by criticism, particularly from within the deaf community, that cochlear implants affect the psychosocial integrity of the prelingually deaf child. The programme is clearly intended as a rolling one, presumably with further publications on greater cohorts lying ahead in time. The authors' intention is to provide a set of investigative tools that are normed against both hearing and deaf populations, so that a more effective statistical model can be elaborated (p.186). In providing substantive detail on the psychosocial outcomes of paediatric cochlear implantation, research in the area and of this type is of critical future importance.

However, the drawing test interpretations might be read as putting a 'hearing spin' on the drawings. It might be suggested that an interpretation of a drawing by a deaf person using normative statements derived originally from similar research on hearing people may be unable to account for the demonstrated greater visual acuity of deaf people. These findings may reflect the fact that psychological tests habitually assume perception to be universal (rather than particular) in nature – as in the test described here. In sum, the analytical tools in this element of assessment might well prove to be insufficiently discriminating, or not 'Deaf aware' in the cultural sense. As a further expansion of a project of this kind, the tests themselves should ideally be normed against a wider range of populations, including those with different modes of communication, perception and interpretation. In other words, there is a call for studies on larger numbers, being rich on demographic detail, so that different subsamples can be matched with those of other studies.

Fortnum HM, Marshall DH, Bamford JM, Summerfield AQ (2002) Hearing-impaired children in the UK: education setting and communication approach. Deafness and Education International 4(3): 123–141.

Population size
    757
Population comments
    Cohort in a subset (n = 12 255) study on 17 657 deaf children (> 40 dB HL)
Demographics
    Not detailed. Deaf population as a whole representative of UK deaf population
Selection criteria
    Sampling based on survey design, included in BATOD survey (1998)
Dependent variables
    Survey assessment of:
    • education setting
    • communication approach
Independent variables
    Gender
    Co-morbidity
    Hearing loss
    Aids to hearing
    Level of support
Method
    Group percentage reporting; linear correlation analysis of identified variables
Results
    '... distribution of educational setting among the implanted children [included in the study] approximates to that of the children with hearing levels of 91–100 dB HL' (pp.129–30).
    That is to say that among children with profound impairments, significantly higher percentages of those with implants than those without implants were placed in a mainstream setting (p < 0.001), with a significantly lower percentage placed in a school for the deaf (p < 0.001) (p.130).
    The pattern of communication approach among the implanted children included in the study also approximated to that of the children with hearing levels of 101–110 dB HL; a significantly higher percentage of those with implants were assigned to the aural/oral approach (p < 0.001), and significantly fewer to the 'sign' approach (p < 0.001), while there was no difference between percentages assigned to the TC approach (pp.130–1).
    In relation to multiple handicap and educational support:
        'The probability of a child being in a setting with a lower implied level of
        support, relative to a child matched on all other variables, was significantly

greater if the child had a lower hearing level (p < 0.001), was older (p < 0.02), possessed a cochlear implant (p < 0.001), did not have another disability (p < 0.001)' (p.136).

While with regard to communication mode:

'The probability of a child using an approach with a lower involvement of signing, relative to a child matched on all other variables, was significantly greater if the child had a lower AHL (p < 0.001), was older (p < 0.02), possessed a cochlear implant (p < 0.001), did not have another disability (p < 0.001), or was female (p < 0.001)' (p.136).

Conclusions

'... children with implant, on average, function similarly to children with hearing levels at the severe/profound boundary who use acoustic hearing aids' (p.138).

There is an effect on educational setting and communication approach of possessing an implant and of gender (p.138).

Observations

With this study the authors suggest that they have constructed a 'reference data-set' against which the impact of future changes and intervention may be calculated (p.123). The study aims to provide a comprehensive and comparatively detailed assessment of the UK deaf school population at a single point in time, 1998. This study reports data on a subsample for whom all included variable data were available, a UK representative population of 12 255, including 757 cochlear-implanted children.

The study finds some support for changes in educational setting following cochlear implantation, but recognizes that over-time assessment is necessary, in particular to separate out the effect on educational setting in early implanted children implanted prior to choice of schooling, and the effect on education setting for children who are implanted during any particular school-setting experience and who may be less likely to change setting (p.138).

The main strength of the study is its reporting on a very large population while covering a significant number of potential variables. However, the survey represents a point in time, and it is therefore not possible for the authors to analyse the effects of education and deafness as an ongoing process.

At the same time, analysis is limited to linear correlations and a brief analysis of co-variation of a number of key variables. There is no attempt to establish cause-and-effect relationships, or to locate the findings into current education policy and process. Hence the conclusions are mostly confirmatory rather than exploratory.

Francis HW, Koch ME, Wyatt JR, Niparko JK (1999) Trends in educational placement and cost-benefit considerations in children with cochlear implants. Archives of Otolaryngology, and Head and Neck Surgery 125: 499–505.

Population size

35 school-aged children without other disabilities with multichannel cochlear implant devices and 10 control children without implants from total communication programmes

Demographics

Age: between kindergarten and 12th grade

Age at CI: range 2–15 years, mean 5.2 years (SD = 3)

CI device: multichannel

No demographics offered for HA group.

Selection criteria

CIs undergoing aural rehabilitation at The Listening Centre at Johns Hopkins University School of Medicine

Multiple disabilities deselected

No selection criteria provided for HA group

Dependent variables
Retrospectively obtained grades corresponding to ages 5, 8 and 11 years
Independent variables
Placement
Method
Statistical comparison of placement and public expenditure
Economic evaluation type: cost-benefit analysis
Study perspective: societal (partial)
Comparator intervention: no intervention
Source of effectiveness data: none reported
Direct costs: charges – preoperative evaluation, hardware, operative fees and two years'
    postoperative (re)habilitation
Indirect costs: changes in education costs
Discount rate for costs and benefits: 5%
Outcome measure: educational cost savings
Currency and price year: US$, 1997
Sensitivity analysis: not conducted
Results

> 'A correlation was observed between the length of cochlear implant
> experience and the rate of full-time placement in mainstream classrooms
> (p = 0.4). There was also a negative correlation between the length of implant
> experience and the number of hours of special education support used by fully
> mainstreamed children (p = 0.03). Children with greater than two years of
> implant experience were mainstreamed at twice the rate or more of age-
> matched children with profound hearing loss who did not have implants' (p.499).

Cochlear implantation results in cost savings of US$30,000-200,000 (in 2001/2 prices
– £24,275 to £161,830 or US$36,497 to $243,312) for children implanted at age 3 years
and US$27,000–192,000 (in 2001/2 prices – £21,847 to £155,357 or US$32,847 to
$233,580) for those implanted at age 5 years.
Conclusions
'Cochlear implantation accompanied by aural rehabilitation [led to] higher rates of
mainstream placement in schools and lower dependence on special educational support
services' (p.499).

'The cost-benefit analysis suggests that a decrease in special education costs is one of
the early societal benefits of cochlear implantation in young children' (p.504).
Observations
This paper is not a true cost-benefit economic evaluation; it would be more appropriately
described as a cost-minimization study. The study does not attempt to attach a value to
benefits in monetary terms, this would require the use of a method such as contingent
valuation or conjoint analysis. An analysis that only considers changes in costs is
misleading for resource allocation decisions since only programmes that are cost saving
would be seen as worthwhile – this ignores the effectiveness of the intervention. In
addition, educational placement is only an intermediate measure of outcome. That is, it
may be an indicator of what a child is likely to achieve but does not actually measure the
end-point outcome of educational qualifications achieved or higher income earned as a
result of improved educational opportunities. The small sample size used in this paper
hinders statistical analysis, since the study does not have enough power to test the full
range of hypotheses stated.

Mainstream education is assumed to be the goal; other provision represents failure, because

> '... severe hearing disability, including poor speech perception, is predictive of
> educational placement in which oral communication and reading skills are less
> likely to develop, further limiting the potential for educational and professional
> achievement' (p.500).

As with other studies, this also finds that by three to five years post implantation, there is a slowing down of the rates of improvement. This is often put down to a ceiling effect in the test measures used (e.g. Blamey et al. 2001; Boothroyd and Eran 1994; Svirsky and Meyer 1999). Francis et al. equally report a diminishing effect. However, they interpret it not as a ceiling, but as a floor effect. It concerns the fact that the number of support hours needed by the cochlear-implanted children was inversely proportional to the duration of cochlear implant experience. However, when the group with more than four years' experience was included (i.e. the entire population of 35), the significance of this relationship was lost (p = 0.09) (p.502). To an extent this may indeed reflect the small numbers involved. However, the authors suggest that:

> 'A smaller reduction in the use of support services after four years of implant experience was most likely the result of a floor effect rather than a slowing of language acquisition or educational independence' (p.502).

Frisch SA, Pisoni DB (2000) Modeling spoken word recognition performance by pediatric cochlear implant users using feature identification. Ear and Hearing 21(6): 578–589.

Population size
48

Demographics
CI device: Nucleus 22 multichannel
CI coding strategies: SPEAK, MSPEAK
Age: range 3.9–10.8 years (mean 7.3 years)
HL: range 97–120 dB (mean 108–113 dB)
Educational programme: oral (23). total communication (25)
Age at CI: range 2.2–8.9 years (mean 5.5 years)

Selection criteria
Selected from population of children followed at Indiana University School of Medicine (no selection details provided)

Dependent variables
PB-K, Lexical Neighborhood Test (LNT; open-set) and minimal pairs test administered 1.5–2 years post-CI

Independent variables
Feature-identification strategies for phoneme perception

Method
Testing a probabilistic model of phoneme recognition, with a performance-based probabilistic confusion matrix produced for each participant. This matrix used as input component to test three models of word recognition: NAM, PCM and SPAMR (for linguistic detail see article)

Correlations between PB-K and LNT scores, and minimal pairs test established (strongly correlated, test accepted). Minimal pairs test then used to produce confusion matrix for vowels and consonants and rescored for word recognition

Results
Open-set word-recognition performance can be successfully predicted using feature-identification scores. Word-recognition ability was best predicted in the model in which phoneme decisions were delayed until lexical access.

> 'Although the SPEAK users generally performed better than MPEAK users, as has been found elsewhere (Parkinson et al. 1998; Skinner et al. 1994), the difference in performance appears to be quantitative, not qualitative. [...] the broader pattern of results indicates that NAM is the most appropriate model of spoken word recognition performance for both groups. The PCM and SPAMR

models appear to be better suited as models of processing nonwords and unfamiliar words' (p.585).

Conclusions

Closed-set feature identification and open-set word recognition focus on different, but related, levels of language processing. The most successful model of performance is consistent with current psycholinguistic theories of spoken word recognition.

'We have some preliminary evidence that the process of spoken word recognition by pediatric cochlear implant users is much the same as in children and adults with normal hearing. Pediatric cochlear implant users are sensitive to the phonetic similarity of spoken words represented in an internalized lexicon, as predicted by current psycholinguistic theories like NAM' (p.587).

'Successful implant users are able not only to discriminate distinct speech sounds, but more importantly, they are able to isolate, discriminate, select, and identify words from a multi-dimensional lexical similarity space' (p.587).

Observations

This is a study of a technical design, in part aimed at assessing psycholinguistic theories of spoken-word recognition for children who use cochlear implants, as compared to the performance of commonly used closed- and open-set speech perception tests. The explanation of what the assessment involved can not be put more succinctly than in the words used by the authors themselves:

'A software simulation of phoneme recognition performance was developed that uses feature identification scores as input. Two simulations of lexical access were developed. In one, early phoneme decisions are used in a lexical search to find the best matching candidate. In the second, phoneme decisions are made only when lexical access occurs. Simulated phoneme and word identification performance was then applied to behavioural data from the Phonetically Balanced Kindergarten test and Lexical Neighbourhood Test of open-set word recognition. Simulations of performance were evaluated for children with prelingual sensorineural hearing loss who use cochlear implants with the MPEAK or SPEAK coding strategies' (p.578).

This article is mainly of interest to those seeking to either improve or build new clinical tests pertaining to speech perception in deaf children; they are referred to the article for its level of description and detailed analysis. In terms of outcome reporting, it suffices to note here that the tests (use of the PB-K in particular is widespread) generally target the same skills in deaf children with cochlear implants as they do in hearing children.

Fryauf-Bertschy H, Tyler RT, Kelsay DM et al. (1997) Cochlear implant use by prelingually deafened children: the influences of age at implant and length of device use. Journal of Speech, Language and Hearing Research 40(Feb): 183–199.

Population size

34

Demographics

Profound deafness (≥ 65 dB – detailed), or scored speech perception tests below chance level

Age at CI: 2–15 years (19 ≥ 5 years)

Age at identification: all ≤ 2.6 years

CI: Cochlear Nucleus 22 multichannel (systems detailed)

Active electrodes: 22

CI use: 3–5 years

Aetiology detailed

Communication mode: total communication

Educational programmes: variety, none residential school

Selection criteria

University of Iowa Implant Center

Grouped by age

6 children deselected: 2 medical complications; 3 non-use of CI; 1 device malfunction

Judged by clinical psychologist

Dependent variables

Speech perception test battery at annual intervals:

1 Monosyllable Trochee Spondee Test (MTS)

2 Four Choice Spondee test from ESP

3 Word Intelligibility by Picture identification (WIPI)

4 Vowel Perception Test (VWP)

5 Phonetically Balanced Kindergarten Word List (PB-K)

Parent Monthly Diary questionnaire (daily use)

Independent variables

Age at CI

Period of CI

CI use per day

Method

One-tail binomial model t-test of variance significance (0 = chance)

Results

The highest incidence of non-use was found in children implanted after age 8 years; there were three non-users and three minimal users. After 24 months all the remaining children but one scored above 50% (MTS). Concerning effects of age at cochlear implantation, when grouped in implant ≤ 5 years and > 5 years, outcomes proved less reliable (lower numbers affect outcomes). The outcomes were more robust for the PB-K, where the difference became statistically significant at the 36-month (p = 0.0217) and 48-month (p = 0.0488) test intervals. Child numbers were not adequate to report on the 60-month test interval.

No significant differences in performance for children implanted before age 5 years at 36/48 month intervals.

The amount of daily use affects all measures of speech-perception performance, but the statistic may be affected by the inclusion of the number of eventual non-users who might have been excluded from the assessment; the correlation was significant at the 36-month (p = 0.0062) and 48-month (p = 0.0497) intervals on the MTS test, and was repeated for all other tests.

Conclusions

Most children derive benefits from cochlear implantation for speech-perception tasks. Some perform well, others derive limited use from their hearing (p.196). Results of this study support the premise that cochlear implantation improves speech-perception abilities in children when the devices are used consistently.

Observations

In their introduction, the authors raise the question as to whether a deaf child should grow up in the hearing or the deaf community. It is argued that the cochlear implant will widen access to the hearing community by providing much greater auditory input than has hitherto been the case, with positive social and psychological consequences arising out of successful spoken-language acquisition (e.g. Osberger 1993). It is relevant to note here also the authors' observation that studies to date are characterized by wide individual variation in performance.

The main reason given by the authors for reporting this study is that in 1997, relatively few studies had reported the speech-perception performance of a large group of children with more than two years' experience of cochlear implantation. This study includes 34 children with three to five years' experience.

There is a wide age-range (2–15 years), with nine children between the ages of 2 and 3:11 at the time of the study. The sample has been disaggregated for age: aged 2–3, aged 4–5, aged 5–7 and aged 8 and over. This seems a good way to report, especially on larger populations, preferably much larger still than is the case here. The demographic reporting is done as a table per child; it is perhaps worth noting that the authors suggest that 'in every case all 22 active electrodes were placed in the cochlea and medical follow-up was uneventful' (p.185).

Furthermore, in comparing the data with those of many other studies, it is worth noting that in this study all children used total communication, although it is noted that their communication skills varied widely (p.185). 'As with many other studies, the test conditions used auditory input via speakers, although with younger children 'live voice' (p.187) was used – the study does not specify whether there was a visual element to the input.

The outcomes seem robust, although the disaggregation reported for age concerns only that between below 5 and over 5 years at implantation; the significance of the findings must therefore be interpreted with the wide overall age range at implantation in mind.

It seems clear from the reported findings that the amount of daily use of the cochlear implant is an important factor in outcome, and here produced a more consistent correlation with performance than does age at implantation. However, it may not be a single factor. It is likely to be a combination of, for example, parental support factors, proper working of the device, the amount of acceptance of the device, and even the level and quality of the rehabilitation service. Nevertheless, the amount of daily use will go some way towards explaining the wide individual variation in performance that exists between cochlear implant users (p.195).

Overall, the authors' assessment of the findings is that most, but not all, of the implanted children derive benefit from their cochlear implant (p.196).

Gantz BJ, Rubinstein JT, Tyler RS, Teagle HFB, Cohen NL, Waltzman SB, Miyamoto RT, Kirk KI (1999) Long-term results of cochlear implants in children with residual hearing. Annals of Otology, Rhinology and Laryngology (Supplement) 184: s33–s36.

Population size
  7
Population comments
  Comparison group (*n* = undetailed) of 'more severely hearing-impaired' (p.35) hearing aid users
Demographics
  Age: range 6–12 years
  Age at CI: range 4–11 years
  No further demographics detailed; no demographics detailed for HA users
Selection criteria
  None detailed, but all were multichannel CI users
Dependent variables
  Speech perception test: PB-K
Independent variables
  Preoperative PB-K scores
Method
  Percentage scores reporting
Results
  'The speech perception skills of this group of children two years after implantation are extremely encouraging. The mean score of 75% on the PB-K word test is similar to that of a small group of children who have a 71 dB PTA...' (p.35).

Conclusions

'... this selected sample of children with residual hearing and limited word understanding with hearing aids achieved significantly greater open-set word recognition with a multichannel cochlear implant than did profoundly deaf children with no preoperative word recognition' (p.35).

Observations

Included despite minimal sample because it confirms results by Zwolan et al. (1997). Both concern a candidacy issue: to implant children with pre-existing speech perception. The term 'long-term' in the title is misleading: data concern a follow-up period of only up to two years post implantation. Moreover, the group is not consistent over time, with different individuals included at different intervals.

This study concerns a small subgroup of cochlear-implanted children in Iowa implant centres who had some residual hearing. The research follows from parental requests for cochlear implants for children with some residual hearing. In summary, the selected sample (n = 7, age range 4–11 at two-year follow-up) of cochlear-implanted children with some residual hearing outperformed matched group of non-cochlear-implanted children with residual hearing, and scored similar to a group of moderate deafness hearing aid users. The limited size of the group, in combination with the large overall age-range, makes the findings difficult to interpret, while the lack of demographic description further undermines the study's findings.

Gantz BJ, Tyler RS, Woodworth GG, Tye-Murray N, Fryauf-Bertschy H (1994) Results of multichannel cochlear implants in congenital and acquired prelingual deafness in children: five-year follow-up. American Journal of Otology 15-S: 1-7.

Population size

54

Population comments

Prelingual children, of which 44 congenital. A separate group of 5 postlingually deaf CIs was also included

Demographics

Age: range 20 months–15:10 years

CI device: Nucleus 22

Aetiology: congenital (44), meningitis (8 out of 10 prelingually deafened)

Electrode insertion: full

No demographic or age details provided for the 5 postlingual children

Selection criteria

Implanted at the Iowa Cochlear Implant Clinical Research Centre, meeting specific selection criteria (not detailed)

Dependent variables

Test battery, speech perception and production:

- MTS
- WIPI
- PB-K word list (modified for age, minimum 25, average 40–45 words)

Independent variables

Aetiology

Prelingual (≤ 24 months), postlingual (≥ 5 years)

Method

Percentage scores, calculation of significance: one-tailed test

Results

MTS

Prelingual, 1-year: 62% mean, 23.6 SD

Postlingual, 1-year: 85% mean

Prelingual, 2-year: 82% mean
Prelingual, 5-year: 91%
Postlingual, 3-year: mastered
BP-K
Prelingual, 1-year (five children only): range 4–25% correct
Prelingual, 4-year (82% of children): limited sound-only word understanding
Prelingual, 5-year: 'similar rates of progress'
WIPI
Not reported

'Results for all tests indicate that the congenitally deaf group (*n = 44) achieved better average speech perception scores on all tests compared to the prelingually deafened group* (n = 10). The detrimental effects of meningitis appear to negate any positive influence afforded by previous auditory stimulation' (p.4).

'In this study, several congenitally deaf children achieved higher scores than some postlingually deafened children. After four years of experience, more than 80% of the prelingually deafened group exhibited limited open-set word understanding' (p.5).

'Experiencing a brief exposure to acoustic input does not appear to be a significant advantage for the group with prelingually acquired deafness' (p.5).

Conclusions

'In summary, prelingually deafened children obtain significant benefit from multichannel cochlear implants as demonstrated by significant improvement over pre-implant levels on speech perception tasks and speech production measures. Prelingually deafened children gain these skills at a much slower rate than postlingually deafened children and adults. Individual speech perception and production scores continued to improve over the five-year follow-up period of the present study' (p.6).

Observations

It is important to note that this study reports a set of 'preliminary findings' (p.s1) on prelingually deafened children between 2 and 13 years of age, thus covering a relatively wide age range. The study investigates the performance of prelingually and congenitally deaf children, in the light of the hypothesis that these children might underperform relative to postlingually deaf children since they have not developed an auditory memory. Hence the study reports on the speech perception and production performance of 54 prelingual and congenitally deaf children with outcomes over a five-year period. The overall aim of the research is to identify appropriate age limits for implantation at the Iowa Cochlear Implant Center (p.s2).

They conclude that the children in the study can gain substantial benefit from multichannel cochlear implants, while some outperform congenitally deaf children (p.s1).

The test battery included the MTS, WIPI and PB-K. Clear ceiling effects noticeable on MTS tests starting at one-year intervals for postlingual children in particular. Outcomes on the PB-K test eventually became statistically significant for age (2–5, 5–7, and 8 years and older) at the 24-month test interval ($p = 0.033/.016$ between groups), remaining significant at the 36-month interval only between the youngest and eldest group ($p = 0.033$).

'The improved speech production in the prelingually deafened group is especially encouraging. [...] One congenitally deaf individual was able to produce 78% of words and 92% of phonemes correctly after six years of experience with an implant' (p.6).

Geers AE (1997) Comparing implants with hearing aids in profoundly deaf children. Otolaryngology – Head and Neck Surgery 117(3/1): 150–154.

Population size
5

Population comments

Matched with 5 HA (> 100 dB) and 5 HA+ (90–100 dB) for age, HL, test scores and socio-economic status

Demographics

Age: range 5.6–13.6 years, average 8.10 years

Hearing loss: profound deafness, PTA thresholds ≥ 100 dB HL

Intelligence: IQ performance score range 90–130, average nonverbal 105

Selection criteria

Restricted to profoundly deaf children ≤ 11 years, born deaf or lost hearing by age 3 years. Selected for group matching criteria on the basis of those selected for CI

Dependent variables

Speech perception and production test battery, including:

• ESP

• WIPI

• PB-K

Independent variables

Device: CI, HA

HA+ ('Gold' users with PTA thresholds between 90 and 100 dB HL; mean 15 dB advantage over CI; last year of study only)

Method

Test score percentages. Calculation of significance over time of independent variables

Results

Speech perception

'... after five years of implant use, speech perception scores of the CI group exceeded those of the HA+ group on all four speech perception measures, but the differences are still not very large or statistically significant' (pp.151–2).

Speech production

At three years,

'... both the CI and the HA+ groups exceeded the HA group but did not differ significantly from each other; however, the HA+ group had the highest average scores at 75% correct for speech imitation and 52% correct for spontaneous phoneme production. When imitation scores for the partial samples were examined two years later, performance of the CI and the HA+ groups was virtually identical at 80% correct' (p.153).

Conclusions

'... it is important to keep in mind that children with hearing losses in the 90 to 100 dB range who receive hearing aids and auditory-oral instruction at an early age perform just as well as children who receive implants at the end of three and even five years of use. [Until] we can document performance changes in implant users that surpass results observed in the HA+ group, we do not recommend an implant for children whose pure tone average thresholds are less than 100 dB in the better ear, regardless of their speech perception scores' (p.154).

Observations

In this study, speech perception, speech production and spoken language skills of 13 age-matched groups of prelingually deaf children, all enrolled in the same educational setting, were compared. Each group consisted of three children, two with hearing aids but different degrees of hearing loss (pure-tone average > 100 dB HL and pure-tone average between 90 and 100 dB HL) and one who had used a Nucleus multichannel implant for three years, as an ongoing concern of the CID's programme of research. A description of the CID's research can be found in Geers and Moog (1996).

This study has been included despite its low sample size (*n* = 5) mainly because it builds meaningfully on studies of the CID population reported by Geers and Brenner and Geers and Moog, both in 1994. This time the HA+ (90–100 dB) group has been included in the study for five years in total, while the tactile aid group has been dropped. The article is of interest because of its findings regarding the group of children with hearing losses between 90 and 100 dB unaided, since these are now increasingly considered suitable candidates for implantation. Indeed,

> 'Because use of a cochlear implant with a young child is both costly and invasive, it is important to determine which children will perform just as well or better with conventional hearing aids' (p.150).

The authors note that children in the HA+ group qualify for cochlear implants under the first criterion established by the US FDA (p.150). Given the findings, however, namely that the cochlear-implanted children in this small sample do not in the slightest outperform the non-cochlear-implanted children with slightly less severe hearing losses, the authors conclude that we lack the evidence to suggest that children in the HA+ group would perform better with cochlear implants, and therefore discourage implanting children in this group. The small sample size marks this conclusion as tentative.

Geers AE (2004) Factors affecting the development of speech, language and literacy in children with early cochlear implantation. Education and Cochlear Implantation (in press).

Population size
136
Demographics
Age at research: 8–9 years
Age at onset: < 3 years
Duration of CI use: ≥ 4–6 years (102 ≥ 5 years or more); 20 no experience with latest speech-processing technology
Age at CI: 2–4 years
CI device: Nucleus 22
Selection criteria
Normal intelligence (no details given)
Monolingual speaking homes (presumably English monolingual)
Sampled from across US/Canada
Dependent variables
Test battery of speech perception, production, language and reading
Independent variables
Communication method
Classroom setting
Rehabilitation
Method
Multivariate analysis. Range of demographic factors used as intervening variables (including IQ, socio-economic status measures, age details and implant characteristics)
Results
Characteristics of the child and the family (primarily nonverbal IQ) accounted for approximately 20% of variance in post-implant outcome. Twenty-four percent was accounted for by implant characteristics, and 12% by educational variables, particularly oral communication mode.
Conclusions
Auditory, speech, language and reading skills achieved four to six years after cochlear implantation were most strongly associated with nonverbal IQ, implant functioning and use of an oral communication mode.
Observations
This study reports that 10 cochlear implanted children (n = 16) implanted before age 5

achieved 50% recognition of words on open list (PB-K). The study included nine minimal and eventual non-users, who all scored below 32% open-set word recognition.

They comment that:

'Possible reasons for poor performance include inadequate device fitting, insufficient cognitive skills, poor motivation, educational, and social environment emphasising manual communication, and limited parental support'.

Geers A, Brenner C (1994) Speech-perception results: audition and lipreading enhancement. Volta Review 96(5): 97–108.

Population size

13

Population comments

Matched with 13 TA and 13 HA for age, HL, test scores and socio-economic status

Demographics

Age: range 2–12 years at start of project

Hearing loss: profound deafness, PTA thresholds ≥ 100 dB HL

Intelligence: IQ performance score range 90–130, average nonverbal 105

Selection criteria

Restricted to profoundly deaf children ≤ 11 years, born deaf or lost hearing by age 3 years. All enrolled at CID, oral/aural communication programme. Selected for group matching criteria on the basis of those selected for CI

Dependent variables

Speech perception test battery, 1, 2 and 3 years after CI

WIPI

PB-K open-set word list

Phonetic Task Evaluation (PTE)

MATRIX

Lipreading enhancement scores

Independent variables

Device: CI, TA, HA

HA+ ('Gold' users with PTA thresholds between 90–100 dB HL; mean 15 dB advantage over CI; last year of study only)

Method

Range of statistical analysis tools

Results

Speech perception performance of all three groups was similar before beginning the study, when all children were tested with hearing aids, indicating detection, but limited discrimination, of speech.

'By 12 months, the median performance of the CI group had reached category 3 [on speech perception categories based on WIPI and PB-K], indicating beginning word recognition based on spectral rather than temporal cues. After two years, the median had reached category 4, indicating vowel identification skill. By three years, 11 of the 13 children with implants differentiated words on the WIPI based on consonant information and four of these recognised three or more words from the open-set PB-K list. This performance compares quite favorably with the speech perception skill demonstrated by the HA+ group...' (pp.99–101).

No such strong development was found for the HA or TA groups (p.101).

Lipreading skills improved significantly for the cochlear implants relative to the two other groups. This effect was strengthened by adding the data for the third year only of HA+.

After 36 months, 11 of the 13 children with cochlear implants were able to identify words on the basis of auditory consonant cues. Feature perception scores reflected an implant advantage in the perception of pitch, vowels and consonant place. Significant lipreading enhancement was achieved after 36 months of implant use, which was comparable to that achieved by profoundly deaf children with 90 to 100 dB HL hearing losses who receive benefit from hearing aids.

Conclusions

Results indicate

'... that the Nucleus 22-channel cochlear implant is superior to either tactile aids or hearing aids for promoting closed-set word recognition skill in some profoundly deaf children' (p.102).

'The high performance levels attained by both the CI and HA+ groups demonstrate that sufficient information is available through hearing aids to children with 90–100 dB HL average threshold levels and through Nucleus 22-channel cochlear implants to children with greater losses to help them understand speech' (pp.106–7).

Observations

In this early part of an ongoing and wide-ranging study (Geers and Moog 1996) looking at a wide range of outcomes in oral education, Geers and Brenner compare a group of 13 cochlear-implanted children in matched triadic groups with different sensory aids, including tactile vocoders and hearing aid users in each triad. This study is significant, in particular for its careful matching of different aid users all drawn from the same oral programme. The authors comment that although significant auditory gains over and above hearing aid users have been reported for cochlear implant users (presumably of comparable unaided hearing loss thresholds), even after two to three years of implant use:

'most prelingually deaf children reported in the literature can understand words only when they are presented in a closed set of choices which differ substantially in suprasegmental or spectral information' (p.97).

Nevertheless, the authors suggest that irrespective of the type of hearing aid used, children in oral programmes develop greater speech perception skills than do children enrolled in programmes that include sign language (p.98).

The authors suggest that the auditory skill performance of the cochlear-implanted children contrasts most sharply with the tactile aid group, who 'did not change speech perception category throughout the next 36 months of device and instruction' (p.101), although across the tactile aid group there were overall improvements noted. On the measures taken by the study, the hearing aid group started out one standard level ahead of the other two groups, but 'the HA group's median performance rarely exceeded the first measured level throughout the duration of the study' (p.101).

As findings show, the cochlear-implanted group steadily progressed over the three years of oral instruction in the CID programme (p.99). A significant difference ($p = 0.001$) existed between the CI and HA+TA groups in post hoc tests measuring percentage enhancement in lipreading-plus-listening advantage, suggesting that the cochlear implants had resulted in the cochlear-implanted children becoming better in lipreading than children with hearing or tactile aids.

Geers A, Brenner C, Nicholas J, Uchanski R, Tye-Murray N, Tobey E (2002) Rehabilitation factors contributing to implant benefit in children. Annals of Otology, Rhinology and Laryngology 189: s127–s130.

Population size

136

Population comments

Subsample from total ($n = 180$) included in the overall CID study

Demographics
Age at testing: range 8–9.11 years, mean 9 years (SD = 6)
Age at onset of deafness: range 0–3 years, mean 4 months (SD = 9)
Age at CI: range 1.10–5.2 years, mean 3.6 years (SD = 9)
Performance IQ: range 65–136, mean 102 (SD = 15)
CI experience: range 3.9–7.6 years, mean 5.6 years (SD = 0.9)
SPEAK experience: range 0–5.2 years, mean 3 years (SD = 1.8)
Number of active electrodes: range 6–22, mean 18 (SD = 2.86)

Selection criteria
Population attending CID summer camp held at St Louis. Selected for age (8–9 years), onset of deafness before 3 years, CI before 5 years, 4–6 years' CI experience, normal intelligence and from English-speaking home environment

Dependent variables
CID test battery: speech perception, speech production, spoken language, speech and sign language, and reading (not detailed)

Communication method
Classroom type
Amount of therapy
Child and family variables (controlled)

Method
Multivariate design used to examine effects of independent variables with intervening variables controlled (intervening variables collected at one point in time, independent variables collected over time)

Results
Child and family characteristics together explained 18% of variance in speech perception factor scores, 15% in speech production, 11% in spoken language, 17% in spoken and signed language, and 20% in reading (p.128). The IQ measure was significant across those outcomes ($p \leq 0.001$–0.05).

Implant characteristics accounted for 26% additional variance in speech perception, 22% in speech production, 23% in spoken language, 21% in spoken and signed language, and 17% in reading (p.128). All correlations were significant ($p < 0.05$).

'Educational variables' accounted for 16% of additional variance in speech perception, 18% in speech production, 10% in spoken language, 5% in spoken and signed language, and 7% in reading, while 'the greater the emphasis on speech and auditory skill development, the better the outcome' (p.129). Mainstreaming correlated significantly with speech production, language and reading.

In combination, the above elements accounted for 54% of variance in outcome; child and family characteristics (mostly IQ) accounted for 18%, implant characteristics for 24% and educational factors for 12%.

Conclusions
Since age at implantation was not found to have an effect on any outcome measure,

'... a sense of urgency about performing implantation in infancy may be unnecessary, or at least deserves further evaluation' (p.129).

Child and family characteristics do not seem to provide a particular (dis)advantage for cochlear implant outcomes, since the more highly educated parents did not have higher achieving children when the IQ was factored out, but there was a tendency for smaller families to have children who had somewhat better overall language development (p.129).

All of the measured implant characteristics (processor, electrode insertion (and MAP), dynamic range and loudness growth) contributed significantly to the overall variance (p.129).

Communication mode was the primary rehabilitative factor associated with outcome performance, while the use of

'sign communication with children with implants did not result in an advantage for overall English language competence, even when the outcome measure included sign language. Oral education appears to be an important educational choice for children who have undergone cochlear implantation before 5 years of age' (p.130).

Observations

This is the latest included addition to reporting from the CID summer programme started in 1996.

The explained variances for IQ and device factors are important, because of their size. The variance explained by IQ is notable, in particular because the study controlled for IQ in the sample selection. Between child/family characteristics (mostly IQ) and device characteristics, 54% of outcome variance is explained, with 12% accounted for by 'educational factors' (primarily communication mode).

It is surprising that, in this study, age at implantation is not a significant predictor of the outcome. This finding contradicts several other studies in the literature and raises questions about the current trend towards early implantation. Other variables like dynamic range, loudness growth, number of electrodes and duration of SPEAK use accounted for 26% of the variance, factors which have not been found that important in other studies. These marked discrepancies with the majority of findings reported in the literature cannot simply be attributed to the weaknesses in the design of the study. The children came from several cochlear implant programmes, although they may not have been entirely representative of the entire population of implanted children as these were children willing to come to the summer camp and participate in extensive everyday testing. However, the outcomes of several tests were combined in a single-factor score without giving details of how this was done and how valid this procedure was, and this may have resulted in statistical complications. It is important that the outcomes of this study are explored by other studies addressing the issues raised.

Geers A, Moog J (1994) Spoken language results: vocabulary, syntax and communication. Volta Review 96(5): 131–148.

Population size

13

Population comments

Matched with 13 TA and 13 HA for age, HL, test scores and socio-economic status

Demographics

Age: range 2–12 years at start of project

Hearing loss: profound deafness, PTA thresholds $\geq$ 100 dB HL

Intelligence: IQ performance score range 90–130, average nonverbal 105

Selection criteria

Restricted to profoundly deaf children $\leq$ 11 years, born deaf or lost hearing by age 3 years. All enrolled at CID, oral/aural communication programme. Selected for group-matching criteria on the basis of those selected for CI

Dependent variables

Spoken language test battery, 1, 2 and 3 years after CI

Spontaneous language sample category analysis:

- SECS
- GAEL
- RITLS
- Peabody Picture Vocabulary Test (PPVT-R)
- Expressive One-Word Picture Vocabulary Test (EOWPVT)

Parent interviews (Meaningful Auditory Integration Scale)

Independent variables

Device: CI, TA, HA

HA+ ('Gold' users with PTA thresholds between 90–100 dB HL; mean 15 dB advantage over CI; last year of study only)

Method
F-statistic and chi-square for linear regressions, and repeated measures ANOVA for multi-variable analyses

Results

'After three years in the study, the average child in the implant and tactile aid groups was developing compound sentences, while the hearing aid group had just mastered kernel sentences' (p.137).

For the formal tests,

'... the increase in percentile ranks achieved by both the TA and CI groups demonstrates that their improvement was much greater than is typical for deaf children their age. [After three years, the CI group] had advanced to the 72nd percentile in expressive language and the 86th percentile in receptive language' (p.141).

In summary, the cochlear implant group exhibited faster acquisition of all language and communication skills. Their average performance, compared to the tactile aid and hearing aid groups, was significantly higher after 36 months of auditory-oral instruction in the areas of expressive vocabulary (re hearing norms), receptive syntax (re deaf norms) and everyday use of the sensory aid. The latter findings were generated from the parent interviews, as was the finding that:

'After three years of experience with a cochlear implant, the CI children were exhibiting auditory behaviours which closely resembled those of the HA+ children, while the TA and HA groups showed relatively little change' (p.146).

Conclusions
'... most of these children used speech effectively to communicate regardless of their sensory aid. [...] For children with cochlear implants, three years of steadily improving auditory skill was sufficient to reach performance of the HA+ group in everyday use of speech' (p.146).

Observations
As part of the rolling programme of study (Geers and Moog 1996), this article reports on the acquisition of English vocabulary and syntax in three sets of pupils over three years – those with cochlear implants, with conventional hearing aids and with tactile vocoders. As in the other reports available that concern the same population (e.g. Geers and Brenner 1994; Geers and Moog 1997), the children with cochlear implants significantly outperformed other pupils matched by hearing loss and age, with performances more comparable to the performance of pupils with conventional hearing aids and unaided hearing losses between 90 and 100 dB. The CID test programme uses a fairly extensive set of testing tools, all pertaining to spoken language (English).

Although this is not reported in detail, it seems from the figures provided that the tactile aid regression lines – at least on the spontaneous language sample, the developmental sentence score and the vocabulary development scores (PVTs) – are very close to those of the cochlear implant group. This is also true for the percentile ranking of expressive language based on the formal test scores.

This consistency in development seems to break down for the receptive language percentile ranking.

Geers A, Nicholas J, Tye-Murray N, Uchanski R, Brenner C, Davidson L, Torretta G (2000) Effects of communication mode on skills of long-term cochlear implant users. Annals of Otology, Rhinology and Laryngology 109(12)s185: 89–91.

Population size
43

Demographics
Onset of deafness: < age 3 years

Age: 8–9 years

CI device: Nucleus 22

Speech processing strategy: SPEAK, MSPEAK

Communication mode: oral (20), total communication (23)

Matched on socio-economic status criteria, except fewer education years of mothers among total communication cochlear-implanted children

Placement: range of public and private placements in the US and Canada

Selection criteria

Children selected for normal distribution of nonverbal IQ and are from English monolingual speaking homes

Dependent variables

Speech perception

VIDSPAC

ESP

WIPI

LNT

BKB

CHIVE

TACL

Speech intelligibility

32 McGarr sentences to 3 naive listeners

Reading

Word Attack subtest of Woodcock Reading Mastery Test

Two subtests of the Peabody Individual Achievement Test (Recognition and Comprehension)

Independent variables

Communication mode: oral and total communication

Method

t-test analysis of differences in mean scores

Results

The detailed scores of significance are listed per outcome in a table, ranging between $p = 0.01$ and 0.04 (p.91), and cannot be replicated here in full.

'The oral children demonstrated a significant advantage in their overall VIDSPAC score and in their discrimination of manner and vowel cues. No difference was apparent in perception of voicing and place cues, which were difficult contrasts for both groups' (pp.90–91).

'Significant differences between the oral and total communication groups were apparent on all closed-set speech perception tests, with the oral children nearly topping out on the ESP and showing a 20% advantage on the WIPI test. Significant differences between groups were also observed on the open-set speech-perception tasks. The oral children exhibited an average 20% advantage over the total communication group on the monosyllable lists of the LNT and a 27% advantage on perception of key words in BKB sentences' (p.91).

Such similar differences are also recorded for speech production intelligibility (p.91).

'A comparison of reading-grade equivalent scores indicated higher average scores for the oral group, but the differences did not reach statistical significance' (p.91).

Conclusions

'... preliminary results indicate that students enrolled in educational settings in which they must depend on spoken language for communication achieve significantly more auditory benefit from an implant than do children whose program includes sign' (p.91).

'The relative benefits of the two approaches for development of reading skills are equivocal at this time...' (pp.91–2).

Observations

This study reports on a sample of 43 8- to 9-year-olds in a longitudinal study concerned with investigating the effects of different programmes and rehabilitation on Nucleus multichannel implant users. The report is a preliminary one and concerns communication mode only.

A wide range of spoken language outcomes is targeted. However, given the inclusion of total communication children, it is unfortunate that the notion of 'language' focuses on the auditory mode and the spoken language in the tests, the findings and the discussion, and the authors' hypothesis seems to equate language with spoken language:

> 'We have hypothesised that those children who rely on speech and hearing throughout the day for communication will develop higher levels of speech perception, speech production, language, and reading skills than children who rely on both speech and sign' (p.90).

The authors report significant positive correlations between oral education and all speech-related outcome. However, it needs to be borne in mind that total communication is much less focused on those targets, and addresses a wider range of communicative options and abilities. This probably accounts for the fact that:

> 'The oral group averaged 81 hours per year of [auditory and speech] therapy, whereas the total communication group averaged 41 hours' (p.90).

Although this variable does not return in later analyses or discussion, it does mean that – for obvious reasons – half the attention is paid to aural rehabilitation among the total communication group, an issue that needs to be considered in the analysis.

The language element of the hypothesis appears to be absent from the research, since only spoken-language (speech perception and production) tests are administered in clinical one-to-one conditions, although the authors seem to consider the TACL a general language measure.

The fact that no differences of significance were found between the oral group and the total communication group on the three measures of reading (p.90) might actually support the notion that comparisons between oral and total communication children on the basis of modally specific language measures are too simplistic.

Gfeller K, Witt SA, Spencer LJ, Stordahl J, Tomblin B (1998) Musical involvement and enjoyment of children who use cochlear implants. Volta Review 100(4): 213–233.

Population size
65

Demographics
Gender: male (33), female (32)
CI device: Clarion, Nucleus 22 and 24.
Coding strategies: MPEAK, SPEAK, F0F1F2
Age: range 24 months–20.6 years (mean 11.2 years)
Age at CI: range 1.6–18 years (average 6.2 years)
Aetiology: prelingual (61), postlingual (3), perilingual (1)
Communication mode: total communication (53), oral communication (12)

Selection criteria
University of Iowa Health Care Department of Otolaryngology children with cochlear implants received over the preceding 11 years. Questionnaires targeted to all parents (n = 73). Return rate 89%. No deselections reported

Dependent variables
Music appreciation: parent questionnaire, scored into four categories of music appreciation

Independent variables
School age: preschool, primary, secondary

PB-K, WIPI speech perception test scores, Short/Long Sentence Test speech production test score and a 'local' global performance measure called a 'clinical performance rating'

Method

General reporting; some percentage scores reported, with case study exemplars of outcome range provided in appendix

Results

A large proportion of these children are involved in some type of formal or informal musical activity. The authors comment that few accommodations are made in formal music classes for children with cochlear implants, so that there is scope for musical enjoyment to be optimized. Although a correlation was established between a measure of language performance and music enjoyment, this concerned a local test of 'clinical performance rating'; no correlation of significance was established for either WIPI or PB-K.

A separation was established between socially motivated music activity (including peer pressure) and self-instigated musical enjoyment. Overall, regarding formal school music lessons, 46% of cochlear-implanted children attended general music class, while 20% played an instrument, 20% participated in a choir and 11% participated in a band; there was no attempt to clarify whether individuals scored under more than one of the categories listed. Informal activity ranged from 63% listening to music to 32% attending concerts.

Category results: clear dislike (8%), no noticeable response (8%), participation primarily socially motivated (25%) and clear evidence of musical enjoyment (60%).

In addition, correlations between speech measures and general attitude toward music show that children who are involved and enjoy music are more likely to be those who demonstrate greater competency with aural/oral skills.

Conclusions

A large proportion of children who use cochlear implants are involved in some type of formal or informal musical activity, despite the fact that the implant has been designed primarily for speech perception. Music involvement is most common during the elementary school years, during which the majority of children participate in regular music education. The most common accommodation is a sign language interpreter for those children using total communication, who can assist the child in following teacher directions and classroom discussion.

Observations

The data are of clear interest because of both the number of cochlear-implanted children targeted in this study and the topic of investigation. Music appreciation may be of psychological interest, and the notion that technical developments in acoustical signal processing in particular might be able to target the sort of range of acoustic information in the near future might give cochlear implant users benefits of music appreciation (p.213).

According to the authors, there is some anecdotal evidence available that suggests that any musical experience that is available to current implanted children is of a much less pleasant and meaningful quality than that available to a hearing person, arising from the speech processing strategies used. Hence the attempt is to investigate this area more systematically. Although it seems that significant numbers of cochlear-implanted children are involved in some type of formal musical activity, few accommodations are made in musical class. Moreover, cochlear-implanted children involved in music are more likely to be those who demonstrate greater competency with aural/oral skills. Of course, rather than a causal relationship, this correlation will be with another factor as cause.

No comparison against a (standardized) hearing population is offered, making interpretation difficult.

Further detailed assessments of the quality of participation will provide greater understanding of, in particular, the breakdown between social pressure (and encouragement) and personal enjoyment.

Gordon KA, Daya H, Harrison RV, Papsin BC (2000) Factors contributing to limited open-set speech perception in children who use a cochlear implant. International Journal of Pediatric Otorhinolaryngology 56(2): 101–111.

Population size

5

Demographics

CI experience: ≥ 2 years, range 34–86 months (mean 56.2 months)

Age at CI: range 9.3–13.3 years (mean 11.8 years)

Duration of deafness: range 9.3–13.3 years (mean 10.7 years)

Gender: male (3), female (2)

Aetiology: congenital (4), meningitis (1)

Home language: 2 children came from ESL (English as second language) homes

Selection criteria

Regression slope approaching zero or a negative value was obtained on the PB-K word list; these children showed no objective improvement in open-set speech perception (PB-K) with at least two years of implant use

Selected from cohort of one single implant centre

Dependent variables

Range of pre-implant factors such as functional hearing, age, speech and language abilities, and educational issues (survey design)

   Post-implant concerns focused on type of therapy provided, at what intervals the therapy occurred and for how long the therapy continued post implant, as well as what type of school placements these children were in and whether English was a second language in the home

Independent variables

Low speech-perception test scores (PB-K) two years post-CI

Method

Pre-implant factors were examined using a graded profile analysis and post-implant factors were assessed in a retrospective chart review. Two control groups, one random (n = 10), one age-matched (n = 5)

Linear correlation analysis (Kruskal–Wallis ANOVA on ranks; Dunn's method of pairwise multiple comparisons).

Results

A greater number of pre-implant concerns were raised in the study group than in randomized controls ($p < 0.01$). Age and duration of deafness were pre-implant concerns in all study group children ($p < 0.005$). A greater number of post-implant concerns were found in the study group than in randomly selected controls (these included factors concerning the technological maintenance and programming, and rehabilitation).

   In both the experimental and age-matched control groups, the consistent concerns identified were both age and duration of deafness.

   'All of the children who ultimately achieved no open-set word recognition skills were implanted at ages beyond 5 years with > 5 years of deafness. Thus, both age and duration of deafness were identified as concerns. Moreover, the five children who did not achieve open-set word recognition were significantly older with longer durations of deafness than a random sample of children who were able to achieve some degree of open-set word recognition' (p.108).

Yet these factors 'alone cannot account for limited speech perception outcomes and should not be used in isolation as a predictor of post-implant performance' (p.109).

Conclusions

The authors concluded that while appropriate selection of candidates for cochlear implantation is important in predicting speech perception outcomes, post-implant follow-up is also essential and must include regular monitoring of equipment, monitoring of stimulation levels with use of objective measures of stimulation levels if necessary, as well as consistent habilitation.

Observations

The authors identified potential factors contributing to poor performance with an implant by studying implanted children who do not develop functional speech perception, identifying five children as developing no open-set word recognition skills after at least two years of implant use. This small population was compared to a randomly selected control group (n = 10) and an age-matched control group (n = 5). Pre-implant factors were examined using a graded profile analysis and post-implant factors were assessed in a retrospective chart review.

Although below the minimum population size considered for this review, this project is a valuable attempt at explaining the wide variance in speech perception outcomes reported by various other authors, in particular focusing on poor performance. Hence, the article is included in this review.

The study used a control group from the larger sample but sampled for normal range test scores and matched for age.

The findings are somewhat disappointing to the extent that they add little to current knowledge. This may be partly explained by the binary scoring of concerns, which does not allow for levels of subtlety to be addressed.

Nevertheless, a few observations stand out. First, although English as home language was not included in the binary quantification of concerns, a non-English home language was used by two of the five children who were underperforming. Although this may very well be pure coincidence in the light of the low numbers, the authors deem it of sufficient interest to suggest that this issue be monitored (p.108).

Second,

> 'While many issues were distinguished, two main factors emerged as potential concerns in the pre-implant phase. All of the children who ultimately achieved no open-set word recognition skills were implanted at ages beyond 5 years with > 5 years of deafness. Thus, both age and duration of deafness were identified as concerns on the pre-implant graded profile analysis. Moreover, the five children who did not achieve open-set word recognition were significantly older with longer durations of deafness than a random sample of children who were able to achieve some degree of open-set word recognition' (p.108).

Despite the inclusion of this article among the reviews here, there are obvious problems in generalizing results concerning just five research children to entire populations of weak performers. This must be kept in mind, especially when comparing this article with results from much larger cohorts in other studies in this volume.

Gstöttner W, Hamzavi J, Egerlierler B, Baumgartner WD (2000) Speech perception performance in prelingually deaf children with cochlear implants. Acta Oto-Laryngologica 120: 209–213.

Population size

31

Demographics

Age at onset: range 0–1 year, mean 0.1 year
Age: range 0.7–9.5 years, mean 4.1 years

Selection criteria

Selected perilingual and congenital children only out of n = 55 implanted children at the University of Vienna's Medical School

Dependent variables

EARS test battery preimplantation then at 1-, 3-, 6-, 12-, 18-, 24- and 36-months following implantation

Independent variables
  Pre implant test scores
Method
  Percentage scores
Results
  'As also observed in other studies speech perception performance varied greatly
  from child to child within our group' (p.211).
  A number of percentage score improvements over time are reported: 30–93% on LiP, 0–
  100% on MTP and Closed-Set Monosyllabic Word Test, 0–97% on Sentence-Level Test,
  and 10–100% on GASP (pp.211–12).
Conclusions
  'The results of our study indicate that speech perception in prelingually deafened
  children implanted with a Combi 40/40+ cochlear implant improves slowly yet steadily
  over time. This was most evidenced on the open-set tests, as the children exhibited more
  dramatic early performances on the easier, closed-set tests' (p.212).
Observations
  This study adds to existing findings, mostly by aligning the situation of cochlear implant
  recipients in Austria with the larger datasets that are emerging from within the US, UK
  and Australia in particular. This research concerns speech perception exclusively,
  reporting on measures taken within the EU context of the EARS programme (Evaluation
  of Auditory Responses to Speech). The key objective with EARS is to evolve a
  standardized measures protocol, so that results will in due course allow for the
  aggregation of European datasets. A later study of the same population is available in
  Baumgartner et al. (2002), also reported in this volume.
  Results as reported may well be robust but are largely confirmatory rather than
  exploratory, so that the conclusion that 'results for the open-set testing measures were
  most encouraging, with some children reaching fairly high levels of speech perception,
  receiving scores as high as 100%' (p.109), is rightly more general in substance.
  As the results reveal, there are clear ceiling effects on most of the tests reported,
  which means that tests were too easy, and that progress over time is affected by the
  ceilings encountered in the EARS protocol. A potential issue with the EARS protocol may
  well turn out to be that, perhaps as a direct result of its focus on standardizing existing
  measures, it is not sensitive to new developments and concerns in the field, but it would
  be premature for us to attempt a categorical assessment. In the current dataset
  relatively few articles report back using the EARS protocols of assessment.
  The scores at three years post-implantation are based on extremely small populations,
  e.g. 5 (LiP), 4 (MTP) and just 3 (Sentence-Level Test), as not all have reached this stage
  yet, while the participating population size was detailed in only half of the tests used.
  This makes interpreting the findings difficult, and generalization problematic.

**Hamzavi J, Baumgartner WD, Egelierler B, Franz P, Schenk B, Gstöttner W (2000)
Follow up of cochlear implanted handicapped children. International Journal of
Pediatric Otorhinolaryngology 56(3): 169–174.**

Population size
  10
Population comments
  Concerns children with cochlear implants, having a range of additional disabilities, from
  mild learning difficulties to autism, hemiparesis and psychomotor retardation, described
  on a case-by-case basis
Demographics
  Gender: male (6), female (4)

Aetiology: congenital (9), meningitis (1)
Age at CI: range 8–77 months (mean 47.2 months)
A per-child demographic table is included

Selection criteria

Vienna CI centre. 10 multi-handicapped out of total number of CIs of 80. None deselected

Dependent variables

EARS. Preoperatively, then at 1-, 3-, 6-, 12-, 18-, 24- and 36-month intervals post-CI

Independent variables

Multi-handicap

Method

Not applicable

Results

Detailed on a case-by-case basis (see example in comments); not generalizable in terms of larger samples.

Conclusions

Providing multi-handicapped children with cochlear implants can result in substantial benefit for both the child and parents. Multi-handicapped children are not contraindicated for cochlear implantation, although not all are considered to be good candidates.

'Based on our experiences, we would not implant children with handicaps such as auto-aggression, severe intellectual deficit associated with severe performance disturbances, or malignant diseases with reduced life expectancy' (p.174).

Observations

This report is included in the reviewed set despite its low sample size for its obvious interest in children with complex needs and the effect on spoken language performance. Because of the low incidence of multiple disability in any dataset, there is only one large sample study on this same topic available, that of Pyman et al. (2000), reporting on 75 motor- and cognitive-delayed children, all with an age at the time of the study of below 5 years – not dissimilar to the population reported here. The Pyman et al. cohort concerned children implanted between 1985 and 1998, hence the devices of some children in that study used older speech-processing strategies than did the children in this study.

However, the two studies clearly arose out of opposing concerns. Pyman et al. were concerned to explain wide individual variation and suggested the notion of delayed milestones, caused by motor and cognitive delays, as a strong factor accounting for underperformance. Other studies have also focused on underperforming children for the same reason (e.g. Gordon et al. 2000). By contrast, the aim of this study was to investigate limitations on cochlear implant candidacy and the hypothesis that deaf children with multiple disabilities might very well benefit from cochlear implantation, even though they may be less likely to match the outcome performance of the cochlear implant population as a whole.

Taking this approach, the question is more aligned with those that challenge existing threshold criteria for implantation. Examples of these are children with amounts of residual hearing and hearing losses just below the threshold criteria for implantation (e.g. Geers and Moog 1997), or very young children currently generally falling below the age of 2. Indeed, many of the concerns, especially those regarding parental expectations and different rehabilitative needs reported here in the introduction (p.169), overlap in the issue of candidacy.

The sample reported on here is a subsample of the total cohort of 80 implanted in Vienna at the time the article was written. Of those, 10 are characterized as having multiple handicaps. Tests included the EARS battery (reported for the general cohort in Gstöttner et al. 2000) and the MTP test. Given both the limited number and individual variation of disability status and level, the authors have sensibly resorted to qualitative per-case description of the results.

In one child, the implant was subsequently explanted because of rejection by the user. One child combines cochlear implant/speech with sign language communication. Other children derived minor to significant auditory benefits from the implant.

No audiological results are reported in this study; instead, more general observations on improvement or changes in behaviour are noted per child, so, for example,

'Child 5: At the time of implantation, her disabilities were not yet discovered (Table 1). The child started phonating two months following the surgery. During the first six months, there was an improvement in her motor development. She started seeking the source of a sound after 18 months, her phonation has become differentiated, and her voice is much more powerful, but she has not yet demonstrated any speech recognition or production.'

There is reason to remain somewhat sceptical of the paper's claim to report both objective and subjective outcomes, although clear gains in speech perception are reported. Given the intensive rehabilitation accompanying these children, results may relate to levels of attention and care. No socio-economic or parental support measures are provided, which might help explain level and quality of attention and care in individual cases. However, the pre- and postoperative measures do present a useful indication of 'value-added'.

Harrigan S, Nikolopoulos TP (2002) Parent interaction course in order to enhance communication skills between parents and children following paediatric cochlear implantation. International Journal of Pediatric Otorhinolaryngology 66: 161–166.

Population size
11

Population comments
Parents of children with cochlear implants

Demographics
Detailed in table (p.164)
Age: range 2.02–6.03 years, mean 4 years
Duration of deafness: range 0.9–5.04 years
Aetiology: congenital (8), acquired (3)
CI experience: range 2–23 months
Communication mode: total communication

Selection criteria
Voluntary participation in course

Dependent variables
Pre-course interaction rating

Independent variables
Post-course interaction rating

Method
Two-tailed t-test comparison of paired (pre- and post-course) rating samples

Results
Parent interaction training appears to have a beneficial effect on the contingency and linguistic appropriateness of parents' communication behaviour (p.164), with the number of parental initiations half those of pre-course results, while the number of responses in the discourse samples doubled; results were statistically significant ($p < 0.05$, p.164).

Conclusions
Parent interaction training courses were found to be well accepted by the parents, proving to be effective in promoting positive changes in parental communication behaviour (p.165).

Observations
This report seems to revisit the material published by Paganga et al. (2001), also included

in the review. It reports the outcomes for a Nottingham course on parent–child interaction for a group of 11 parents, with much the same conclusions attached. Course and research focus on discourse initiations and responses, underpinned by the hypothesis that by following the course (which was set up to achieve just this) parents would change discourse strategy from a predominance of initiation to a greater number of responses, in video-taped discourse interactions at home.

It is worth noting here as a minor criticism, also valid for the Paganga text, that course satisfaction was measured only by attendance record. Otherwise, the intervention and applied research design are straightforward and effective.

Harrison RV, Panesar J, El-Hakim H, Abdolell M, Mount RJ, Papsin B (2001) The effects of age of cochlear implantation on speech perception outcomes in prelingually deaf children. Scandinavian Audiology 30(53): s73–s78.

Population size
70

Demographics
Age range: 2–15 years
CI: Nucleus multichannel
CI use: up to 5 years
Aetiology: congenital 78%

Selection criteria
All children of Toronto implant programme who were followed (and tested at regular intervals) for up to five years post implant (70 out of 120) were considered. Those aged < 2 years and those implanted at Toronto but followed elsewhere were excluded

Dependent variables
Speech perception test scores:
- closed sets: TAC and WIPI
- open sets: GASP and PB-K

The number of children varies between tests (n = 82–58)

Independent variables
Age at CI

Method
Optimal binary partitioning of the population into two age groups according to maximum split in outcome at a particular age. Repeated measures analysis of variance to calculate statistical significance

Results
Optimal split for PB-K scores is age 8.4 years. The scores of children below 8.4 are significantly better (p = 0.003).
Significances confirmed on other tests (Gasp p = 0.004; WIPI p = 0.001; TAC p = 0.01). Optimum age splits for WIPI and TAC 4.4 years, for GASP 5.6 years.

Conclusions
'We find very robust differences in average performance of younger implanted children compared with older implanted children...' (p.75).
'Our results do suggest that when one poses a question about the advantage of early versus late cochlear implantation, one should take into account the complexity of the outcome measure task that is being used to assess performance' (p.77).
'... the optimal age of implantation split is not a universal value but depends on the complexity of the outcome measure test' (p.75).

Observations
This is a valuable article, in that it explores the relationship between the level of complexity of outcome measures (and presumably what they measure) and the notion of an 'optimum' age of implantation. Combined with a large cochlear implantation sample

(*n* = 70), the resulting report and its conclusions are of significance to developments in the entire field of assessing the spoken language outcomes of paediatric cochlear implantation. The article also focuses on findings elsewhere that early implantation produces greater improvements over time, using a wholly different method of analysis (see below) to calculate differences based on age of implantation. The authors aptly summarize the issue with reference to other studies as follows:

'Nikolopoulos et al. (1999) looked at the correlation between age and speech perception outcome measures in 126 children who were implanted before the age of 7 and followed up to four years post-implant. They found a strong negative correlation between age at implantation and speech perception that only became apparent 3–4 years following implantation. On the other hand, Gantz et al. (1994) in their five-year follow-up study of 59 children, found that age at implantation between 2 and 13 years has little influence on speech understanding abilities. Osberger et al. (1999) determined speech perception results in 58 children from 2 to 17 years after 18 months of follow-up and found significant improvement in performance over all test measures over time. One of the difficulties with looking for age of implantation effects on speech understanding is in the general heterogeneity of the patient populations' (pp.76–7).

The study concerns a retrospective analysis on prelingually deaf children exclusively, who were followed for up to five years consecutively post implantation. A number of closed-set (TAC, WIPI) and open-set (PB-K, GASP) tests were administered. A binary partitioning algorithm was used to divide the dataset on the basis of age at implantation. This means that for each measure a statistic providing the maximum performance level is located at an exact age at implantation point:

'The data in every outcome measure are sorted by the age variable and a sequence of splits defined at unique age values is performed. For each split the data are partitioned into two groups: those children whose age is below that value form one group, and those whose age is greater than or equal to that value form the other group. Splitting of the data is based on the concept of reducing heterogeneity in the response distribution by separating the children into two subsets based on ages that are more homogeneous when they are split than when they are combined. A measure of heterogeneity is deviance [...] The maximum drop in deviance identifies the optimal split which is the age cut-off that best separates the age groups' (p.76).

The outcome of the research is both intriguing and significant. The authors note that the 'critical age' of implantation depends on the level of complexity of the outcome tasks set to children with implants. Closed set tasks have a distinctly lower optimum split at age of implantation (age 4.4 years) than does the PB-K open-set task (age 8.4 years).

However, these cut-off criteria and results depend also on the population studied and the number of children in each age band. For example if only seven children are implanted between 3 and 4 years of age, it will be very difficult for any statistical analysis to have the power needed to reveal that these children outperform the older implanted children. As a consequence the study will not show that there is any difference between such groups.

Hildesheimer M, Teitelbaum R, Segal O, Tenne S, Kishon-Rabin L, Kronenberg Y, Muchnik C (2001) Speech perception results – the first 10 years of a cochlear implant program. Scandinavian Audiology 30(52): s39–s41.

Population size
    81
Population comments
    Plus group of 39 adults (mean age at CI 44 years, range 17–68)

Demographics

Age at CI: 1.6–16.6 years, mean 5 years

No further details given

Selection criteria

None provided

Dependent variables

Open and closed set scores (Hebrew)

HeSPAC, CVC words (Hebrew AB), two-syllable words, and words in sentences

Independent variables

Age (paediatric versus adult implantation)

Method

Percentage test scores

Results

Category scores (pattern perception only, closed-set perception only and open-set) were similar between groups. On average, children attained maximum performance levels more quickly than adults (0.6 versus 0.5–1 year), but as a group maximum performance was reached after two years. A qualitative difference existed between children and adults in their perception of the various contrasts (p.40).

Conclusions

Average open-set score results of adults were similar to those of the children.

Observations

This study has limitations on demographic description and the reporting of findings. The conclusion is both unsurprising and very general, and lacking in detail. Of interest mainly because of its attempt to compare the outcomes of cochlear implants in children with those in adults, which has obvious consequences for any test design and administration. It is also the only report included in the review reporting on a Hebrew-speaking population. Of significance also is the large sample size ($n = 81$), which have been followed for up to five years at the time of writing.

The tests administered have reportedly been adapted for age, but no details are given in the short report. The main conclusion is that children and adults attain comparable results on the closed- and open-set tests administered, although it took the adult population ($n = 39$) slightly longer. The paediatric cohort continued to improve over the full five-year time span.

Hodges AV, Dolan Ash M, Balkany TJ, Schloffman JJ, Butts SL (1999) Speech perception results in children with cochlear implants: contributing factors. Otolaryngology – Head and Neck Surgery 121(1): 31–34.

Population size

40

Demographics

Age: range 2–14 years, mean 6 years

CI use: range 3 months–5 years, mean 2.1 years

CI device: Nucleus Spectra (27), Nucleus MSP (7), Clarion 1.2 (6)

Aetiology: congenital (34), prelingual (2), perilingual (4)

Educational settings: range

Communication mode: oral (19), total communication (21)

Language background: English not native language for one or both parents (11)

Socio-economic status: range detailed

Selection criteria

Children implanted at the University of Miami Ear Institute between 1990 and 1995 ($n = 58$). Deselections are explained

Dependent variables
Speech perception test scores:
- ESP
- Minimal Pairs test
- NU-CHIPS
- PB-K

Chart review by specialists
Parent questionnaire (socio-economic status measures)

Independent variables
Communication mode
Length of implant use
Age at surgery
Type of device
Family socio-economic status
Bilingualism in the home
Type of school setting
Participation in therapy

Method
Multiple-regression analysis of independent variables correlated with speech perception test scores

Results
Results show that communication mode with an r value of 0.67 ($p < 0.0001$) is the most highly predictive factor of speech perception performance. School setting ($p < 0.002$), socio-economic status rank ($p < 0.008$) and participation in private therapy ($p < 0.008$) also exhibited strong positive relationships with performance on speech perception measures.

Conclusions
Those who used some form of oral communication scored significantly higher on a battery of both closed- and open-set speech-perception tests; the strongest relationship proved to be communication mode.

Observations
The authors undertook a wide-ranging analysis of factors affecting speech-perception scores. Half of the children were in oral programmes, the other half in total communication programmes. The age range of the cohort is considerable. The authors conclude that oral children outperform total communication children, a conclusion they recognize as being inconsistent with other reports (p.31). Hence they analysed seven more factors, nevertheless confirming that communication mode is most significantly correlated with attainment.

It is important to note that only auditory speech perception is measured, eliminating visual cues for both the oral and total communication subjects.

The fact that bilingualism scored weakly on regression against test results is perhaps explained by the test procedure, since it too is a language-dependent measure (p. 34). Otherwise,

> 'These factors show that children in higher socioeconomic groups, those who attend private schools, and those who receive private therapy also score higher on speech perception measures.'

Huang WH, Huang TS (1997) Speech perception performance of prelingually deafened children and adolescents with Nucleus 22-channel cochlear implant. Advances in Oto-Rhino-Laryngology 52: 224–228.

Population size
8

Demographics
Detailed in Table 1 (p.226)

Age at implantation: range 6–18 years
Age: range 6–18 years
Age at onset: range 6.0–18.0 years
Gender: male (4), female (4)
Active electrodes: range 13–22

Selection criteria

None detailed; implanted at the Chang Gung Memorial Hospital, Taipei, Taiwan

Dependent variables

Speech-perception tests (bespoke):
• vowel identification
• consonant identification
• tone perception
• speech pattern perception
• closed-set word identification
• closed-set sentence identification
• open-set speech recognition
Tests conducted in a sound-proofed room

Independent variables

Prior achievement

Method

T-test analysis of percentage scores

Results

Report significant effects ($p < 0.05$) in 'most items', except vowel, consonant, tone and open-set sentence tests. The teenagers of group B showed more modest gains than the younger children with implants of group A (p.225).

Conclusions

Results of the investigation matched anticipated outcomes by revealing a significant effect in stimulus dynamic range among subjects (p.228).

Observations

This article is included here because it covers Mandarin, a tone language. As the authors note:

'Generally speaking, it would seem that a tone language should be markedly more difficult to discriminate when the feature of tone is eliminated by simulating a mild hearing-impaired condition after receiving cochlear implant surgery' (p.224).

In Mandarin Chinese, tone distinguishes lexical meaning through pitch variation using four fundamental voiced frequencies or 'tones'; grammatically they represent suprasegmental phonemes (p.224).

Unfortunately the study suffers from time limitations, being restricted to just 12 months postoperative follow-up, and a small sample of only eight, divided into those aged 6–12 years (group A) and those aged 13–18 years (group B) (p.225).

Although significant effects are reported (as group functions) for some of the tests, these effects do not include tests measuring vowels, consonants or tone, and cover lexical-level (as opposed to sentence level) outcomes only (p.225), hence no new findings were generated. However, it is of clear wider interest for the researchers to extend their research into children with implants using Mandarin Chinese to cover much larger samples being tracked over much longer periods of time, exactly because of the role of tone in Mandarin.

Other factors must also be addressed in future studies, such as controlling for maturation alone, correcting for artificial statistical effects due to random grouping for age, disaggregating mean group results in order to account for individual variation, including real-life measures in addition to laboratory tests, and so on. This report will be of interest to manufacturers looking at speech processing strategies.

Hutton J, Politti C, Seeger T (1995) Cost-effectiveness of cochlear implantation of children: a preliminary model for the UK. Advances in Otorhinolaryngology 50: 201–206.

Population size
Nil – assumptions and published sources
Demographics
Current age: not reported
Age at onset: not reported
Age at CI: not reported
Duration of deafness: not reported
Life expectancy: lifetime (until 70 years old)
Setting UK
Method
Economic evaluation type: cost-utility analysis
Study perspective: societal (partial)
Comparator intervention: non-implanted
Source of effectiveness data: assumed
Direct costs: average cost of implantation (covering preoperative assessment, implantation, major/minor complications, medical follow-up and clinical rehabilitation) and lifetime support costs (including continued rehabilitation, routine follow-up visit and test, and special equipment for daily living)
Indirect costs: changes in education costs
Discount rate for costs and benefits: 6%
Outcome measure: assumed improvement in quality of life
Currency and price year: £, price year not stated
Sensitivity analysis: educational costs were tested (the extra educational costs per annum for the non-implanted were £7,500 in the base case, range £5,500–£13,200 in the sensitivity analysis and for implanted children were £1,000 in the base case with a range of £500–£1,800 in the sensitivity analysis
Results
The paper assumes an average quality of life improvement of 0.6 to 0.7, such that with a net gain of 3.66 QALYs discounted at 6%, the cost-per-QALY for PCI in children in the UK was £16,214.
Conclusions
'This is by no means a high figure in comparison with other clinical interventions' (p.205).
Observations
This early paper raises a number of interesting questions regarding the true health-utility impact of implantation, the educational costs/benefits, how much extra support the implanted will need in mainstream to perform better or do they in fact achieve better results in special school education? Some of the answers to these questions still remain uncertain. The paper does rely on a large number of assumptions reflecting its early publication date and the lack of empirical data at that time.

Illg A, von der Haar-Heise S, Goldring JE, Lesinski-Schiedat A, Battmer RD, Lenarz T (1999) Speech perception results for children implanted with the Clarion cochlear implant at the Medical University of Hanover. Annals of Otology, Rhinology and Laryngology 108: 93–98.

Population size
167
Population comments
Grouped in < 7 years and 7–15 years of age, and subgroups of < 4 years (average 2.7 years) and 4–7 years (average 5.5 years)

Demographics

Age at CI: 15 months–15 years, average 6.5 years

CI device: Clarion

Encoding strategy: CIS

Age at onset: 'before learning oral speech and language' (p.93)

Aetiology: 'most commonly meningitis or congenital' (p.93)

Selection criteria

All Clarion users implanted at between 1994 and 1997

Dependent variables

Speech perception test battery at 3, 6, 12, 18 and 24 months post implantation

Closed-set

Pattern Perception Test

Two-syllable Word Test

Monosyllable Word Test

Minimal Pairs Test

Open-set

TAPS Word Test (comparable to GASP)

Monosyllable Word Test (comparable. to PB-K)

GASP Sentence Test

Common phrases (Mr Potato Head Task for younger children)

Independent variables

Pre-implantation speech perception scores

Method

Test scores and Wilcoxon correlation statistic

Results

Percentage scores listed in tables (pp.94, 95).

Closed-set

> 'In general, the results were very good for both groups, although the improvement
> as a function of time differed between the younger and older children. [...] The
> results for the three tests were similar in that the scores improved steadily to
> about 80% to 85% by two years postimplantation' (pp.94–5).

Younger children have better scores on average, showing 'a very steep improvement
curve on the PP, two-syllable, and monosyllable tests' (p.95).

Open-set

The overall scores were comparatively lower than for the closed-set tests, but showing
improvements over time; the older group plateaued after the first year at around 40%
and 45% scores (p.96). The GASP test was the only test in which the older children had
higher final scores than the younger children (p.96).

Analysis of the subgroups (< 4, and 4–7 years) reveals the same trends as with the
closed-set tests, the younger group attaining ±10% higher scores; but similar for GASP
and Mr Potato Head tasks (pp.96–7).

Conclusions

'... deaf children between the ages of 1 and 15 can benefit from a cochlear implant' (p.97).

'Younger children achieve more rapid gains than older children, who tended to plateau
between 12 and 18 months postimplantation' (p.98).

Observations

This study is significant because of the large number of cochlear-implanted children
participating (*n* = 167). The study utilizes a range of tests in both closed- and open-set
speech perception. The study under-reports demographic detail, test administration and
score analysis.

The population is broken down into age groups without reasons being given for the
age-boundary decisions, so that some findings may result from a seemingly random
methodological imposition; it might have been more appropriate to analyse the effect of
age at implantation as a continuous measure.

It should also be noted that the group, although large, extends across a significant age range, including children at the pre-verbal stage right through to 15-year-olds. For a number of tests, and for all tests at the 24-month interval, the number involved drop to n = 10, for unexplained reasons.

In addition to this, the plateauing effects of the older age-group remain unanalysed and undiscussed, and no measures are in place to consider the reasons for this result. In comparison to many other more recent studies reported here, the 24-month period of assessment may be considered as short and inconclusive, although of course the plateau effects are reported for the 12-month interval postoperative results. Nevertheless, the data are in agreement with many other studies reporting on speech-perception outcomes.

Incesulu A, Vural M, Erkam U (2003) Children with cochlear implants: parental perspective. Otology and Neurotology 24(4): 605–611.

Population size
28
Population comments
Parents of cochlear-implanted children
Demographics
Gender: male (19), female (9)
Age: range 2–13 years, mean 5.07 years (SD = 2.33)
CI use: range 12–30 months, mean 19.5 months (SD = 5.95)
CI device: multichannel
Placement: mainstream (7); mainstream plus rehabilitation centre visits (7); full-time special school (13)
Selection criteria
Minimum of one year post implantation. Return 27/28 sent
Dependent variables
Parents' closed-question questionnaire; same format as the model used in Nottingham cochlear implant programme
Independent variables
CI
Method
Reporting percentage categories of selected questions
Results
'... only seven parents recommended the use of sign language as well as verbal communication to support the speech and language development right after the implantation for a short time.'
'Most parents (21/78%) strongly agreed that their child had needed more help from the family since he had cochlear implant.'
'The majority of parents (26) strongly agree that communication with the child by speaking than by signing is easier than before.'
Conclusions
'This study revealed that cochlear implantation is a long, complicated stressful process for both family and professional staff in the implant centre.'
Observations
Of limited interest, partly because of the confusing and selective reporting. For the Nottingham questionnaire, external validation and standardizing the administration of the questionnaire has since been undertaken, and details have been published.

The suggestion that open-format questionnaire results cannot be coded may spring from unfamiliarity with qualitative research methods. In any case, one would imagine that open-format questionnaires are useful for giving fuller information about cochlear

implantation and its outcomes, especially given some of the contested areas of meaning
and choice of outcomes, and the relatively exploratory nature of this area of investigation.

**Inscoe J (1999) Communication outcomes after paediatric cochlear implantation.
International Journal of Pediatric Otorhinolaryngology 47(2): 195–200.**

Population size
80
Population comments
Population not detailed ('a large group', p.195); reference is made to 80
Demographics
Age: range 1–9 years
Age at onset: < 4 years
Aetiology: 50% congenital
Selection criteria
Classified as 'pre-verbal' – presumably a reference to a set of spoken language test
scores conducted at the candidacy stage, but the term is not further detailed
It is probable that no CIs were deselected, since the text makes reference to the inclusion
of some CIs with complex needs (p.199); no categorical statement was found
Dependent variables
Early communicative behaviour assessments, consisting of parent questionnaire,
criterion-referenced rating scales and a profile of speech skills: PPECS; SECS; SIR; PALS
Independent variables
CI
Method
Quantification of information obtained, represented as accumulated percentage scores
Results
PPECS
'By the one year interval, the results on 80 children show 50% of them had established
abilities in using and responding appropriately to spoken language, and more than 25%
had progressed in interaction and conversation skills. By the three year interval 80% of
the 35 children had established abilities in using and responding to spoken language. An
unsurprising slightly slower rate of progress is noted in the linguistically more complex
areas of verbal interaction and conversation' (pp.196–7).
SECS
'By the one year interval 45% of children were able to learn new words readily and 22%
of children were able to combine verbs and nouns into phrases and sentences. Three
years after implantation only 10% of children in this sample were using sentences with
more than one verb form' (p.198).
SIR
'Before implantation 85% of selected children were pre-verbal or relied on sign language
as the primary means of everyday communication. The remaining 15% were mainly, but
not exclusively, deafened children. The subsequent rate of progress in speech
intelligibility over five years complements the PALS data.
  'By the three year interval, 55% of the children were considered intelligible to an
experienced listener. By the five year interval 33% of the children were considered
intelligible to all, and an additional 50% were rated as intelligible to both experienced
listeners and those with limited experience of the speech of a deaf speaker. A total of 11%
were rated as still using sign language as their main form of expressive language, and
6% could not use intelligible connected speech' (p.199).
PALS
'By the three year interval over 75% of the children in this sample had attained
functional language status at receptive and expressive language levels, prosodic or voice

skills were also well advanced and a delay in attaining a phonological or rule based speech sound system was noted, as anticipated' (p.200).

Conclusions

'Progress was seen in the responses to and uses of spoken language as the children's main mode of functional communication after three years; verbal receptive and expressive language development, and in speech intelligibility over five years' (p.200).

Observations

The study arose out of a concern that no appropriate test designs were available for the age group of the cochlear-implanted children sampled. Therefore, four assessment measures were selected to demonstrate the rate of spoken language. Three out of four of the assessment outcomes included most of the children implanted, i.e. congenitally deaf and deafened children aged between 1 and 9 years. At the time of implantation, the majority of these children were unable to carry out a performance test of language with reliability.

This study is of obvious interest because of the size of the sample (n = 80) and the fact that this concerns all very young children (or rather, they are classified as being at the pre-verbal stage at the time of implantation). However, the sample size is in doubt because actually there is no categorical statement regarding sample size to be found anywhere in the text. The paper reports on four assessment measures used in the analysis of spoken language development post implantation. They concern a pragmatics profile of everyday communication skills (parental interview), the scales of early communication skills (criterion-referenced rating scale presumably used by rehabilitation professionals), the speech intelligibility rating scale (as above) and the profile of actual speech skills, covering five linguistic areas of competence. All of these are relatively conventional measures (some available commercially) used as a matter of course at the Nottingham paediatric rehabilitation service.

The observation that speech skills for some, but by no means all, of the sample improve over time raises further questions about the reasons for such differences.

It may also be a mistake to group 'pre-verbal' and sign language using children together (p.199); we cannot revisit any relevant modal distinctions in a post hoc assessment because modality is left unmeasured and unassessed.

Kelsay DMR, Tyler RS (1996) Advantages and disadvantages expected and realised by paediatric cochlear implant recipients as reported by their parents. American Journal of Otology 17: 866–873.

Population size

50

Population comments

Parents of deaf children

Demographics

CI population

Age: 2.1–16.7 years

CI device: Nucleus 22

Age at onset: prelingual deafness

Selection criteria

Targeted CIs from Iowa implant centre. Non-response and response variation over time accounted for

Dependent variables

Parent questionnaire, not detailed, sent yearly over three years

Independent variables

CI experience (in one-year intervals over three years)

Method

Qualitative assessment; mainly offering percentage subtotals across category responses

Results

'Preimplantation, parents were realistic in their expectations of how a cochlear implant would affect their children's lives' (p.868).

The parental ratings of the cochlear implant outcomes show steady increases across the intervals [but see comments on the longitudinal element].

'Three years postimplantation benefits reported included perception of environmental sounds (61% of parents), speech perception (78%), and speech production (74%). Postimplantation, 36%, 24% and 52% of the parents had no disadvantages to report at the one, two, and three-year intervals, respectively' (p.866).

'Improved communicative competence may also have contributed to parents responding at the two-year postimplant interval that their children were more independent' (p.869).

'Only a few parents expected or noted postimplant advantages in their child's educational achievement, language development, psychological well-being, and behaviour' (p.871).

Conclusions

'Subjective questionnaires, such as the one used in the present investigation, may be a valuable clinical tool when evaluating a child as a candidate for a cochlear implant [,] would complement the type of objective information that professionals share with parents who are considering a cochlear implant for their child [and] may also be useful for evaluating a child's progress with a cochlear implant' (p.872).

Observations

The study concerns measuring parents' perspectives on the effects of cochlear implantation on their children. There is a lack of description of both the questionnaire and the research sample of parents. Nevertheless, the study is of value for both the sample size (but see comments below) and the line of questioning. See also Kluwin and Stewart (2000).

The authors did not track the same population of parents throughout the study. Note also the finding that only a few parents noted changes in educational achievement or language development.

As the authors suggest, the study is limited in value because differences in responses over time may be influenced by the different sets of parents participating at each interval. This is particularly significant when it is suggested that:

'Only one parent participated at all four test intervals because his child received his implant during the initial year the questionnaire was administered' (p.869).

The authors then go on to detail significant migration in and out of the study over the time frame (p.869). This certainly means that it becomes problematic to interpret the longitudinal element of the findings, which is otherwise inviting, in particular because of the homogeneity of the data and the positive development of responses over time, and in part because the authors seem inclined this way themselves in their discussion.

Another issue to consider is the time of the first questionnaire. The authors suggest that:

'Parents in this study were counseled regarding advantages and disadvantages of cochlear implant use before they made a decision to proceed with cochlear implantation for their child. The questionnaires used in this study were given to parents the day before their child's surgery.' (p.871).

There is, of course, an issue when specialists counsel parents on what would be 'realistic expectations' (p.868) for the implant outcomes, but then also interview these parents on their hopes for the outcomes of the implant. This is problematic as the definition of realistic expectations is shaped by professionals outside any dialogue with parents themselves.

This identifies a central issue, namely that both interview design (used for investigative purposes rather than for rehabilitative purposes) and interview administration over time should, in the interests of independence, not be controlled by the centres or 'specialists' responsible for implantation. At the very least a disinterested party should pilot the questionnaire.

In the light of the above it is, finally, also worth noting the four cases of non-use of cochlear implant. The authors note that three out of four non-users '... were adolescents. The fourth child lived in a community and attended a school programme with a strong anti-implant position' (p.871). Otherwise,

> 'Parents of the four children who eventually discontinued using their cochlear implants did not differ significantly from the group as a whole in terms of their expectations of cochlear implantation' (p.868).

Kiefer J, Gall V, Desloovere C, Knecht R, Mikowski A, von Ilberg C (1996) A follow-up study of long-term results after cochlear implantation in children and adolescents. European Archives of Oto-Rhino-Laryngology 253(3): 158–166.

Population size
19

Demographics
Onset, aetiology and age at CI listed per child in table
Age at onset: range, pre- to post (14 years); prelingual (14)
Aetiology: unknown (7), hypoxia (2), meningitis (9), cytomegalic (1)
Age at CI: range 3–18 years, mean 8.7 years
CI device: Nucleus 22 (17), Med-EI single-channel (2)
Placement: regular schools, individual auditory training sessions (18); 6 taught German
    Sign Language in addition

Selection criteria
Implanted at the University of Frankfurt. No selection criteria detailed

Dependent variables
TAPS, in auditory mode only

Independent variables
Prior achievement on tests

Method
Individual scores

Results
Phoneme detection on the TAPS test reached ceiling (completion) after one-year interval (p.160). Post- and perilingually deafened children obtained best results on phoneme identification, showing clear progress even during year 4 (p.160).

A range of scores characterized the population on the pattern perception task, with most scoring 100% over time, and two failing to score or scoring below 40% (p.160). All children using their implants for at least four years scored close to 100% in all three subtests.

For speech identification, 16 scored above chance in at least one closed-sentence word test, 11 scoring above chance in the closed-set sentence test (p.162).

For speech recognition, open-set sentence recognition was observed in seven children, with the mean score at 55%.

As a composite result, the percentage of children scoring above chance, and the level of scoring, both increased as a factor over time. Strongest correlations existed for age at onset, duration of deafness and time post implantation, while age at implantation was not significantly correlated with test results (p.163). Correlation statistics are detailed per test in tables (p.165).

Conclusions
'... after at least one year of experience all children benefited from their cochlear implants' (p.165).

'Statistically the most relevant factor accounting for differences in the results is the duration of implant use in all groups [...] Age at onset was found to be another relevant factor' (p.165).

Observations

The authors suggest that long-term tracking of results of paediatric implantation is necessary. They report here on such data up to five years postoperatively, but the mean follow-up across the population reported is much more modest, 28 months (p.158). The results suggest that all children tested at the four-year test interval had developed open-set sentence understanding, with duration of implant use the most relevant factor among those measured (p.158). For prelingually deaf children, duration of deafness and age at implantation correlated negatively with the results (p.158).

The study reports on 19 children, but it is not clear how many children reached the five-year interval reported, so that the results of the statistical analyses remain unclear. The age range is wide, 3–18 years at the time of implantation, with all children apparently being administered the same test. Moreover, the 18-year-old might have skewed the age at cochlear implantation and duration of deafness results in this relatively small sample of children.

As with similar studies, the absence of non-implanted comparison or control groups means that the results cannot simply be attributed to cochlear implantation, as opposed to the benefits of prior learning (in the case of older children), rehabilitation and/or schooling, or maturation alone or in combination.

Kirk KI (1998) Assessing speech perception in listeners with cochlear implants: the development of the Lexical Neighborhood Tests. Volta Review 100(2): 63–85.

Population size
28

Population comments
Experiment 1, 28; Experiment 24, 19; Experiment 5, 20

Demographics

Experiment 1
CI device: Nucleus 22
Age at onset: mean 1.4 years (SD = 2.3)
Age at CI: mean 7.2 years (SD = 2.7)
CI use: average 3 years (SD = 2.4)
CI encoding strategy: F0F1F2 (2), MPEAK (26)

Experiment 2, 3 and 4
Same criteria as Experiment 1; demographic characteristics similar

Experiment 5
Age at onset: mean < 6 months
Age at CI: ± 5 years
CI use: average 3.5 years
Age: mean 8.5 years
Communication mode: oral (12), total communication (8)
Encoding strategy: MPEAK (8), SPEAK (12)
CI: Nucleus 22

Selection criteria
Selected from among the group of cochlear implant users followed at Indiana University School of Medicine
Criteria: CI use one year; demonstrated some closed- or open-set spoken word recognition

Dependent variables

Experiment 1
LNT, test scores

Experiment 2
   LNT versus MLNT test scores
Experiment 3
   Parent questionnaire tracking word familiarity on all three tests
Experiment 4
   Recorded LNT, MLNT scores
Experiment 5
   Single speaker, multi-speaker test conditions
Independent variables
Experiment 1
   PB-K test scores
Method
   Simple linear statistical analysis of test score outcomes
   For the recorded version tests, repeated measures of variance were computed to assess
      effects of lexical difficulty, test list and test session. Pearson product moment
      correlations were computed between individual scores to determine test-retest
      reliability
Results
Experiment 1
   On average, the 28 children correctly identified 30% of the LNT easy words, 23% of the
   LNT hard words and 14% of the PB-K words. Mean phoneme identification scores were
   45% correct for the LNT easy words, 46% for the LNT hard words and 37% for the PB-K
   words. Statistical analysis revealed that the percentage of words and phonemes correctly
   identified was significantly higher for the LNT than for the PB-K. Phoneme recognition
   did not differ between the LNT easy and hard word lists. (pp.67–8).
Experiment 2
   Word recognition scores were significantly higher for the multisyllabic stimuli on the
   MLNT (51%) than for the monosyllabic stimuli on the LNT (39%). In addition, word-
   recognition scores were significantly higher for the lexically easy words than for the
   lexically hard words. In contrast, phoneme scores did not differ significantly between the
   MLNT (64%) and the LNT (60%) (p.69).
Experiment 3
   Post hoc analysis indicated that the LNT words were rated as most familiar, followed by
   the MLNT words and then the PB-K words.
Experiment 4 (recorded test)
   On average, the children with cochlear implants correctly identified 67% of the
   phonemes on the lexically easy MLNT words compared to a mean of 60% for the lexically
   hard MLNT words. Correlation analysis demonstrated that test–retest reliability is quite
   high for the LNT and MLNT.
Experiment 5
   Four low scorers in single-speaker condition eliminated from study to avoid floor effects
   (two oral, two total communication). There was a main effect of talker condition: mean
   word-recognition performance was significantly lower in the single-talker condition
   (34%) than in the multiple-talker condition (42%). Only one child had significantly higher
   word-recognition scores in the single-talker condition than in the multiple-talker
   condition (pp.76–7).
Conclusions
Experiment 1
   PB-K may underestimate spoken-word recognition by children with profound deafness. (p.68).
Experiment 2
   Children with cochlear implants are able to use the linguistic redundancy in multisyllabic
   stimuli to aid them in spoken-word recognition (p.69).
      The results demonstrate that spoken-word recognition by children with cochlear
   implants is influenced by the lexical characteristics of the stimulus items. Children with

cochlear implants were significantly better at identifying multisyllabic words than monosyllabic words (p.70).

Experiment 3

Poor performance on the PB-K may result, in part, because children with profound deafness are unfamiliar with the test items (p.71).

Experiment 5

The authors noticed a great deal of individual variability in test scores (20–60% single, 20–70% multiple-talker). Discrepancy in single versus multiple-talker condition results might relate to procedural differences (p.78).

In summary, children with cochlear implants organize and access words from memory in a manner similar to listeners with hearing, and they are sensitive to the indexical characteristics of the speech signal.

Observations

This report contains a helpful critique of the PB-K test, suggesting that 'phonetic balance' has been demonstrated to be less a requisite than age-appropriate measures (child age, language level) (pp.63–4). The author quotes Fryauf-Bertschy (1997), needing to reduce the word list for young cochlear-implanted children because of inappropriate items. Second, the test is 'unnatural' (clinical) in its administration, hiding stimulus variability (p.64).

Two new measures of spoken-word recognition for children with sensory aids, the Lexical Neighborhood Test (LNT) and the Multisyllabic Lexical Neighborhood Test (MLNT), developed at Indiana University School of Medicine, are here being further evaluated. One important new feature of these tests is that they provide information about the underlying perceptual processes supporting spoken-word recognition in listeners with hearing loss. At the same time the tests are based on a contemporary theory model of spoken word recognition (NAM) (p.65). This study summarizes data concerning the word familiarity, inter-list equivalency and test–retest reliability of these two measures. Test items on the LNT and MLNT were selected from the CHILDES database (age-appropriate vocabulary) for ages 3–5 years.

The article reports on the results of the test administered to a cohort of 28 children with an average experience of cochlear implantation of three years, and with an average age at cochlear implantation of 7.2 years and a mean age (experiment 2) of 8.2 years. The LNT is contrasted with other tests, notably the PB-K. Results suggest that the PB-K test may underestimate the word-level skills of the cochlear-implanted cohort tested, and that some items on the PB-K test are inappropriate. On both tests there was significant individual variation in achievement.

It would be helpful to standardize scores against a very significant sample of hearing children, because in the absence of 'normal' spoken language development data the test score interpretations remain locked in uninterpretably 'delayed' levels of spoken language acquisition. The fact that both LNT and MLNT score better than PB-K has nothing to say about such norm-referencing.

Moreover, the tests are spoken-language vocabulary tests, and do not necessarily reflect real language conditions (let alone multimodal conditions) in any meaningful way.

Kirk KI, Hay-McCutcheon M, Sehgal ST, Miyamoto RT (2000) Speech perception in children with cochlear implants: effects of lexical difficulty, talker variability, and word length. Annals of Otology, Rhinology and Laryngology 109(12): 79–81.

Population size

28

Demographics

Presented in table for oral and total communication groups
Age at onset: mean 0:1 and 0:6 years respectively
Age at CI: mean 5:0 and 4:3 years respectively

Age: mean 8:2 and 8:8 years respectively
CI use: mean 3:3 and 4:5 years respectively
Hearing loss: unaided PTA mean 108 and 114 dB respectively

Selection criteria
No selection criteria given

Dependent variables
Talker variability
Lexical difficulty

Independent variables
Speech perception:
- LNT
- MLNT

Method
Paired t-tests to evaluate separate effects, and 2-way repeated measures ANOVA with talker condition and word length as independent variables

Results
'The results demonstrate that lexically easy words are recognised with significantly greater accuracy than lexically hard words ($p < 0.002$). Further, the effects of lexical difficulty were significant regardless of talker condition or length of the stimulus words. For both the LNT and MLNT, word recognition was significantly higher in the multiple-talker condition than in the single-talker condition ($p < 0.04$). The results also demonstrated that multisyllabic words were identified with significantly greater accuracy than monosyllabic stimuli ($p < 0.002$). The effects of word length do not depend on the number of talkers presenting the stimuli' (p.81).

Conclusions
'The present results demonstrated that all three factors − lexical difficulty, stimulus variability, and word length − significantly influenced spoken-word recognition by children with multichannel cochlear implants (p.81).

Observations
This article concerns a study on lexical difficulty and talker variability in clinical one-to-one test administration conditions. The authors claim that spoken-word recognition by cochlear implant recipients has been assessed traditionally with the PB-K word lists. They note two problems with the PB-K: children being unfamiliar with some of its test items, and it yielding little insight into factors that influence spoken-word recognition − such as talker variability (p.79).

They suggest that research has shown that, in listeners with hearing, the lexical characteristics of the stimuli and the presence of talker variability influence word recognition. In response, the researchers developed a protocol to assess the effects of both on the performance of cochlear implant users using the LNT and MLNT tests. Their lists were recorded by different speakers, and their intelligibility assessed by a panel of hearing listeners who scored 97% words correct. A single-talker and a multiple-talker version of each of the lists were produced from the digital files (p.80).

Testing was therefore conducted via audition only to the group of 28 cochlear-implanted subjects, aged 5 and over (mean 8:2 years). Results suggest that both lexical difficulty and talker variability affect outcomes (p.81), making comparisons between studies more difficult.

Kluwin TN, Stewart DA (2000) Cochlear implants for younger children: a preliminary description of the parental decision process and outcomes. American Annals of the Deaf 145(1): 26−32.

Population size
35

Population comments
Parents of cochlear-implanted children

Demographics
No demographic detail was obtained because of a prior existing confidentiality agreement

Selection criteria
Random sample based on an initial list of 150 CIs over five-year period provided by a large, university-based implant programme. Sixty-five randomly selected were targeted (target n = 50); 35 were located/responded

Dependent variables
Telephone interview; open-ended series of questions listed on p.28

Independent variables
Not applicable

Method
Responses were coded and categorized into Likert scales by two individuals; responses scored by a third

Results
Two types of decision sequences are followed. One type of parent has initial and primary contact through a medical practitioner, uses that source of information exclusively and is motivated by a desire for a 'normal' communication situation. The second type of parent learns about implants from another parent, family member or teacher. This individual will seek other sources of information and is most often motivated by the child's lack of communication skill.

Most parents reported improvements in communication skill following cochlear implantation (p.30). Children whose spoken language skills improved were less likely to be described as having any negative changes resulting from cochlear implantation than the children who used signs and gestures (p.30).

Conclusions
Generally, from parents' perspective, language and speech rather than improved social skills or social contact are the primary benefits of the implant.

> 'The decision to have the child receive an implant appeared to have been driven by three things: a desire for 'normality', access to medical advice, and the availability of insurance. [...] In the case of the implant process, there is the clear pairing of a medical problem with a medical solution' (p.31).

> 'The parents' frequent use of the word normal indicated that early implant options are presented inside the envelope of grief and confusion that accompanies the initial diagnosis. [...] this pairing of two events, diagnosis and remediation without sufficient information, has implications for late 'success' rates' (pp.31–2).

Observations
This study contributes a different, qualitative method for parents.

The authors conducted a preliminary telephone interview study of a random sample of 35 parents whose children had received cochlear implants through a large-scale implant programme. Parents were asked about their child's pre-implant and post-implant communications skills, how they learned about implants, and how they arrived at the decision to have their child receive an implant. Results of the interviews suggest, at least for this programme, that two types of decision sequences are followed. One type of parent has initial and primary contact through a medical practitioner, uses that source of information exclusively and is motivated by a desire for a 'normal' communication situation. The second type of parent learns about implants from another parent, family member or teacher. This individual will seek other sources of information and is most often motivated by the child's lack of communication skill. Generally, from parents' perspective, language and speech rather than improved social skills or social contact are the primary benefits of the implant.

This study was based on random sampling among the parents of a large implant programme, and telephone interviewing. The returns of telephone interview approaches are typically low, and this research reports 35 cases. The conclusions are general, and describe a pattern occurring in the authors' assessment between pre-implant expectations and post-implant outcomes. The research provides a useful addition to other research in this area, but the conclusions would benefit from a more detailed assessment over a much larger and wider sample.

The authors note, as is reflected in the range of texts reviewed here, that past work is:

'... biased by a specific focus on a limited set of dependent measures and the use of small samples. [...] These studies have produced a volume of information that includes recurrent assertions such as the following: that children under age 5 years are more likely to benefit from an implant; that the amount of daily use predicts the quality of speech recognition or speech production; that between six months and two years of use are required before results are noticeable; and that the age of onset of hearing loss conditions users' success rate, or at least their rate of improvement' (pp.26–7).

They suggest there are also methodological weaknesses pervading the research:

'... most frequent limitations being self-selection of children, use of clinical samples, and use of narrowly defined outcome measures' (p.27).

However, the authors recognize that bias is difficult to avoid, and it affects their own study in that self-selection may equally be a characteristic of questionnaire returns.

'By the time we were finished, we had tried to contact 75 families and succeeded with only 35. In other words, only half of the families of the children with implants were actually available to us. This was a sample biased toward those who maintained contact with the programme' (p.32).

Based on responses from this set, the authors consider that results in cochlear implantation may reflect outcomes of other types of medical intervention, being successful most specifically for a rigorously selected subpopulation of highly motivated individuals.

'Like so many other treatments and procedures, implants may be effective with only a specific population under specific training conditions' (p.32).

The authors therefore argue for proper definitions of both 'success' and 'failure' to be established, and that a range of research tactics be addressed to both these issues.

Knutson JF, Boyd RC, Goldman M, Sullivan PM (1997) Psychological characteristics of child cochlear implant candidates and children with hearing impairments. Ear and Hearing 18(5): 355–363.

Population size
69
Population comments
All were candidates for cochlear implantation
Demographics
PTA: > 95 dB HL
Aetiology: congenital (59)
Age at onset: before 18 months (59); after (10)
Gender: male (33), female (36)
Age: range 2.5–15 years (mean 5.9 years)
Families socio-economic status: wide range, not detailed
Control group of deaf non-CI candidates drawn from separate hospital location (not matched for age: older)
Selection criteria
The children had been consecutively referred for a Nucleus multichannel cochlear

implant and seen at the Department of Otolaryngology-Head and Neck Surgery at the University of Iowa Hospitals and Clinics (Implant Candidates)

Dependent variables

Psychological instruments test battery; range of intelligence tests (detailed); parental questionnaires

Independent variables

Comparison between CI-candidates and non-CI candidate deaf children

Method

Single correlations using chi-square. Multi-variable regression analysis using ANCOVA

Results

Although the comparison group evidenced more externalizing and social problems than the implant group, the means of both groups fell well within the normal range. Similarly, although mothers of the implant group rated their child's home as characterized by more positive and supportive interactions than did mothers of the children in the comparison group, both group means were well within the average range. On measures of intelligence, the two groups also did not differ.

No statistically reliable differences between the group of implant candidates and the comparison group were identified on any of the eight MCPS scales. Moreover, the means of both the implant and BTNRH samples were well within normal range on all eight scales, with only three of the 16 means being greater than 0.5 standard deviations from the normative population means. Both group means on the Conformity scale, however, were approximately 0.7 standard deviations below the general population mean.

Home environment

Within this relatively restricted range, only one statistically significant group difference was found, with the implant group having a higher mean score on the affiliation scale than the BTNRH group ($p < 0.05$). This score indicated that the implant group mothers described their homes as being slightly more affiliative and emotionally warm than did the mothers of the comparison group.

Conclusions

Overall, the study indicated that children with hearing impairments and their families who were seeking cochlear implants are not significantly different from children with hearing impairments whose parents were not seeking a cochlear implant. The results provided no support for the notion that children with hearing impairments from families seeking a cochlear implant for their child evidence more behavioural deviance than children with hearing impairments whose parents have not sought an implant.

Observations

This is a relatively straightforward investigation, analysing the hypothesis that CI-candidate children are in some ways socio-psychologically dissimilar from those for whom no implant is being sought. A sample of children, consecutively referred for a cochlear implant at the University of Iowa Hospitals and Clinics, was contrasted on a number of standardized psychological measures with a cohort of children from Boys Town National Research Hospital, who had hearing impairments and whose families had not sought a cochlear implant. The authors report no such differences, using a battery of assessment tools standard in psychology to test the hypothesis. The sample concerns candidate clients of the Iowa Cochlear Implant Centre.

The authors comment that in many respects, the present findings argue for embracing a null hypothesis, an action that is not generally approved in contemporary science. However, support of the null hypothesis in this study seems appropriate and the findings, say the authors, strongly suggest that there is no support for those making assertions that denigrate the psychological status of families seeking cochlear implants for a child with profound deafness.

The report seems to be aimed mainly at dispelling claims from within the deaf community. See also Knutson, Boyd, Reid, Mayne and Fetrow (1997) for related observational work on early communication in a smaller subsample of cochlear implant candidate children.

Knutson JF, Boyd RC, Reid JB, Mayne T, Fetrow R (1997) Observational assessments of the interaction of implant recipients with family and peers: preliminary findings. Otolaryngology – Head and Neck Surgery 117(3/1): 196–207.

Population size
31 parents of cochlear implant candidates; in addition a control of 22 non-CI deaf, broadly matched
9 peer-group entry procedure; in addition, a control group of 9 non-CI, significantly older (mean 9.9)

Demographics
Parent interaction
Onset of deafness: congenital (84%)
Age: 2–12 years, mean 5.9 years
Peer-group entry procedure
Age: ≥6 years (mean 6.9 years)
CI use: 8–36 months (mean 17.8 months)

Selection criteria
The children had been consecutively referred for a Nucleus multichannel cochlear implant and seen at the Department of Otolaryngology–Head and Neck Surgery at the University of Iowa Hospitals and Clinics (Implant Candidates). Invited participation based on contact list

Dependent variables
Child–parent interaction
Interpersonal Process Code (IPC) locally developed for hearing populations
Peer-group entry
Likert-scaled categories on Peer Interaction Code (PIC) developed locally for the study

Independent variables
Child–parent interaction
CI candidacy
Peer-group entry task
CI/non-CI

Method
Specially developed coding schemes; for parent interaction videotaped activity normed against larger hearing population. In some instances, Pearson correlation coefficient, in some ANCOVA multiregression analysis
Inter-scorer reliability and agreement established for both experiments

Results
Child–parent interaction
'The only statistically reliable difference between the mothers of the two groups was with respect to the occurrence of positive social interaction, with the implant [candidacy] mothers showing an overall rate of 1.02 acts per minute and the [non-candidacy] mothers showing a rate of 0.48 acts per minute' (p.199).
 When compared to the normed hearing data: '... the mothers of the deaf children displayed a rate pf physical behavior that is more than twice that of the normative hearing group. The mothers of the deaf children displayed an overall rate of verbal behavior that is approximately 25% greater than the comparison group, and their social interactions were approximately twice that of the comparison group. [...] The children have a similar pattern with respect to overall physical behaviors' (p.200).
 In terms of quality of interaction: '... the deaf children tended to be more physically positive and the hearing children had more positive social interactions' (p.200).
Peer-group entry task
It is relevant to note that this task concerned entry into a pre-established play context of two hearing peers. The time frame actually being recorded and coded is ten minutes.

'Of the 18 children who participated in the peer-group entry task, only 12 actually entered within 10 minutes of being introduced to the peers' (p.205).

In terms of quality of entry: 'Eight children were classified as entering unsuccessfully and 10 were classified as entering successfully' (p.205).

For entry ratings ANCOVAS, successful entry was negatively correlated with cochlear implantation (p.205), but the authors suggest that the lower mean age of the cochlear-implanted group will largely explain that effect. The same goes for their findings that children without implants had interaction characterized as more friendly, accepting, cooperative and successful in entry than had those with implants (p.205).

Conclusions

Child–parent interaction

'One potentially important finding is the lack of systematic differences between hearing families with a deaf child who seek a cochlear implant and hearing families of a deaf child who choose not to seek an implant [and] suggest that those families seeking an implant are not distinguishable on objective indexes of psychological function or parenting' (p.201).

This finding replicates that by the same main author (Knutson, Boyd, Goldman and Sullivan 1997).

Peer-group entry task

'... the data suggest that the implant candidates and recipients are decidedly immature with respect to social interactions with hearing peers' (p.206).

But note that this concerns findings on hearing peers only.

'Clearly the data indicate that parents and educators cannot merely place profoundly deaf children with age-matched hearing peers and hope for successful social engagement' (p.206).

Observations

With this study, the authors are attempting to assess the value of an observational system of interactions between implant candidates and users with family and peers as a more independent vehicle of outcome reporting than parent questionnaires (p.197). The authors use specifically targeted assessment tools, one of which is a 'peer-entry task' in which the child is introduced into a prior established playgroup of peers, to measure the interaction that results and the time lapse until interaction and/or play occurs. The playgroup concerned two hearing peers. Successful peer-group entry is reportedly low for both candidates and non-candidates. However, it should be noted that the follow-up period was comparatively short, 8–36 months.

See also Knutson, Boyd, Goldman and Sullivan (1997) for related work on the psychological characteristics of cochlear implant candidates, on a larger sample.

Knutson JF, Wald RL, Ehlers SL, Tyler RS (2000) Psychological consequences of pediatric cochlear implant use. Annals of Otology, Rhinology and Laryngology 185: s109–s111.

Population 24
Demographics

Gender: boys (13), girls (11)

CI device: Nucleus

Age at CI: mean 5.6 years (range 2-13 years)

Placement: 'most' attended mainstream schools, usually with the aid of sign language interpreters (p.109)

Selection criteria

Drawn from ongoing study at University of Iowa

Dependent variables

Psychological measures, 36-month follow-up

Three tests of general intelligence:
- Hiskey-Nebraska Test of Learning Aptitude
- Leiter International Performance Scale
- Wechsler Intelligence Scale

Parent questionnaires
CBCL
Speech perception
MTS
WIPI
PB-K
Low-verbal monosyllabic and spondee ESP, four-choice vowel recognition measure

Independent variables

Psychological change following cochlear implantation

Method

Correlation co-efficient (not detailed)

Results

'The children were classified according to whether their WISC-III Verbal or Performance IQ scores evidenced a 0.5 SD or greater change across the follow-up period. The WISC-III population norms indicate an SD of 15 points; therefore children who gained at least eight IQ points were classified as "improved", and children who lost at least eight IQ points were classified as "deteriorated". Children for whom any change in IQ was less than eight points were classified as "unchanged". [...] 56% of the children evidenced a 0.5 SD or greater increase in Verbal IQ, and 46% evidenced a 0.5 SD or greater increase in Performance IQ. No children evidenced deterioration in IQ across the follow-up period' (p.110).

Conclusions

'... the results of this study are most usefully framed within the context of varying levels of adaptive functioning rather than in terms of pathology' (p.110).

'Maternal reports of externalising behavior [...] and total behavior problems were negatively correlated with a wide range of speech perception measures at 36 months' (pp.102–3).

'[Therefore] no evidence of negative psychological sequelae of cochlear implantation was found' (p.111).

Observations

The study is concerned with suggestions that cochlear implant use reduces the academic, social and emotional difficulties in deaf children, with counter-claims being raised from within the deaf community. Because of the paucity of evidence, the claims concern mostly conjecture (p.109). The authors hypothesize that audiological benefits could afford some psychological benefits to cochlear implant users. The study's objective is to:

'... assess the presence and direction of psychological changes after pediatric cochlear implantation and to determine the relationship between audiological benefit and psychological change.' (p.109).

The authors found no correlation between cochlear implantation and negative psychological sequelae. The study is a relatively straightforward one, mostly concerned to dispel conjecture arising from within quarters hostile to cochlear implantation.

Koch ME, Wyatt JR, Francis HW, Niparko JK (1997) A model of educational resource use by children with cochlear implants. Otolaryngology – Head and Neck Surgery 117(3/1): 174–179.

Population size

42

Demographics

No demographics detailed

Selection criteria
Enrolled in the Listening Center's Johns Hopkins programme of aural rehabilitation
Dependent variables
Cost
Independent variables
Placement
Method
ERM, which models placement and resource
Results
'The matrix illustrates that small increases in educational independence can result in significant annual savings in educational expenses' (p.176).
'Annual savings of $17,900 can be realized by moving a child from a full-time state school for the deaf to a self-contained class in a regular school, even allowing for $8,100 in annual assistive support' (p.176).
Conclusions
'Initial cost-benefit projections based on observed advancement toward educational independence indicate a favorable net present value of the implant (cost savings minus cost)' (p.178).
These cost-benefit projections will need to be supplemented with measures of the impact on quality of life and future educational and vocational options to determine the overall cost-effectiveness of cochlear implants in children.
Observations
This study concerns the modelling of the cost of educational resources required by cochlear-implanted children, measured on a scale ranging from 'educational dependence' to 'educational independence', where the latter equates with full mainstream education. The conclusion is that cochlear implants produce a net gain in educational resource savings. However, despite elaborate modelling of costs versus benefits, the assessment is based on gains in hearing being likely to result in a shift in placement (reduced expenditure of 'special' educational assistance, in this case support for audition) and the assumption that the desired outcomes of deaf education should be spoken language and access to 'normal' hearing provision.

The authors track 42 cochlear-implanted children (aged 4–11 years) receiving aural rehabilitation through the Listening Center at the Johns Hopkins Hospital through educational progress and changes in support. In line with the health outlook, educational placement is aligned along a continuum of 'independence' (the relative need for educational crutches) for successful participation in healthy, hearing, spoken language education.

They suggest that '... figures indicate that costs per student in residential settings are more than fivefold greater than those associated with educationally independent "mainstream" settings' (p.176). However, this may not reflect the different populations appropriately and indicate the difficulties of the economic model when it applies a medical model of care to education.

Lachs L, Pisoni DB, Kirk KI (2001) Use of audiovisual information in speech perception by prelingually deaf children with cochlear implants: a first report. Ear and Hearing 22(3): 236–251.

Population size
27
Demographics
Age: range 4.2–7.10 years
CI experience: 2 years
Age at onset: range 0–1.8 years

Age at CI: range 2.2–5.8 years (average 4.5 years)

PTA: 112 dB HL

Active electrodes: range 8–22

Educational programme: oral (12), total communication (15)

Selection criteria

CI experience 2 years. No further details given

Dependent variables

Common Phrase Test (CPT) under three presentation conditions: auditory (AU), visual alone (V) and audiovisual (AV)

LNT and MLNT and PB-K to assess open-set speech recognition performance

Independent variables

Speech reception test scores ('auditory measures')

Method

First report

Results

Children who were better at recognizing isolated spoken words through listening alone were also better at combining the complementary sensory information about speech articulation available under audiovisual stimulation. In addition, children who received more benefit from audiovisual presentation also produced more intelligible speech, suggesting a close link between speech perception and production, and a common underlying linguistic basis for audiovisual enhancement effects. Finally, an examination of the distribution of children enrolled in oral communication (OC) and total communication (TC) indicated that OC children tended to score higher on measures of audiovisual gain, spoken-word recognition and speech intelligibility.

The range of scores in all presentation conditions varied considerably. In the auditory-alone condition, scores varied from 0% to 90% correct. Similarly, in the visual-alone condition, scores ranged from 0% to 80%. Audiovisual scores varied across the entire possible range.

'Almost half of the children tested had higher visual-alone scores than auditory-alone scores. Thus, gains in the audiovisual condition might be better described as gains observed over visual-alone rather than auditory-alone performance' (p.242).

'For most children, audio-visual performance did not differ from the simple sum of performance in the audio-alone and visual-alone conditions. Thus, there does not appear to be a super-additive effect of audiovisual integration during the perception of highly familiar test sentences, such as those on the Common Phrases Test' (p.242).

'... average, naïve adult listeners could correctly identify 17.13% of the words produced by these children on the elicited sentence production task. The speech intelligibility scores ranged from 2% to 45%. Although this may seem like very poor performance, it is important to emphasize here that these judgments were made by naïve adult listeners. Trained clinicians, such as those who administered our auditory-alone tests, have much more experience with the speech of deaf children and have little difficulty understanding their responses' (p.243).

Conclusions

The relationships observed between auditory-alone speech perception, audiovisual benefit and speech intelligibility indicate that these abilities are not based on independent language skills, but instead reflect a common source of linguistic knowledge, used in both perception and production, that is based on the dynamic, articulatory motions of the vocal tract. The effects of communication mode demonstrate the important contribution of early sensory experience to perceptual development, specifically language acquisition and the use of phonological processing skills. Intervention and treatment programmes that aim to increase receptive and productive spoken-language skills, therefore, may wish to emphasize the inherent correlations that exist between auditory and visual sources of information in speech perception.

> 'Teaching hearing-impaired children about language in general does not appear to be sufficient for building the kinds of representations most advantageous for auditory speech perception. Rather, emphasis on the underlying linguistically relevant articulatory events that produce speech, by training orally and aurally, leads to improved ability in the perception and production of speech' (p.247).

Observations

The authors suggest that relatively little research has been focused on the nature of the audiovisual skills involved in speech perception and production outcomes. They speculate that skills here concern specific linguistic knowledge about the dynamic articulations of the vocal tract, underpinned by a combination of visual and motor elements in the development of speech production skills. Given the method followed (auditory-only and audiovisual test conditions), it is hardly surprising that oral communication children were observed to outperform total communication children. However, it does provide apparent support for the combination of audition and perception in the development of spoken language skills. The authors nevertheless note language delays in all cochlear-implanted children and severe language delays in some.

A finding pointing to visual acuity in two of the children is put down to 'inhibition', rather than possibly indicating a propensity for an additional language modality, when the authors note that:

> 'Interestingly, for two of the children, the visual-alone score was higher than the AV score, suggesting the possibility that for these children, additional auditory information may produce inhibition and reduce performance' (p.242).

A final note on spoken language delays:

> 'Although they are delayed in their auditory and spoken language development relative to their normal-hearing peers, many of these children appear to be making large gains in language development (Svirsky, Robbins, Kirk, Pisoni, & Miyamoto 2000). However, other children are not so fortunate and they seem to have much more difficulty making use of the degraded auditory information provided by their implant' (248).

Lea RA, Hailey DM (1995) The cochlear implant: a technology for the profoundly deaf. Medical Progress through Technology 21: 47–52.

Population size
Nil – data from published sources
Demographics
Current age: not reported
Age at onset: not reported
Age at CI: not reported
Duration of deafness: not reported
Life expectancy: 10-year lifespan used
Setting Australia
Method
Economic evaluation type: cost-utility analysis
Study perspective: payers
Comparator intervention: no intervention
Source of effectiveness data: assumed
Direct costs: selection costs, surgery/implantation, rehabilitation and maintenance costs
Indirect costs: none
Discount rate for costs and benefits: not indicated

Outcome measure: Quality of Well-Being scale (QWB)
Currency and price year: AUS$, price year unclear
Sensitivity analysis: not conducted

Results

The cost per QALY of PCI for children ranged from AUS$9,400 to $18,800 depending whether the utility gain assumed on the QWB was 0.15 or 0.075. For adults it ranged from AUS$15,067 to $30,135 per QALY.

Conclusions

'This preliminary assessment indicated that should cochlear implantation result in, say, a 10 percent increase in quality of life, the costs per QALY might be in the order of $14,000 for children and $22,000 for adults. Cost per QALY of these magnitudes have often been regarded as representing good to reasonable value for money' (p.50).

Observations

An early paper attempting to estimate the cost-utility of paediatric cochlear implantation in Australia. The study relies on a number of assumptions and it is not clear how they decide which levels of quality-of-life gain to use. The paper also makes a statement that education costs were excluded because they were believed to be common to both implanted children and children with hearing aids.

Lenarz T, Lesinski-Shiedat A, von der Haar-Heise S, Illg A, Bertram B, Battmer RD (1999) Cochlear implantation in children under the age of two: the MHH experience with the Clarion cochlear implant. Annals of Otology, Rhinology and Laryngology 108: 44–49.

Population size

9

Population comments

The study reports on 12 children, but post-implantation test results are only available for 9 children

Demographics

CI experience: range 3–24 months, mean 11 months
Age at CI: range 11–23 months, mean 18 months
Duration of deafness: range 0–12 months, mean 6 months
Aetiology: congenital (10), meningitis (2), infection (5), ototoxicity (1)
CI device: Clarion multichannel

Selection criteria

Children implanted at Hanover. Implanted under the age of 2 (*n* = 61), and using a Clarion device (*n* = 12). No deselections were made from that sample

Dependent variables

Test battery comparable with that used in Clarion trials in the US:
• speech perception
• closed-set: TAPS
• open-set: TAPS, GASP and Mr Potato Head

Independent variables

Preimplantation scores

Method

Pattern of scores over time of assessment. No statistical analysis attempted, perhaps due to the small sample and falling numbers over the time-frame, with nine at three months post implantation to just three at 18 months post implantation

Results

Results reveal a general improvement in auditory performance over time for all children. Closed-set scores exceeded chance at the six-month postoperative interval, with a steady improvement over time. Open-set scores also increased, but with a six-month delay; scores above chance were first observed at 12 months postoperatively. Smallest gains were on the (more difficult) GASP test (p.47).

Conclusions

Results support the concept that early implantation minimizes the effects of auditory deprivation on the development of the auditory system. Further follow-up is necessary, and results should be compared to those of populations implanted at an older age (p.48).

Observations

The results here are not controversial. The article focuses mostly on overall issues of implantation in very young (below age 2 years) deaf children, and also covers surgical issues, so that the outcome reporting is only part of the motivation behind the article. Because of both the short follow-up (18 months) and the small number of children included in the later assessments (three children at the 18-month postoperative test interval), these results are rightly considered to be tentative and inconclusive by the authors.

Lesinski A, Battmer RD, Bertram B, Lenarz T (1997) Appropriate age for cochlear implantation in children: experience since 1986 with 359 implanted children. In: Honjo I, Takahashi H (eds) Cochlear Implant and Related Sciences Update: Advances in Otorhinolaryngology 52: 214–217.

Population size

359

Demographics

None detailed

Selection criteria

Children implanted at the Medical School of Hanover

Dependent variables

Speech perception tests, not detailed

Independent variables

Prior performance

Comparison between two consecutively implanted cohort groupings (implanted 1986–1992, and 1993)

Age at implantation (below age 4 and over age 4)

Method

Group percentage score comparisons

Results

Children implanted under the age of 4 years developed a larger vocabulary than did those implanted over age 4 in both groups I and II; the same result is reported for 'two-word' and 'poly-word' sentences (p.215).

Conclusions

'The development of open-set understanding with a cochlear implant in children is dependent on the age at implantation as well as on the preoperative and postoperative rehabilitation program [...] This study demonstrates that an appropriate age for implantation is under 4 years of age' (p.216).

Observations

The specific purpose of this study was to correlate the postoperative performance over time with the age at implantation, in order to determine appropriate guidelines for age for implantation. There had been an earlier attempt at informing this problem in Hanover (see Meyer et al. 1995). This study intended to disaggregate the population into two cohorts, one cohort with children implanted on or before age 4, the other cohort with those implanted later.

However, there are problems in the methodology. The authors split the population not by age at implantation, but by date of implantation: 'group I' covers children implanted until 1992 (whatever their age), while 'group II' covers children implanted during 1993 (whatever their age). This disaggregation undermines the originally intended comparison; instead of controlling for age at implantation, the authors controlled for date of implantation. As a consequence, the results reported do not disaggregate within the two groups, those implanted before or after 4 years of age. Instead, the performance of an undisclosed number of children implanted under 4 years of age in group I is contrasted with the performance of a similarly undisclosed number of children also implanted before age 4 in group II.

Since there is no demographic description, either for characteristics of group I versus group II, or in terms of numbers of those implanted below aged 4 or above aged 4, the results produce mixed-variable figures which are difficult to interpret. The data reported seem to suggest that those implanted in 1993 outperformed those implanted before 1993 over a postimplantation period of two years on test measures which are not clearly identified.

Lesinski A, Hartrampf R, Dahm MC, Bertram B, Lenarz T (1995) Cochlear implantation in a population of multihandicapped children. Annals of Otology, Rhinology and Laryngology 104(166): s332–s334.

Population size
108

Population comments
A group of 108 candidates with multiple disabilities, from 569 candidates in total

Demographics
None detailed

Selection criteria
Account of the multi-handicapped referrals to the Hanover Medizinische Hochschule

Dependent variables
Not applicable

Independent variables
Not applicable

Method
Description

Observations
This is a completely descriptive article, focusing on implant candidacy of children with complex needs. In very general terms, the report outlines the extended assessment period accompanied by rehabilitation training prior to implantation, and in even more general terms it discusses the relative notion of 'success' in considering implanting deaf children who have additional disabilities.

Of the 108 children with complex needs referred to (19% of the total referrals), 28.7% had meningitis as their cause of deafness, versus 21.5% of the children without secondary handicaps (p.332).

The children were initially generally broken down into two categories of additional handicap: neuropsychiatric and medical disorders. In practical terms, however, it proved more useful to consider individuals' potential for deriving benefit from a cochlear implant and the medical possibility for one (p.332).

'One of the significant results of [an approach combining auditory training and ongoing psychological and neuropædiatric evaluations in the assessment period] was learning that children with problems additional to deafness appeared to have a bigger secondary handicap than was actually the case. That is, deafness was often the more significant factor in the multi-handicapped child, although at first, it seemed that the secondary handicap was worse' (p.332).

Because of the skills and focus of the combined rehabilitation during the assessment period, children who eventually did not receive an implant nevertheless often improved in audition and speech (p.333).

'We found [...] that deaf children demonstrated a pseudo-handicap if adequate opportunities were not provided for evaluation and preoperative training' (p.333).

'We have learned that an intense training and evaluation period offers different possibilities for both pre- and post-cochlear implant recipients, as well as for the specialists working with them' (p.333).

'... the multi-handicapped child will usually show different progress in auditory and speech skills' (p.334).

Lesinski A, von der Haar-Heise S, Battmer RD, Cords S, Goldring J, Lenarz T (2000) Performance of German-speaking children with the Clarion cochlear implant. In: Waltzman SB, Cohen NL (eds) Cochlear Implants. New York, USA: Thieme (art.11e), pp. 215–16.

Population size
70

Population comments
None

Demographics
Age at onset of deafness: prelingual
No further details provided

Selection criteria
Subsample from 168 implanted at Hanover since 1994. No sampling method detailed

Dependent variables
US Clarion test battery here focused on speech perception: TAPS and GASP closed- and open-set items. Single point-in-time assessment, 12 months postoperatively

Independent variables
Age at implantation

Method
Percentage reporting. Sample subdivided by age of implantation into three groups (1–4, 4–9 and 9–14 years at implantation)

Results
The speech development was faster in young children when implanted before age 4, based on group mean results. All three age groups tended to improve over time (p.215).

Conclusions
The expectation is that the children will continue to improve beyond the 12-month postoperative assessment (p.216).

Observations
This is a brief research summary and is therefore lacking in demographic detail. However, the testing and population are straightforward, and findings are in line with those reported elsewhere. There will be value in tracking the population over a longer period of time.

Lutman ME, Tait DM (1995) Early communicative behaviour in young children receiving cochlear implants: factor analysis of turn-taking and gaze orientation. Annals of Otology, Rhinology and Laryngology 104: 397–399.

Population size
47

Population comments
Declining at intervals of 3, 6 and 12 months to 32, 25 and 20

Demographics
Age at CI: not detailed
CI use: 12 months
Aetiology: not detailed
CI device: Nucleus multichannel, plus one Med-El single channel

Selection criteria
Age-matched, range 2–5 years
Selected from one implant programme (Nottingham)
One persistent non-user of CI excluded

Dependent variables
Measures of communicative behaviour, including:
- vocal auditory turn-taking
- gaze orientation

Independent variables
CI
Age

Method
Quantitative video analysis. Factor analysed using Blom method and repeated measures analysis; correlation with age

Results
Vocal auditory turn-taking and gaze orientation explained 72% of variance. No differences could be demonstrated between children with congenital and acquired deafness.

Conclusions
All children adopted primarily a vocal/auditory style, in vocal turn-taking in particular (consistently above 50%) after cochlear implantation. Looking behaviour is substantially unchanged by the provision of a cochlear implant, and may be innate (the tendency to look at the speaker increases only slightly over time).

Deviations from the expected pattern may indicate inappropriate processor adjustment, device malfunction or inadequate support.

Observations
The authors imply that turn-taking strategies are heavily dependent on auditory proficiency, although this is not necessarily the case. Presumably levels of residual hearing, hearing status of the parents and deaf or hearing environment are also clear factors. The study reports on an investigation into the nature of turn-taking among a group of very young (2–5 years) cochlear implant users in a hearing environment. Among the 20 children, 72% of variance in turn-taking measures was explained by vocal-auditory turn-taking and gaze orientation. The aim of the study was to assess the performance of a video-analysis assessment technique that concentrates on measures of turn-taking in pre-verbal cochlear-implanted children; the study builds on earlier work not entered into this review because it predates 1994.

Recordings in this technique consist of five minutes' conversational interaction with a known (hearing) adult. These recordings are transcribed by one of the authors following a written protocol. The recordings were repeated at three-month intervals.

The reported analysis concentrates predominantly on the 'pre-verbal' elements of turn-taking, considering visual strategies to be part of early spoken-language developments. A more general view of language development, including the role and potential of sign language in the language development patterns of deaf children, can usefully draw on the exclusively spoken language predictions reported here (e.g. Dauman et al. 1996; Preisler et al. 1997; McConkey Robbins et al. 1999).

McConkey Robbins AM, Bollard PM, Green J (1999) Language development in children implanted with the CLARION® cochlear implant. Annals of Otology, Rhinology and Laryngology 177: s113–s118.

Population size
    23
Demographics
    No description offered
    CI device: Clarion
    Age: average age at 6-month interval 46 months (p.116)
    Communication mode: limited number in the total communication group (p.116)
    Age at onset: prelingually deaf, almost all of them congenitally deaf (p.116)
Selection criteria
    No criteria detailed
Dependent variables
    Spoken language development:
    • Reynell Developmental Language Scales (RDLS)
Independent variables
    Communication mode: oral, total communication
    Preoperative RDLS scores
Method
    Score comparisons; repeated measures analysis of variance with test interval as the within-child variable and communication mode as the between-children variable
Results
    Results revealed a significant improvement in receptive ($p < 0.001$) and expressive ($p < 0.001$) spoken language over the test interval. Mean receptive age equivalent was 20 months preimplantation and 29 months at the time of testing. For receptive age equivalence the scores were 19 and 28 months respectively (p.115).
    No significant difference was observed for communication mode (p.115).
    Although not found to be statistically significant:

> 'For the 23 implanted children, the average rate of improvement for receptive language during this period was 140% (SD = 130). The average rate of improvement for expressive language was 139% (SD = 110). Thus, the average rate of language progress for the implanted children (i.e. 140%) was approximately 40% faster than expected for their normal-hearing peers of the same language age.' (p.116).

Conclusions
    'Significant increases in average age-equivalent scores in the first six months of Clarion use were measured in this group of 23 children. This finding is consistent with previous reports demonstrating that multichannel cochlear implants enhanced children's language development over time' (p.116).
    'Nonetheless, even though the children showed significant increases in their language scores after implantation, their absolute language levels were still substantially delayed compared to those of their peers with normal hearing of the same age – a finding also reported by others. The average age of these children at the six-month interval was 46 months. In contrast, the mean language ages of these children were 29 months and 28 months for receptive and expressive skills, respectively, at the six-month interval' (p.116).
    'The average learning rate of 140% in the implanted children indicates a faster rate of language learning than that seen in normal-hearing children of the same language age (but who would be of younger chronological age)' (p.116).
Observations
    The authors note that the spoken-language deficits of profoundly hearing-impaired

children typically become more pronounced as they grow older, falling further behind their hearing peers over time,

'presumably because the later-evolving linguistic skills require more complex syntactic forms, increased vocabulary, and more abstract concepts than early-emerging skills' (p.113).

The authors intend to measure the rate of spoken-language development in cochlear-implanted children, and they criticize spoken-language development tests standardized on hearing populations and providing age-equivalence scores because

'this type of analysis failed to provide comprehensive information on the change in language skills relative to the child's abilities prior to implantation' (p.113).

The authors propose a multisensory approach to measuring spoken language, including testing across modes, i.e. including signs, speech and audition, in their measure of language development (p.114).

'Thus, the most appropriate method to assess spoken-language skills in children who use total communication is with signs in addition to speech and audition, given that these communication modes reflect their exposure to language in everyday situations' (p.114).

This methodological assessment can be contrasted with those studies that compare oral and total communication children in auditory-only test conditions.

They propose to measure the rate of spoken-language growth over time (p.113), as is commonplace in paediatric cochlear implantation studies reported in this volume. For such studies, the authors note that it has been observed that cochlear-implanted children were observed to match the spoken-language development rates of hearing peers, being faster than those of non-implanted profoundly deaf peers (cf. Robbins et al. 1997; Miyamoto et al. 1997), although absolute language scores remained below those of hearing peers for all deaf children.

The study focuses on two issues, spoken-language changes that occur in children implanted with the Clarion device, and an examination of postoperative language changes as a function of preoperative communication mode (p.114). The examination of language subskills revealed development in some, but not development in all language subskills in the sample of cochlear-implanted children (pp.113–14).

Unfortunately the RDLS administration reported here concerns only six months' postoperative scores, leaving the children very little time to get used to the implant and benefit from the rehabilitation; the six-month score was compared to the preoperative score on the same test. In one analysis, the rate of improvement was expressed as the score difference divided by the test interval. A shortcoming of the study as reported here is that there is no demographic description of the population, nor are there any details on sampling criteria.

The authors, concluding that no statistically significant differences were found in results between oral and total communication children, note that:

'... users of total communication actually may be at a disadvantage for demonstrating language benefit from a cochlear implant, because manual forms of English do not contain the phonetic code of the language. [...] In addition, there may be deficiencies in the way a manual language is constructed and employed that hinder a total communication child from learning aspects of auditory-based English' (p.118).

Moreover, children with more limited auditory potential with hearing aids are typically placed in total communication programmes (p.118).

McConkey Robbins AM, Green J, Bollard P (2000) Language development in children following one year of Clarion implant use. Annals of Otology, Rhinology and Laryngology (Supplement) 185: s94–s95.

Population size

18

Demographics

Age at onset: prelingual

CI device: Clarion

Communication mode: interventions not controlled (p.94)

Age at CI: mean 3:3 years, range 2–5:5 years

Preoperative PTA: mean 111 dB HL, range 95–120 dB

Encoding strategy: CIS

Selection criteria

Two investigational centres, no sampling details given

Dependent variables

Preoperative RDLS scores

Independent variables

Language development:

- Reynell Developmental Language Scales (RDLS), administered in child's preferred communication mode at 6-month (McConkey Robbins et al. 1999) and 12-month interval

Method

Absolute age-equivalent score comparison, and rate of development (scores divided by test intervals)

Results

A significant improvement in receptive and expressive language development at all intervals ($p < 0.04$ between 6 and 12 months). The average growth rate of receptive spoken language during the entire 12-month period was well above that of hearing peers (138%), but was faster over the first six months (138%) than over the second six months (110%). Expressive spoken-language growth rates (98% over the 12-month period) were roughly equivalent to those of hearing peers, slowing down from 140% at six months postoperative interval to 51% at 12 months.

Conclusions

'The rate of language learning was more accelerated during the first six months than during the second six months of implant use, especially for expressive language skills' (p.95).

Developmental psychologists' notion of 'equilibration' periods of accelerated growth typically being followed by less growth, may help to explain the levelling-off effect in spoken language learning (p.95).

'Even with the marked improvements observed in the language skills of the children in this study, the language levels of the implanted children remain delayed compared with those of their peers with normal hearing of the same chronological age...' (p.95).

Observations

Replicates and builds on results reported in McConkey Robbins et al. 1999. Spoken-language development rates reported for the second six-month postoperative interval represent a clear drop relative to those reported for the first six months postoperative scores. On expressive language especially, the accelerated improvement rate drops sharply, from 140% to 51%: from a faster rate to a rate roughly half that of hearing peers (p.94).

As in the earlier study, the report suffers from a lack of demographic and sampling criteria descriptions.

McConkey Robbins AM, Kirk KI, Osberger MJ et al. (1995) Speech intelligibility of implanted children. In: Clark and Cowan (eds) International Cochlear Implant, Speech and Hearing Symposium, pp. 399–401.

Population size

61

Population comments

Comparison groups of HA users: 'Gold' (n = 14) 90-100 dB HL, 'silver' (n = 8) 101-110 dB HL, 'bronze' (n = 28) > 110 dB HL

16 of the bronze HA users were subsequently implanted

Demographics

Age at onset: prelingual, < 3 years, mean 0.6 months

CI device: Nucleus multichannel

Age at CI: average. 5.4 years

Communication mode: oral, total communication, 'about half' (p.400)

Selection criteria

None detailed

Dependent variables

Speech intelligibility measure up to 3.5 years postoperatively

Monsen sentence test: 10 sentences repeated after an examiner's spoken model

Children under 6 used picture-prompted list from BIT (Beginner's Intelligibility Test)

Scored by experienced listeners

Independent variables

CI, non-CI

Method

Correlation co-efficients

Results

'There was a gradual improvement over time in speech intelligibility for the CI children. After only 6 months to 1 year of experience with their device, the intelligibility of the CI children was significantly better than in the pre-CI condition (p = 0.001). Intelligibility scores of each successive interval were also significantly greater than those of the preceding interval (p < 0.02). The scores of the CI children after 1.5 to 2.0 years remain lower than those of the silver HA group. After that time, however, the CI children surpass the silver HA group. [...] After 3.5 or more years of CI use, the speech of the CI children was about 40% intelligible, compared to 72% intelligible for the gold HA group' (p.400).

Error bars indicate wide individual distribution among the cochlear-implanted children, with some approaching the scores of gold users, and some therefore scoring significantly below the average scores reported (p.400).

Conclusions

'... gold HA children are not candidates for a CI at the present time' (p.400).

'... these data also indicate that on average, more than two years of device experience is needed before the advantage of the CI, relative to silver HA benefit, will be observed in pediatric children' (p.400).

Observations

This study compares the development of speech intelligibility in 61 cochlear-implanted children to those of much smaller groups of hearing aid users. The hearing aid users were only tested at one single point in time, while the same cochlear-implanted child could contribute two scores to one postoperative interval, since 'following the pre-CI interval, data from pairs of consecutive intervals were combined' (p.400).

Results indicate improvements over time, eventually overtaking 'silver' hearing aid users, but remember that the scores of the hearing aid users were taken at a single point in time, therefore the results disregard improvements over time for hearing aid users.

Cochlear-implanted children never matched the outcomes of gold users who were recorded at a single point in time.

The study suffers a lack of demographic and sampling criteria description, making comparative interpretation difficult, while the results are further weakened by the methodological step of combining interval periods. The results mainly argue for measuring over-time improvements for all comparison groups as well as cochlear-implanted children in investigations of meaningful over-time benefits of cochlear implant use.

McConkey Robbins AM, Osberger MJ, Miyamoto RT, Kessler KS (1995) Language development in young children with cochlear implants. Advances in Oto-Rhino-Laryngology 50: 160–166.

Population size
15

Demographics
Age at onset: prelingual (mean 0.9 years)
CI device: Nucleus multichannel
Age at CI: mean 5.6 years
Age at testing: mean 6.1 at 6-month and 6.8 at the 15-month postoperative interval
(these figures reflect different populations being tested at different intervals)

Selection criteria
Not detailed

Dependent variables
Language development:
• RDLS (Reynell Developmental Language Scale)

Independent variables
Age at implantation
Prior achievement

Method
The effect of maturation alone was statistically controlled using a predictive measure of normal language development (p.162). Scores reported are group-mean plotted scores

Results
Receptive language skills improved with cochlear implant use over the 15-month test period to a greater extent than would be predicted through maturation alone; for expressive skills, there is an eight-month difference between the scores at the 15-month post-implant interval (p.163).

Conclusions
The use of a cochlear implant promoted both receptive and expressive language development to a greater extent than would be predicted through maturation alone, while the longer the children used their implants, the greater the difference between the observed and the predicted scores (p.165).

Observations
The authors note that language development data (on communication abilities) may be used as part of selection criteria, and then serve as a baseline assessment in measuring postimplantation progress; this is one of the most common reasons for the bulk of research conducted on cochlear implantation outcomes. The authors note that, in their research laboratory, the formal RDLS test results reported in this study are only one element in a wider battery of assessment tools which also includes informal measures. This is a small-scale study, and an early one in our dataset. There is some under-description, in particular with regard to demographic detail, where only group means are reported. Reporting should, ideally, include range, especially where children and language are concerned The time-frame of 15 months is short, which in particular affects the

comment that no plateauing effect was noticeable, followed by a prediction of continued improvement. Other reports have suggested plateau effects anywhere up to four to five years post implantation.

McConkey Robbins AM, Svirsky M, Kirk KI (1997) Children with implants can speak, but can they communicate? Otolaryngology – Head and Neck Surgery 117(3): 155–160.

Population size
23
Population comments
Control of 89 deaf non-CI
Demographics
HAs
Age: range 16–95 months
HA: hearing aid or tactile aid
CI suitability: all were potential candidates
Age at onset: early; congenital (62), 0–2.11 years (27)
Communication programme: total communication (61%), oral (39%)
CIs
Age at onset: congenital (11), < 3 years (12), average 10 months,
Age at CI: average 4.11 years
Communication programme: total communication (14 = 60%), oral (9 = 39%)
CI device: Nucleus
Encoding strategy: FOF1F2 (5), MPEAK (11), SPEAK (7)
Well-matched for age at onset across CI/HA and total communication/oral
Selection criteria
No details provided on sampling or selection criteria
Dependent variables
Reynell Developmental Language Scales (Revised) test scores for English language ability
For CI, at pre-implant, and at 6 and 12 months post-CI
Independent variables
Communication programme: total communication, oral
Method
2-way repeated measures analysis of variance
Results
'Twelve months after implantation, the [CI] children demonstrated gains in receptive and expressive language skills that exceeded by seven months the predictions made on the basis of maturation alone. Moreover, the average language development rate of the children with implants in the first year of device use was equivalent to that of children with normal hearing. These effects were observed for children with implants using both the oral and total-communication methods' (p.155).

This pattern was statistically significant for both receptive and expressive language skills (based on Reynell test scores only).
Conclusions
Results suggest 'that the cochlear implant promoted both receptive and expressive language development to a greater extent than would be predicted by maturation alone. In addition, the findings show that the longer the children used the implants, the greater the difference between the observed and predicted scores' (p.159).
Observations
This research reports on a single language development measure (Reynell Language Development Scales) in a group of cochlear-implanted children aged between 1 and 7 years. Although the title suggests that the report will contrast the ability for speech production with the ability to communicate, the results are based on the results of one test in a clinical

one-to-one controlled test administration design (the Reynell test), and thus does not allow a comparison between speech skill and functional communication ability.

The children without implants provided cross-sectional language data used to estimate the amount of language gains expected on the basis of maturation, suggesting that deaf children are predicted to make half or less of the language gains of their hearing peers. These predicted scores were then compared with actual scores achieved by the children with implants six and 12 months after implantation.

The authors do not comment on the fact that, according to their own findings, the increased gains from cochlear implantation are modest when compared to the normal development scores of the normed population of 1319 hearing children (see, for example, Figures 3 and 4 on pp. 157-8). Although the rate of increase might be similar to that of hearing children, there continues to be a significant delay, making the cochlear-implanted children more like 'slightly less deaf' children, e.g. perhaps like severely deaf children. Given that spoken language ability is targeted, a clear comparison between these data (hearing children and cochlear-implanted children scores) would have offered a useful measure of communicative functioning.

The scores reflect 6- and 12-month postoperative data only, rather than a longitudinal assessment.

The authors consider that the similar progress made by oral and total communication cochlear-implanted children might be explained by

'the possibility [...] that the cochlear implant has a global, multisensory effect on language learning. This would be consistent with the recent findings of Quittner et al. (1994), who reported increases in selective visual attention in children after cochlear implantation, and with anecdotal reports by parents and children...' (p.159).

McDonald Connor C, Hieber S, Arts HA, Zwolan TA (2000) Speech, vocabulary, and the education of children using cochlear implants: oral or total communication? Journal of Speech, Language, and Hearing Research 43(5): 1185–1204.

Population size
147

Population comments
In two groups: total communication (66), oral (81)

Demographics
Age: range 2–10 years
Age at onset: before age 2.5 years
CI: Nucleus 22 (MPEAK or SPEAK encoding strategies) or newer (including Clarion, Med-El Combi 40+, Nucleus 24M)
Postoperative speech detection thresholds: range 15-30 dB HL (stable over time)
CI experience: range 6 months–10 years
Educational placement: oral (81), total communication (66)

Selection criteria
CIs implanted at the University of Michigan Medical Center (UMMC)
Prelingually deaf (before age 2.5 years); between ages 2 and 10 years when receiving CI; demonstrating normal nonverbal cognitive abilities (as assessed by resident clinical psychologist)
Children who changed programme postoperatively during the first three years of CI were excluded from the study

Dependent variables
Yearly interval test battery:
* consonant production accuracy (Arizona Articulation Proficiency Scale: Revised)
* receptive spoken vocabulary (Peabody Picture Vocabulary Test-R/III)

- expressive and productive vocabulary (spoken and signed) (Picture Vocabulary subtest of Woodcock Johnson Test of Cognitive Ability)

Independent variables

Prior achievement (over time). Range of factors including:

- age at CI
- preoperative speech detection thresholds
- type of CI
- full or partial electrode array

Method

Two-level hierarchical linear modelling to analyse performance increases against chronological age for each of the outcome variables. However, interpretation of results beyond six years postimplantation must be considered tenuous because these intervals include a smaller set of children

Results

The authors report over-time improvement of consonant-production accuracy and expressive and receptive vocabulary, regardless of oral or total communication programme. Furthermore, there appeared to be a complex relationship among children's performance with the cochlear implant, age at implantation and communication/teaching strategy employed by the school. Controlling for all variables and across the entire population, children in oral programmes demonstrated an on average superior consonant-production accuracy, with significantly greater improvements over time ($p < 0.001$). However, there was no such programme-related difference for children implanted before age 5.

There were no total communication/oral programme differences in vocabulary development. However, total communication cochlear-implanted children achieved significantly higher receptive vocabulary scores if implanted before age 5.

Implantation during preschool resulted in higher gains relative to implantation during primary.

'Overall, the younger children were when they received their implants, the greater their consonant-production accuracy was over time' (p.1199).

The same comment is repeated for vocabulary development (p.1200). The total communication group demonstrated superior scores and rates of growth on the expressive vocabulary measure (spoken and/or signed) when compared to the oral communication group if they received their implants during their preschool or early elementary school years. There was no significant difference if the children received their implants during middle elementary school. Regardless of whether children were in the oral communication or total communication group, children who received their implants during preschool demonstrated stronger performance, on average, on all measures over time than children who received their implants during their elementary school years.

'Receptive vocabulary development rate of growth was less than the growth rate of the test standardisation sample (PPVT-III) of children with normal hearing, and the gap in expected scores increased over time' (p.1200).

Although expressive vocabulary growth rates approached those of the test standardization sample, this result is confounded by the fact that children were permitted to respond to the test in sign language, while (in the oral group) the examiner might not have understood (or heard correctly) the responses given – a reference to persisting speech skills problems (p.1200).

Conclusions

'Although vocabulary and oral language skills have been positively associated with reading and academic skills for children with normal hearing [...], this association has not been studied adequately for children with cochlear implants. Thus, it is the authors' opinion that it is inadvisable to make recommendations regarding academic placement based on the results of this study or solely upon whether the school program uses an oral or a total communication teaching approach' (p.1201).

'Age at implant consistently affected all of the outcomes measures. [...] Children with incomplete active electrode arrays and/or higher preoperative aided SDT achieved significantly lower speech scores than children with complete arrays and lower preoperative SDT' (p.1201).

'Children who used newer technology [...] achieved higher [consonant-production accuracy and expressive vocabulary] scores, on average, than children using the Nucleus 22' (p.1201).

One explanation for this is that children with newer technology were also more recent candidates, and likely to have been implanted at a younger age. But, 'The results of this study indicate that children in both [oral] and total communication educational programs benefit from using cochlear implants in terms of consonant-production accuracy, receptive spoken vocabulary, and expressive spoken and/or signed vocabulary. However, a number of important factors systematically affect performance, including preoperative aided SDT levels, the potential for and achievement of a complete active internal electrode array, device type, and age at implant' (p.1202).

Observations

The study examined the relationship between teaching method, oral or total communication, used at children's schools and children's consonant-production accuracy and vocabulary development over time. This study is significant in both the sample size (147 children), the range of tests included (especially in the light of the relatively narrow range of independent variables targeted), and its very detailed and clearly recorded programme of statistical analysis. Levels of significance in correlations are not reported here because they concerned ranges across different types of statistical comparison. The research concerned the relationship between teaching programme (oral or total communication) and the cochlear-implanted children's consonant-production accuracy and vocabulary development over time. The range of dependent measures is small, and focuses on spoken language outcomes. The study uses hierarchical linear modelling, controlling for each of the independent variables in turn.

One other noteworthy characteristic concerns the sample population, ranging in age between 2 and 10 years. It is a relatively wide range, including early preschool right through to the end of elementary school, although this allows for the very useful disaggregation between preschool and elementary school cohorts; indeed, the research very usefully reports on the children disaggregated into preschool, early elementary and middle elementary groups. In terms of the outcomes reported, although there was variation in the statistical significance of the correlations observed, the tendencies reported cut across this disaggregation.

Overall, the authors found little support for 'over-and-above' benefits of either oral or total communication programmes, but in contrast to some articles included in this review the authors claim some distinctive advantages of total communication over oral education. The introduction, incidentally, provides a useful summary of the literature concerning such programme-based differences (p.1186).

The authors attempt to explain the total communication results by way of the following assessments:

'The benefits of early language exposure are well documented for children with normal hearing (Locke 1993) and for children with hearing loss (Meyberry 1993). If the benefit of early language stimulation is amodal, sign language input may provide early language stimulation when spoken language is inaccessible because of deafness (see also Petitto and Marentette 1991). Thus, the apparent advantage of total communication programs for children who receive their implants before the age of 5 may have less to do with the program type and more to do with early language stimulation' (pp.1201–2).

'Very few (n = 3) of the participants attended programs that could be described as bilingual-bicultural, and only one attended a residential school for one year.

Thus, our investigation does not assess children's implant performance with regard to these programs' (p.1202).

'The findings also point to the complexity of studying children with cochlear implants and the dangers of making simple dichotomous comparisons without adequately considering the multifaceted variables, both known and unknown, that can affect children's long-term outcomes' (p.1202).

These statements demonstrate the need to discriminate between various research reports in assessments with respect to their relative methodological worth, their internal validity, as well as in direct comparisons of outcomes reported.

Meyer TA, Svirsky MA, Kirk KI, Miyamoto RT (1998) Improvements in speech perception by children with profound prelingual hearing loss: effects of device, communication mode, and chronological age. Journal of Speech, Language, and Hearing Research. 41(4): 846–858.

Population size
74

Population comments
Control groups n = 58 of HA (34) and HA+ (24), broadly matched for characteristics

Demographics
Onset of deafness: range 0–3.0 years
CI fitting: range 1.6–5.7 years
Aetiology: unknown (61%), meningitis (32%), other (7%)
CI device: Nucleus 22, SPEAK, MPEAK
No socio-economic details included (helpful especially with communication mode)
Demographics are detailed in a breakdown for communication mode, so are only summarized here
NB: since 13 of the HA group were subsequently implanted (and included in the CI group) the two participant groups are not mutually exclusive. Because of significant population migration over time, and significant loss of numbers as an effect of time, there are issues in reading effects longitudinally

Selection criteria
Not detailed

Dependent variables
Minimal pairs test
Common Phrases Test
Tested preoperatively and at (varying) six-month or one-year intervals up to 8.5 years post implantation

Independent variables
HA and HA+ scores over time as regression line

Method
HA data analysed using linear regression analysis of speech perception scores as a function of age at testing

Results
Across all groups, oral communication mode outperformed total communication mode, but 'one would have to be careful not to generalise the result to infer that a particular mode of communication is superior to another' (p.856). As Powers et al. (1998) concluded, the measures hide a number of underlying variables not measured here; so results for communication mode will not be summarised here. [See Observations]
'mean performance on the Common Phrases Test improved with increasing implant use under all three presentation modalities [A, V, AV]' (p.853).

In the auditory-only condition
Oral communication
'... scores for the children using cochlear implants remained approximately 20% less than the predicted scores for the children in the HA90–100 group' (p.854).
Total communication
'... they approached the average score for the HA90–100 group (35%) by approximately four years of implant use' (p.855).
Results that concern the auditory-visual condition testing
Oral communication
'... by five years postimplant, the mean score for the children using cochlear implants was approximately 90% and essentially equivalent to the predicted score for the HA90–100 group' (p.855).
Total communication
'... they reached the levels of the HA90–100 group by approximately four years of implant use' (p.855).

In general, speech perception scores for the children using implants were higher than those predicted for a group of children with 101–110 dB HL of hearing loss using hearing aids, and they approached the scores predicted for a group of children with 90–100 dB HL of hearing loss using hearing aids.

Conclusions

'... it is apparent from the present study that children with prelingual profound hearing loss obtain higher speech perception scores with a cochlear implant than they do with a hearing aid if the amount of residual hearing is 101–110 dB HL. Thus, in terms of improvements in overall communication skills, our data suggest that children with profound hearing loss with enough residual hearing to be classified in the HA101–110 group would benefit more from a cochlear implant than a conventional hearing aid, and at least some of the children with 90–100 DB HL of hearing loss might benefit more from a cochlear implant than from a hearing aid' (p.857).

Observations

This study is one of a kind in measuring speech-perception outcomes exclusively in a comparison between groups using different types of aid to hearing. The study expands on an earlier study by Miyamoto et al (1994), who compared the speech perception skills of two groups of children with profound prelingual hearing loss. The implanted group was tested longitudinally. The group using conventional hearing aids was, however, tested at a single point in time. In the present study, speech perception scores were examined over time for both groups of children as a function of communication mode. So in this case the comparison is once more between cochlear implant users and hearing aid users, the latter disaggregated further into one group with profound (101–110 dB HL) and one group with less profound (90–100 dB HL) hearing loss. It should be noted that the latter hearing-aided group was only measured at one single point in time, not at intervals over time as was the case with the cochlear implant users, who were regularly assessed for a period of up to 8.5 years.

This study is notable for its transparent and detailed reporting and straightforward analysis. The article includes a clear introduction which provides an account of change over time in the kind of comparative testing done in published work up to 1998:
• first of CI users at points over time
• then CI users over time compared with non-CI at a single point in time
• then CI users over time compared with non-CI over time
• now CI users over time compared with 'Equivalent hearing loss' HA+ users over time.

This assessment of developments in the research on paediatric cochlear implantation outcomes can be contrasted usefully with descriptions in Blamey et al. (2001) and McDonald et al. (2000). The reported findings seem again to align with those more recently in Blamey et al. (2001), and those earlier in Geers and Brenner (1994), that cochlear implant users end up scoring on a par with HA+ (90–100 dB HL) after about five years post implantation on both speech-perception and production measures. The authors show a more detailed awareness of issues surrounding communication mode and placement than is characteristic of the research reported generally, for example in their comment that:

> 'In particular, it is possible that at least part of the differences in speech perception scores for children in oral versus total communication programs was related to factors we did not control such as socio-economic status and cognitive skills. At least for the children who use hearing aids, it is likely that the amount of residual hearing a child has plays a role in selecting the type of educational setting for that child. [...] Speech perception is usually tested under the auditory-only mode; thus, the children who are educated in oral programs may have a performance advantage on these tests compared to children who are educated in total communication programs' (p.586).

See Hodges et al. (1999) for a particular example of highlighting such advantages through research design.

Meyer V, Hertram B, Lenarz T (1995) Performance comparisons in congenitally deaf children with different ages of implantation. Advances in Oto-Rhino-Laryngology 50: 129–133.

Population size
71
Demographics
Age at onset: congenital (*n* = 71), ≤ 2 years (*n* = 45), >2 years (*n* = 22)
Age at implantation: 2–3 years (*n* = 20), 4–6 years (*n* = 30), 7–13 years (*n* = 21)
For the congenital group:
Experience of deafness: 2–3 years (*n* = 20), 4–6 years (*n* = 30), 7–13 years (*n* = 21)
CI use: detailed as a function of the experience of deafness above with range, mean and SD
Selection criteria
Not detailed
Dependent variables
Hanover Hearing Test, including speech perception and speech production subtests
Independent variables
Age at implantation
Age at onset (congenital or otherwise)
Method
Group mean percentage reporting
Results
Youngest children reach the best scores on the closed-set monosyllable word subtest; no differences are observed for the two-syllable closed-set word subtest (p.131). On the open-set results, it is reported that the young children perform as well as the older ones (p.132).
Conclusions
In all three subtests younger-implanted congenitally deaf children reach 'nearly the same or better' (p.133) scores on average as older-implanted congenitally deaf children.

> 'Now we think that it is allowed to conclude that young deaf born children should be operated on as soon as possible if we can exclude usable hearing rests [sic]' (p.133).

Observations
Excluding the tables, this is a two-and-a-half page report on the application of the Hearing Test (HHT) to investigate the effect of age at implantation, with the conclusion that implantation should be 'as early as possible' (p.133). As with a later attempt at drawing the same conclusion (Lesinski et al. 1997), this study is characterized by a

consideration of the over-time performance of a large group on just a handful of test elements representing one outcome measure alone: speech perception. In this case, discussion is limited to one- and two-syllable closed-set word recognition and one open-set word test, as a single point-in-time measure in which the narrow differences in score distribution, especially when reporting is being limited to group-mean percentage scores, provide very little scope for serious interpretation.

A number of weaknesses characterize the study. First, there is a lack of demographic reporting and sampling detail, which hampers the generalizability of the modest outcomes. Additionally, there is no attempt at statistical modelling of results; instead, there is an interpretation of results which seems particular rather than general. For example, while as suggested all score differences are modest, and furthermore show no consistency between subtests, in two of the three subtest results the younger-implanted children are actually outperformed by the two other older-implanted age groups, while the conclusion suggests implantation at as early an age as possible. It is not only that this conclusion seems predetermined in the light of the results; it is entirely likely that the outcome distributions are themselves an artefact of the random disaggregation of the population into age at implantation cohorts. Equally, the findings may or may not be statistically significant; or even if they were there is no argument presented here that any hypothetical correlation would be accounted for by age at implantation as opposed to a multitude of other factors not measured here. In addition, even apart from the above objections, there is no over-time measure being reported, so that outcome distributions do not present us with a consistent – and therefore reliable – trend in language development. The authors have also not attempted to control for the effect of maturation alone, assuming instead that outcome scores are attributable to the implant.

Finally, we draw attention to the inclusion of 67 deafened children in the initial description who are left out altogether in both the analysis and the focus of the article. Hence we have included only the 71 congenital children in our review, whereas the introduction to the article might lead one to assume that a total of 138 children were included in the study reported.

Miyamoto RT, Kirk KI, Svirsky MA, Sehgal ST (1999) Communication skills in pediatric cochlear implant recipients. Acta Oto-Laryngologica 119(2): 219–224.

Population size
33

Population comments
3 groupings: age at CI < 3 years (n = 14), between 3 and 3.11 years (n = 11) and between 4 and 5 years (n = 8)

Demographics
Age at onset: mean range across groups 0.2–0.7 years
CI use: mean range 0.0–2.3 years
Age at testing: mean range 4.5–4.7 years
PTA: mean range 109–115 dB
No other demographics detailed

Selection criteria
Implanted at Indiana University. Implantation prior to age 6, age between 4 and 5 years, and use of either SPEAK or CIS processing strategies. No individual deselections detailed

Dependent variables
Speech perception tasks:
• GAEL-P
• Mr Potato Head Task (assembling body parts)
• speech intelligibility task
• local procedure: being asked to repeat 10 simple sentences

Language tasks:
  • PPVT
  • Reynell Developmental Language Scales

Independent variables

  Age at CI
  Placement (oral versus total communication)

Method

  Correlation coefficients between task results and independent variables (F-statistic)

Results

Speech perception

  Age at CI (p = 0.001) and communication mode (p = 0.002) both significantly influenced GAEL-P closed-set word identification. The Mr Potato Head task confirmed these results (p = 0.004 and p = 0.008) for both age at CI and communication mode (p.221).

Speech intelligibility

  Only main effect of communication mode was significant (p = 0.02). Scores ranged from 20% mean for oral children to 4.2% among total communication children.

Language measures

  Results on PPVT task produced no significant main results. Overall, all three groups showed delayed receptive vocabulary, performing at a level roughly half their chronological age (scores ranging from 0.45 to 0.7, where 1 is chronological age). In the Reynell test results there was a significant effect of communication mode (p = 0.05) in favour of oral communication (p.222).

Conclusions

  '... both age at implantation and communication mode have significant effects on the development of a number of communication skills in profoundly deaf children. [Children] implanted prior to the age of 3 years had higher spoken word recognition and speech intelligibility than children who were implanted after that time' (p.223).

Observations

  This study is a useful assessment and addition to other studies reported here, in particular for its narrow range of age (all children were 4 years old at the time of testing) and its narrow range of age at onset (between 2 and 7 months). In these characteristics the study reports spoken language development outcomes in a very clearly defined group of cochlear-implanted children. However, a number of observations are appropriate.

  The researchers regard the 'Mr Potato Head' task as an open-set speech perception task. However, given the clear boundaries on both topic (assembling limbs, etc., on to a toy) and the context of a fixed number of elements that are visually available, the task is perhaps more appropriately considered a closed-set speech perception task. Incidentally, Dawson et al. (1998) criticized the task for demonstrating clear ceiling effects for children age 3–4 (as opposed to 2-year-olds).

  The outcomes are affected by the artificial disaggregation of the children according to age at cochlear implantation. Not only does the number across the three sample groups drop from 14 (42% of total) to eight (24%), there has been no attempt to correct for subsample size variation. The children in the most recent cochlear implant group (4–5 years) have had only one test administered, while the groups with longer experience will have had more experience of test conditions repeated at six-month intervals. Moreover, children implanted most recently will have had very much less time to derive benefits from their cochlear implant. To summarize, given the current age range of the group (4–5 years), the relatively modest size of the (sub)samples and the modest average experience of cochlear implants across the children, the results reported can only be tentative and not as general as implied in the conclusion.

Miyamoto RT, Kirk KI, Todd MA, Robbins AM, Osberger M (1995) Speech perception skills of children with multichannel cochlear implants or hearing aids. Annals of Otology, Rhinology and Laryngology 104: 334–337.

Population size
24
Population comments
Comparison groups of HA children: 'gold' users (n = 16), and 'silver' users (n = 14)
Demographics
Demographics listed per group (p.334). For CI children:
• PTA: mean > 110 dB HL
• Age: mean 5.7 years, SD = 1.6
• Age at onset: mean 0.9 years, SD = 0.9
• Age at CI: mean 5.7 years, SD = 1.5
• CI use: mean 0.3 years, SD = 0.3
• CI device: Nucleus multichannel
Selection criteria
Not specified
Dependent variables
Speech perception in six-month intervals up to five years: MTS, in auditory only and auditory + visual test administrations
Independent variables
CI, non-CI comparison
Over-time improvements in two combined intervals
Method
No statistical analyses
Results
At the early interval, test-scores of the cochlear-implanted children on closed-set tasks were roughly equal to those of the 'silver' hearing aid users, while the 'gold' users scored higher. The cochlear-implanted children's speech perception improved substantially by 2.5 years average implant experience, while at the late interval the cochlear implant and 'gold' users' performance was significantly better than that of the 'silver' hearing aid users on all three measures. The 'gold' hearing aid users remained superior to the cochlear-implanted group on the consonant and word-recognition tasks (p.336).

On the open-set task, both 'gold' hearing aid and cochlear implant child groups outperformed the 'silver' hearing aid group over time. Although the 'gold' users performed significantly better than the cochlear implant users at the late interval, in auditory-plus-visual modality the performance became similar (p.336).
Conclusions
'... after an average of 2.5 years of CI use, the speech perception skills of the CI children have surpassed those of the silver HA group (about 15% to 30% better), and are similar to those of the gold HA group on selected measures (i.e. closed-set vowel recognition and open-set phrase recognition in the auditory-plus-visual modality)' (p.336).
Observations
The study resembles those of McConkey Robbins et al. (1999, 2000), but reporting on a wider period of data, however, some of the children entered the study after implantation. The authors set up comparison groups of hearing aid users on the basis of unaided threshold measures; the study continues earlier research comparing cochlear-implanted children with hearing aid 'gold' users, reported in Miyamoto et al. 1994, in which the hearing aid users were tested at one single point in time relative to the over-time measures of the cochlear-implanted group (p.334), a characteristic also noted for the earlier McConkey Robbins studies.

As with the McConkey Robbins studies, some children entered the study after they had received an implant, so for those children no preimplantation data were available, while some were available only for yearly (rather than six-monthly) test intervals. Consequently, the available pre-implant data were combined with the six-month postoperative interval data in the construction of a 'baseline' dataset. The authors suggest that this should not artificially inflate the average performance at the early interval because typical improvement kicks in 12 months postoperatively (p.335). It should be noted that earlier large gains have been reported, for example in a McConkey Robbins study, where a drop in performance between six-month and 12-months was noted (McConkey Robbins et al. 2000). Similar confusion reigns over the hearing aid groups, some of whom were tested more than once, some of whom were tested only once (p.335).

The 'late' interval contained data from the cochlear-implanted children's most recent evaluation, ranging from 1 to 5 years (p.335), which, given the available evidence of improvements over time, represents a limited measure of outcome.

The results demonstrate that cochlear-implanted children outperform 'silver' hearing aid users and approach the performance of 'gold' hearing aid users over time (average 2.5 years). But given the method of combining test intervals and mixing available over-time data with single point-in-time data, combined with the variation in group size and the low overall numbers involved, and the lack of detailed demographic description, there remain question marks over the robustness of the findings reported. Even so, the results are in keeping with those of other studies reported here.

Miyamoto RT, Svirsky MA, Robbins AM (1997) Enhancement of expressive language in prelingually deaf children with cochlear implants. Acta Oto-Laryngologica 117(2): 154–157.

Population size
23
Population comments
23 children with cochlear implants and an overlapping cohort of 37, later introduced into the assessment; 89 hearing aid users to provide predicted scores. The 37 were a group that was entered into the analysis at a later point. No details given on this second group, or why they were entered late, nor is there any detail in the reported analysis at which point they entered the data
Demographics Age: range 1.5–8 years, average 4:2 years
Age at CI: average 50 months
CI device: Nucleus 22
Onset of deafness: < 3 years
Communication mode: total communication (14), oral (9)
Encoding strategy: MPEAK, SPEAK, F0F1F2
Selection criteria
No details on sampling or selection given
Dependent variables
Reynell Developmental Language Scales (normed against hearing population) administered preoperatively, and at six-month intervals up to 2.5 years post implantation
Independent variables
Age
CI experience
Method
Over-time RDLS scores (regression line) of hearing aid group used as prediction
2-way repeated measures ANOVA to measure effect size of interaction between testing interval and scores

Results

At the 12-month post-implant interval, the observed mean language score was significantly higher than the predicted score, so whereas:

'Expressive language skills of prelingually deaf children without cochlear implants were shown to progress at less than half the rate of peers with normal hearing, a finding that is consistent with other published reports. In contrast, the rate of language learning for the group of implanted children was essentially equivalent to that of normal-hearing peers; that is, the implant children made approximately one year of language growth in one year's time. This trend was maintained over time in the implanted children who were followed for up to 2.5 years post-implant' (p.156).

Although the mean group data were extremely encouraging, wide inter-child variability was observed.

Conclusions

Early implantation (before age 3) might be beneficial to profoundly deaf children because the language delays at the time of implantation would be much smaller.

'It is clear that further research is needed to characterize the performance of implanted children over longer periods of time. In particular, the wide inter-child differences need to be explained' (p.157).

Observations

This research compares a narrow range of spoken-language outcomes in cochlear-implanted children with those in an audiologically matched group of non-cochlear-implanted deaf children. Results from this group of 89 unimplanted children provided cross-sectional data which suggested that profoundly deaf children without implants, on average, could only be expected to make five months of expressive language gain in one year. However, at some point in the reporting, a different sample size group of cochlear-implanted children is introduced that makes it difficult to assess the overall merit of the study. The study reports on one single measure, the Reynell Developmental Language Scale.

The findings are in line with those reported elsewhere; in particular, the authors report wide individual variation, a general language delay in comparison with hearing peers and improvements over time for the cochlear-implanted children at a rate in which the delay relative to their hearing peers remained constant (p.154). Results concern over-time analysis of a period of 2.5 years post implantation and a relatively modest population size of 23 children. Findings are affected by the wide age range (1.5–8 years) and average age at implantation of 50 months, suggesting a relatively wide range of experience with cochlear implants across children.

This study demonstrates a more general problem in the research literature where the general notion of 'language' is equated with spoken language. For example, the authors here suggest specifically that their aim is not merely to measure 'speech' (production, perception), but 'language development'. Children in total communication environments, by the very nature of the provision, are most likely to develop language based on both sign and speech forms of communication, so the RDLS assessment is not likely to be appropriate for them, as they may fluctuate towards the gestural end of the modal continuum during their language development. In this case, the majority of children providing the prediction regression used for the cochlear implants (p.154) would normally use a multi-mode (sign/speech) rather than a committed mode of communication, while 14 out of 23 cochlear implant users are themselves enrolled in total communication programs (p.155).

It means that for those total communication children, only a partial measure of language development may actually have been scored, which will have had consequences for the regression line on which the assessment is based.

Molina M, Huarte A, Cervera-Paz FI, Manrique M, Gracia-Tapia R (1999) Development of speech in two-year-old children with cochlear implants. International Journal of Pediatric Otorhinolaryngology 47(2): 177–179.

Population size

8

Demographics

(Spanish language)

Age: 2 years

Aetiology: genetic (3), ideopathic (4), meningitis (1)

Age at onset: birth (7), 1 year (1)

PTA: range 108–130 dB HL

CI device: Nucleus 22

Encoding strategy: SPEAK

Educational placement: regular kindergarten with logopedic support

Selection criteria

Enrolled in early stimulation programmes

No auditory benefits

Implanted at University of Navarra

Dependent variables

GAEL-P (pre-sentence level grammatical analysis of elicited language test for age 3-6 years) six months, and 1 and 2 years after CI

Independent variables

CI

Method

Not applicable

Results

'Six months after surgery children increase babbling and start specific vowel production. After one year, they begin to develop two-word production. After two years of cochlear implant use, they begin to produce phrases with verbs' (p.178).

Includes increase of babbling, uttering single words and increase of vocabulary.

'As long as the children make progress in psychomotricity, bucco-facial ability, and auditory perception and discrimination, they progressively develop a better articulation of phonemes. Articulatory errors decreased from 42% at the age of 1.5 years to 23% at the age of two years' (pp.178–9).

'Concerning the oral language and in particular the spontaneous language, some aspects should be remarked in early implanted children. They increase their expressive language with a progressive extinction of gestural support. The children learn spontaneously words and daily phrases not worked out and finally progressively abandon lip-reading as a mode of communication' (p.179).

Conclusions

'The importance of early cochlear implantation in children with profound bilateral sensorineural hearing loss should be noted, because of the favourable results in comprehensive and expressive language and the integration in the world of sounds' (p.179).

Observations

This Spanish study is included here merely for its reporting on Spanish-speaking children, despite reporting on only eight children in total. The study design is simple and straightforward, reporting only the GAEL-P test across a number of time intervals. The research is mostly concerned to align outcomes in Spain with those reported in the international literature, and is otherwise unproblematic and characteristic of the type of projects reported elsewhere. It also concerns an article that starts with a clear set of prior assumptions regarding language status and language development in deaf children.

These assumptions are as likely to have affected the research project as they are likely to restrict the rehabilitation options of the children reported in the study:

'Auditory deprivation in children causes important adverse effects in speech development, acquisition of knowledge, and the affective area. The use of multichannel cochlear implants permits to restore the auditory capacity and therefore affects directly the children's language and speech development' (p.177).

The GAEL-P test reported here is probably not age-appropriate for the children in the study; in addition to GAEL-P it might be advisable to use, for example, Tait's video analysis with children aged 2 instead, since at least some of their communicative ability is likely to be pre-verbal. None of the results amounts to an account for natural, age-equivalent language development. No substantial evidence for typical language development is reported, even though this is claimed. Results confirm speech production outcomes reported elsewhere for early paediatric implantation.

Mondain M, Sillon M, Vieu A, Tobey E, Uziel A (1997) Speech perception skills and speech intelligibility in prelingually deafened French children using cochlear implants. Archives of Otorhinolaryngology, and Head and Neck Surgery 123: 181–184.

Population size
64
Population comments
Decreasing over four years to 7
Demographics
CI device: Nucleus 22
Onset of deafness: congenital (50); prelingual ≤ 18 months (15), mean 1.6 years
Age at CI: mean 3.11 years
Selection criteria
Children implanted at the Montpellier University Paediatric Cochlear Implant Centre
Selection criteria for implantation included '... being involved in an education programme with
   a strong auditory and oral component, and to have strong family support systems' (p.182)
Dependent variables
Speech perception
Phoneme detection, closed-set word and sentence recognition, and modified open-set (MOS) recognition at preoperative and six-month postoperative intervals up to 4 years post implantation.
Speech intelligibility
Sample recordings played to 40 student volunteers; a subset of 16 cochlear-implanted children involved.
Independent variables
CI experience
For measure of intelligibility: speech recognition
Method
Percentage scores. Correlation with age using Pearson coefficient
Results
Speech recognition
Average scores improved steadily over time. Closed-set word and sentence identification reached 100% accuracy by 48 months (n = 7). Modified open-set recognition scores averaged 67.9% by 42 months, 80% by 48 months (n = 7) (p.181).
Speech intelligibility
After one year 4.2%, and 30.7, 55.2 and 74.2% after four years (p.181).
   There was not found to be a significant correlation between speech intelligibility scores and speech perception scores over time.

Conclusions
'Speech perception scores appear to increase with experience using a cochlear implant. Overall speech intelligibility appears to steadily improve with increased experience and appears to be poorly related to perceptual performance on MOS recognition tasks' (p.181).

Observations
This research is primarily of interest for its reporting on French language children and its significant sample size. Beyond these two characteristics the research in both method and reporting primarily confirms the results of this French cohort to be in line with results reported in the international literature. The study is of a straightforward design, measuring speech perception and speech-production skill in a controlled one-to-one test administration design.

The speech recognition tasks are substantially based around closed-set tests; otherwise, the results confirm existing trends.

There is a problem with interpreting the speech intelligibility task, since it is not a true measure over time. For this measure, 16 children were grouped into having one, two, three and four years' experience of their cochlear implant.

Therefore, the projection of 'development over time' is an artificial effect. This matters first because of the very limited size of the group. Second, individual children might (and indeed seem to have) varied greatly in terms of skill level. Moreover, there is unlikely to have been a 'true' one-year gap of performance difference between groups.

Overall percentage scores given are greatly affected by individual extreme performances and cannot be generalized safely. For example, one child's performance (with two years' cochlear implant experience) was below 10%, while two of four children with three years' experience of their cochlear implant scored below 40%, while the four children with four years' experience of their cochlear implant all have scores over 60%.

Moog JS, Geers AE (1999) Speech and language acquisition in young children after cochlear implantation. Otolaryngologic Clinics of North America 32(6): 1127–1141.

Population size
22

Demographics
Age: range 6:4–10:10 years
Age at CI: range 2:4–9:4 years
CI device: Nucleus multichannel
Encoding strategy: MPEAK, (changed to) SPEAK
CI use: range 1–7+ years

Selection criteria
All children of this age at the Moog Oral School implanted for one year or longer

Dependent variables
Test battery
Speech intelligibility
 • picture-SPINE
Speech production
 • PPVT-III
 • PB-K
 • One Word Expressive Picture Vocabulary Test
 • Test of Language Development–Primary
 • Clinical evaluation of language fundamentals
Reading
 • Gates MacGinitie Reading Tests
 • SAT

Independent variables
Oral education

Method
Correlation coefficient between scores and age at implantation
Results
After four years' average use of an implant (range 1–7 years), PB-K scores ranged from 4 to 84% correct (p.1135). On the SPINE speech intelligibility measure all but three of the cochlear-implanted children scored 90% or better, defined as 'Excellent intelligibility: naïve listeners can understand most of the child's speech at first introduction', while scores of the standardization sample of profoundly deaf children averaged 74% (p.1135).

On the spoken language measure all but one of the children scored within two standard deviations of hearing children of their age, representing greatly improved performance for the cochlear-implanted children (p.1136).

For reading, all but four of the 22 cochlear-implanted children scored within 80% of the hearing peers, an improvement relative to the 50% scores averaged by typical profoundly deaf children, and a level 'considered exceptionally good for profoundly deaf children' (pp.1136–7).

The correlation between PB-K score and age at implantation was significant ($p < 0.001$); receiving an implant prior to age 5 is suggested to be crucial for optimal auditory benefit gains. PB-K scores also correlated with all other measures, reflecting the importance of audition on spoken language performance and reading measures (p.1138).

Conclusions
'The children who achieved the best auditory skills were those who were implanted by 4.5 years of age. Children who achieved the best auditory skills developed language and reading skills that equaled those of their normal-hearing age mates' (p.1139).

'Even when the educational program is very high quality, however, there is still a range in children's auditory performance with an implant that cannot be attributed to differences in age at implant or amount of auditory training' (p.1139).

Observations
Length of implant use ranged widely from 1 to 7 years without giving data at specific intervals. Pre-implant performance was not included in some of the tests used and other important demographic details of the children, such as aetiology of deafness and age at onset of deafness, were not included. The sample concerns children enrolled in highly selective US oral education, and is not representative of the target population.

The authors suggest that, for the general population of deaf children, severe deficits in language constitute the major factor accounting for delayed reading abilities of deaf individuals, the delay increasing as test items place increasing demand on comprehending complex sentences and paragraphs, although the claim is here that oral education produces marked benefits (p.1127). Results suggest that children benefiting from a cochlear implant show clear improvements in this specific type of schooling. However, there is no comparative element to the study, and given the highly particular nature of both the educational environment and the population, in combination with a lack of clear demographic detail, this makes the findings difficult to contrast with findings reported elsewhere.

Nakisa MJ, Summerfield AQ, Nakisa RC, McCormick B, Archbold S, Gibbin KP, O'Donoghue GM (2001) Functionally equivalent ages and hearing levels of children with cochlear implants measured with pre-recorded stimuli. British Journal of Audiology 35(3): 183–199.

Population size
31
Population comments
Comparison group of hearing children ($n = 40$) and HA users ($n = 22$), average hearing level 92 dB (range 55–113 dB)

Demographics
Gender: male (19), female (20) – unselected sample
CI device: Nucleus 22 multichannel
Encoding strategy: MPEAK
Age at onset: birth (21), < 2 years (10)
Communication mode: oral (11), total communication (20)
Further details listed in outcome data table (p.191)

Selection criteria
Recruited via the Nottingham Paediatric Cochlear Implant Programme, subset of children attending follow-up appointments. No exclusions detailed. Five attempted the test but failed a criterion level of performance

Dependent variables
Speech-perception task, pre-recorded via computer (auditory only), with picture mapping to auditory input
Level-A of the Iowa Matrix Test

Independent variables
Age
Hearing level
Aided hearing threshold

Method
Bayesian statistical techniques in preference to conventional curve-fitting procedures to enable a priori knowledge to constrain the fitting procedure (p.189)

Results
Scores were higher with greater duration of implant use ($p < 0.01$), with a younger age at implantation ($p < 0.01$) and with a shorter duration of deafness prior to implantation ($p < 0.05$); children using spoken language exclusively scored higher ($p < 0.05$) than children using total communication, while four other variables (age, age at onset, average pre-implant hearing level and average pre-implant aided threshold) did not correlate with outcome scores (p.189).

Cochlear implant use and young age at implantation accounted for 47% of variance in matrix scores, with no other variable accounting for significant additional variance (p.189). Accordingly, children were split according to age (≤ 4 and > 4 years) and cochlear implant use (≤ 2.5 years, > 2.5 years) (p.190).

Functionally equivalent age
'The functionally equivalent ages of the implanted children ranged from 0.75 to 6.25 years, with a mean of 3.4 years. Ten children achieved scores within the range expected for hearing children of the same age. These children either had used their implants for more than 2.5 years and/or were aged 4 years or younger at the time of implantation. On average, however, functionally equivalent ages were 3.9 years below the chronological ages of the children (ranging from 0.5 years above to 8.7 years below' (p.190).

Significant effects were observed for duration of implant use ($p < 0.01$) and age at implantation ($p < 0.05$) (p.190).

Functionally equivalent hearing level (n = 25)
Average functionally equivalent hearing loss improvement was established at 94 dB (range 7–121 dB), an average improvement over pre-implantation levels of 23 dB. Again there were significant effects for duration of implant use ($p < 0.01$) and age at implantation ($p < 0.05$) (p.190).

Functionally equivalent aided thresholds (n = 28)
Twenty-seven children scored at levels numerically higher than expected for children with similar hearing levels using acoustic hearing aids, averaging 45 dB (range 5 dB to 93 dB) aided response, representing a 55 dB average improvement over preimplant levels (p.193). Again age at implantation and duration of CI use were found to be statistically significant ($p < 0.05$ and $p < 0.01$) (p.193).

Conclusions

Five detailed conclusions summarizing data are reported, as per findings.

'... transformations showed that: (1) mean FE age (3.4 years) lagged mean chronological age (7.4 years), but some implanted children performed within the range expected for children with normal hearing of the same age; (2) mean FE AHL was 94 dB compared with a mean pre-implant AHL of 117 dB; (3) mean FE aided threshold was 45 dB(A) compared with a mean pre-implant aided threshold of 99 dB(A)' (p.183).

Observations

This research uses a computer-based (pre-recorded) speech-perception measure to test the age equivalence across three groups of tested children, one hearing group, one hearing-aided group and one cochlear-implanted group, at a single point in time. Results indicate that cochlear-implanted children outperform hearing-aided children, but that there remains a gap between hearing and cochlear implant performance, although some implanted children scored within the normal hearing range. Wide distributions characterize the results, leading to large confidence intervals for the findings.

The article records a detailed background on research concerning both functionally equivalent age and functionally equivalent hearing levels (pp.184–6).

The results map the cochlear implant children against hearing peers for functional equivalent age, hearing loss and aided thresholds, confirming that '... implantation of appropriate candidates leads to functionally better hearing than would be expected with acoustic hearing aids' (p.183).

This research continues comparisons of functional equivalence between cochlear-implanted children and matched deaf and hearing comparison groups, contributing a computerized test of speech perception which allows for standardized, controlled, consistent test administration across children and populations.

Nevins ME, Chute PM (1995) Success of children with cochlear implants in mainstream educational settings. Annals of Otology, Rhinology and Laryngology 104: s100–s102.

Population size
16
Demographics
None detailed
Selection criteria
None detailed
Dependent variables
Support protocol using observer check list and teacher interviews
Independent variables
Placement: mainstream
Method
No statistical analyses
Results

Of 16 children reported on via this protocol, all but two children were reported to be performing in the top half of their class, while five of the 16 were rated by their teachers as being both socially and academically successful in the classroom (p.101).

All but two children continued to receive speech-language therapy at least three times a week for 30 minutes. Four children received services in some form or another from a certified teacher of the deaf (p.101).
Conclusions

Children with cochlear implants placed in the mainstream are for the most part experiencing social and academic success. Careful placement and continued monitoring are essential elements of mainstream success (p.102).

Observations

The authors report that cochlear-implanted children show a significant trend toward 'less restrictive' (p.100) educational environments (mainstreaming), making these transitions earlier than non-implanted children. Experience suggests to the authors that once a receiving school is identified and a child is placed in the mainstream, he or she is seldom followed up with the same intensity that was in evidence prior to the placements decision. They consider it naive to expect that comprehensive pre-mainstreaming evaluation ensures subsequent social and academic success (p.100).

A programme at the Clarke School for the Deaf routinely contracts with local school districts to provide support to the mainstream placement, with the suggestion that this model is essential to ensure successful mainstreaming. Such across-placement support is likely to be more typical of the support schemes run via implant support services in the UK, so that a perhaps more typically US situation is being tackled here.

The protocol being described utilizes an observer checklist form and teacher interviews conducted by the implant centre's educational consultant.

The results suggest that successful placement in the mainstream is possible and does occur.

The report has only limited demographic description and information on the placements involved, which does not help in comparative assessments of the summary findings. The text is useful for the more detailed description of some reported case studies.

Nikolopoulos T, Archbold S, Lutman ME, O'Donoghue GM (2000) Prediction of auditory performance following cochlear implantation of prelingually deaf young children. In: Waltzman SB, Cohen NL (eds) Cochlear Implants. New York, USA: Thieme, pp.216–217.

Population size

103

Population comments

Sample size dropping to 29 at three-year test interval

Demographics

Age at CI: range 21 months–6.11 years, mean 4.3 years)
Onset of deafness: range 0–2.9 years (mean 6.7 months)
Duration of deafness: range 0.2–6.8 years (mean 3.8 years)
Aetiology: meningitis (42), congenital (53), other causes (8)
Electrode insertion: > 20 (90), 10–20 (7), < 10 (2)
CI device: Nucleus multichannel
Processor: MSP, upgraded to Spectra

Selection criteria

Unselected sample, representing all children implanted at Nottingham Cochlear Implant Centre

Dependent variables

CAP (Categories of Auditory Performance) pre-implantation and at 1, 2 and 3 years post implantation

Independent variables

Pre-implantation test scores
Age at implantation
Duration of deafness

Method

Stepwise multiple regression, CAP measure as dependent variable, supported by nonparametric Spearman Rank correlation analysis

Results

At 24 months age at implantation (p = 0.03) and duration of deafness (p = 0.01) were significantly associated with test scores, and at the 36- and 48-month intervals only age at implantation (p = 0.01, p = 0.04) was significantly correlated with CAP (p.217).

Conclusions

CAP outcomes are consistent with the published literature. The demonstration of age at implantation as a predictor of outcome has important consequences for cochlear implant practice, since it indicates that earlier implantation generally yields greater benefits (p.217).

Observations

Despite being a brief summary of the research carried out, the study is rich in demographic and methodological description. The sample size is substantial (although dropping to 29 after three years of study) and the results are consistent with those reported elsewhere. The study was also concerned to demonstrate the effectiveness of CAP as an observational face-validity measure of auditory potential in young children who are unable to participate in formal testing.

Nikolopoulos TP, Archbold SM, O'Donoghue GM (1999) The development of auditory perception in children following cochlear implantation. International Journal of Pediatric Otorhinolaryngology 49-s1: 189–191.

Population size

103

Population comments

At one year post CI; 77, 52, 30, 21, 11 children at 2-, 3-, 4-, 5- and 6-year interval

Demographics

CI experience: up to 6 years post-CI
Age at onset: prelingual deafness, < 3 years
Age at CI: < 8 years
Aetiology: congenital (77, 58%), other causes (11, 8%)

Selection criteria

Consecutively implanted; no deselections

Dependent variables

CAP

Independent variables

Not applicable

Method

As other Nottingham research: same population
One implant centre, consecutively implanted sample

Results

Prelingually deaf children showed significant improvement in the auditory perception with implant experience. Eighty-two percent of children who reached the six-year interval could understand conversation without lip-reading. The respective percentage in the four-year interval was 70%.

Conclusions

The long-term results of cochlear implantation reveal that the majority of prelingually deaf children, when implanted before the age of 8 years, will develop significant auditory perception.

'The relative paucity of children at the five-year interval is typical of many series and highlights the difficulties faced by all paediatric implant teams who, of necessity, have to measure outcomes over such long periods. Accepting the small sample size in the long-term follow-up, their results were very encouraging, showing significant auditory perception following cochlear implantation' (s191).

Observations

This study arose out of the observation that outcomes in speech perception in cochlear-implanted children reveal improvements extending over significant lengths of time, so that it is imperative to repeatedly measure such improvements over time, necessitating an ongoing programme of data-collection and analysis.

The study reports clear improvements in speech perception outcomes over a period of six years post implantation, although the lack of comparison groups means that this cannot be attributed unequivocally to the implant.

Using a general spoken-language perception assessment in a questionnaire format that can be completed easily by non-specialists, it is reported that 82% of the cochlear-implanted children 'could understand conversation without lip-reading' six years post implantation. It is clear that such results are significant, and result directly from a range of factors combined in the implant process.

O'Donoghue G, Nikolopoulos TP, Archbold SM (2000) Determinants of speech perception in children after cochlear implantation. The Lancet. 356(9228): 466–468.

Population size

40

Demographics

Age at implantation mean 52 months (range 30 months to 7 years).
Age at onset of deafness mean 11.8 months (range 0–34 months), below 3 years
Multichannel implant system
Gender 60% male ($n = 24$), 40% female ($n = 16$)

Selection criteria

Consecutively implanted, no deselections

Dependent variables

Connecting discourse tracking (CDT) at three, four and five years after implantation. Age-appropriate texts

Independent variables

Age at implantation
Number of inserted electrodes
Aetiology (congenital or meningitis)
Mode of communication (oral or 'total')
Socio-economic status

Method

Correlation analysis and repeated-measures ANOVA

Results

The mean number of words per minute perceived increased on average for the sample of children from 0 before implantation to 44.8 (SD 24.3) five years after implantation.

Age at implantation was a significant covariate ($p = 0.01$), and mode of communication was a significant 'between individuals' factor ($p = 0.04$).

Conclusions

Young age at intervention and oral communication mode are the most important determinants of later speech perception in young deaf children after cochlear implantation.

Observations

This small but detailed report targets a number of key variables affecting outcomes in paediatric cochlear implantation, namely age at implantation, number of inserted electrodes, communication mode and socio-economic status. Age at implantation and communication mode together accounted for 43% of variance reported in the findings.

Because only speech perception was measured, although it is not the predominant target outcome in total communication programmes that combine different language modes, this is likely to contribute to the 'advantage' of oral communication mode given a restricted view of language outcome.

Age range is still very wide, from 34 months to 7 years, and the authors suggest that disaggregation by age group in larger studies is necessary to control for maturation and language ability factors. In this study, however, the subsample numbers would have been insufficient to generate reliable correlation outcomes.

O'Neill C, Archbold S, O'Donoghue GM, McAlister DA, Nikolopoulos TP (2001) Indirect costs, cost-utility variations and the funding of paediatric cochlear implantation. International Journal of Pediatric Otorhinolaryngology 58: 53–57.

Population size
Nil – data from published sources
Population comments
Profoundly deaf children with an unaided hearing loss of greater than 95 dB
Demographics
Age at onset: not available
Age at CI: 4 years (assumed)
Duration of deafness: not available
Life expectancy: 75 years (assumed)
Setting Nottingham Cochlear Implant Centre, UK
Method
Economic evaluation type: cost-utility analysis
Study perspective: societal
Comparator intervention: no intervention
Source of effectiveness data: derived from published literature
Direct costs: costs included assessment, rehabilitation and maintenance
Indirect costs: local authority education costs
Discount rate for costs and benefits: 6%
Outcome measure: assumed utility gain based on published adult value
Currency and price year: £, 1997/8 (£1 = US$1.45)
Sensitivity analysis: none conducted
Results
Cost per QALY was estimated by education authority type. Net discounted cost per QALY gain was £17,809 (in 2001/2 prices – £21,196 or US$31,868) in London authorities, £16,207 (in 2001/2 prices – £19,290 or US$29,003) in Metropolitan authorities, £15,022 (in 2001/2 prices – £17,879 or US$26,881) in Unitary authorities and £12,049 (in 2001/2 prices – £14,341 or US$21,562) in County authorities.
Conclusions
'We have demonstrated that variations in the cost-utility of paediatric cochlear implantation has the potential to produce anomalous purchasing of the intervention in the UK. We have also argued that this can be avoided (while continuing to use CUA information) if a ring-fenced budget for the intervention is considered' (p.57).
Observations
The study assumes that implantation results in educational cost savings, that is with an implant the profoundly deaf child has the same educational costs as a severely deaf child. It also assumes the utility gain, lifespan and age at implantation.

O'Neill C, O'Donoghue GM, Archbold S, Normand C (2000) A cost-utility analysis of pediatric cochlear implantation. The Laryngoscope 110: 156–160.

Population size
Nil - data from published sources
Population comments
Profoundly deaf children with an unaided hearing loss of greater than 95 dB
Demographics
Age at onset: not available
Age at CI: 4 years (assumed)
Duration of deafness: not available
Assumed life expectancy: 71 years
Setting Nottingham Cochlear Implant Centre, UK
Methods
Economic evaluation type: cost-utility analysis
Study perspective: societal
Comparator intervention: no intervention
Source of effectiveness data: derived from published literature
Direct costs: charges to health authorities by year. Year 1 covered assessment and implantation, years 2 and 3 rehabilitation and maintenance and year 4 onwards maintenance only
Indirect costs: local authority education costs
Discount rate for costs and benefits: 0 and 6%
Outcome measure: assumed utility gain based on published adult value
Currency and price year: £, 2000 (£1 = US$1.60)
Sensitivity analysis: none conducted
Results
Cost per QALY £10,341 (US$16,546) (in 2001/2 prices – £11,345 or US$17,057) (discounted) and £2,532 (US$4,051) (in 2001/2 prices – £2,773 or US$4,169) undiscounted. Utility gain equalled 0.23 per annum and summed 16.33 QALYs over a child's lifetime.
Conclusions
Paediatric cochlear implantation is a cost-effective intervention for profoundly deaf children.
Observations
The study assumes that implantation results in educational cost savings, that is with an implant the profoundly deaf child has the same educational costs as a severely deaf child. It also assumes the utility gain, lifespan and age at implantation.

Osberger MJ, Fisher L, Zimmerman-Phillips S, Geier L, Barker MJ (1998) Speech recognition of older children with cochlear implants. American Journal of Otology 19(2): 152–157.

Population size
30
Demographics
Age at cochlear implant ≥ 5 years (mean oral 8.6 years, total communication 9.8 years)
Age at onset ≤ 3 years (mean oral 0.5, total communication 1.4)
Bilateral profound sensorineural hearing loss (pure-tone average ≥ 90 dB)
Clarion multichannel CI
Mode of communication: oral (19), total communication (11)
Selection criteria
No mental retardation
English as primary language

Enrolled in clinical trial for Clarion CI (FDA monitored)

No sampling strategy is given, although some form of sampling did take place

Dependent variables

Speech recognition (ESP/GASP/PB-K) at 3 and 6 months after CI

Independent variables

Mode of communication (oral, total communication)

Method

Repeated measures analysis; no statistics approach detailed. Percent scores and standard deviations given, plus measure of significance

Results

Oral children significantly outperformed total communication children on four out of five measures. Median scores for oral children were close to test ceilings six months after cochlear implantation (p.152).

Conclusions

Significant benefit from cochlear implant compared with conventional hearing aids. Greatest benefit for children using oral communication (p.152).

Observations

This study reports on research which used the population of Clarion recipients in the US as a target for sampling. The purpose of the study was to determine whether prelingually deaf children, implanted after the age of 5, would derive more benefit from cochlear implants than from acoustic hearing aids. It is suggested that previous research had demonstrated limited benefits for recipients of this kind. It was further hypothesized (although no reason is provided for this) that children in oral programmes would outperform children in total communication programmes.

First, a few guiding remarks should precede further assessment:

- although mean ages are given, no scale is detailed for the age range
- children seem to have been selected, but no real sampling approach is detailed
- statistical reporting lacks reference to method
- no detail on, e.g. socioeconomic differences, gender, ethnicity or prior achievements, which, as the authors comment, typically affects in particular placement (p.157).

Despite these provisos, the findings on speech perception are straightforward. With regard to placement, however, the reported findings are likely to be affected by test administration, since it was conducted in auditory mode exclusively. The authors report findings on placement in both results and conclusion, while acknowledging weaknesses in their assessment with regards to placement in the text.

Osberger MJ, Geier L, Zimmerman-Phillips S, Barker MJ (1997) Use of a parent report scale to assess benefit in children given the Clarion cochlear implant. American Journal of Otology 18: s79-s80.

Population size

60

Population comments

Parents of cochlear-implanted children; after six months $n = 23$, unexplained

Demographics

Age: 2–15 years

CI device: Clarion Multi-Strategy

Onset of deafness: prelingual (undefined)

Selection criteria

All 60 prelingual children out of $n = 124$ implanted with the Clarion device. Presumably based on Advanced Bionics client list

Dependent variables

Three- and six-month post-implantation parent survey (closed question): 'Meaningful Auditory Integration Scale' (MAIS)

Independent variables
CI preoperative outcomes of MAIS
Method
Percentage reporting
Results
'After 6 months of Clarion use, 91% of the children frequently or always responded or always alerted to a variety of sounds in the environment. Moreover, slightly more than half of the children frequently or always responded to their name in noise, and showed curiosity about sounds' (p.s80).

'Six months postoperatively, about two thirds of the children frequently or always recognized routines in the home or school based on auditory signals, distinguished between the voices of at least two talkers, and discriminated speech from non-speech stimuli' (p.s80).
Conclusions
'After implantation, the children showed improvements in three skill areas: bonding to the device, spontaneous alerting to sound in everyday situations, and ability to derive meaning from sound in the environment' (p.s79).
Observations
This article reports on a study using structured interviews to address the 'limitation of traditional evaluation measures' (p.s79), and draws on interviews with 60 parents of deaf children, taken from the client list of Advanced Bionics' Clarion implant in the US. The Meaningful Auditory Integration Scale (MAIS) was used to determine improvements in auditory skills as reported by the parents of those implanted. In the analysis of the interviews, a four-point Lickert scale scoring system was used. Categories of assessment included bonding with the device, being alert to sound and deriving meaning from sound.

In their conclusion, the authors report improvements across all three areas for all children, as reported by their parents. Whatever the nature of the original study, the reporting in this article is lacking in detail across all elements of the study. It remains unexplained why after only three months (between three- and six-month measures) the population dropped from 60 to only 23, i.e. just one-third of the original population. In a comparison between the Clarion device and other aids, the authors chose to compare the Clarion against two much older types of cochlear implant: a single-channel 3M/House device and the Nucleus FOF1F2 implant, which uses an older processing strategy.

Moreover, the three- and six-month reporting is likely to be within a post-implant 'honeymoon period' of getting used to the device, and may not reflect appreciation over a longer period of time.

One key characteristic of this type of research — especially where the research is conducted by professionals who provided access to the intervention in the first place — is the need for independence. There is often a possibility that parents with an interest in reporting positive findings (following a commitment to a cochlear implant operation in a very young child in particular) respond positively when information is requested by professionals who have a clear interest in reporting positive findings. Although these comments do not by any means invalidate the data, the method does point to the need for clear, demonstrably independent research.

Osberger MJ, McConkey Robbins AM, Todd SL, Riley AI (1994) Speech intelligibility of children with cochlear implants. Volta Review 96(5): 169–180.

Population size
18
Population comments
9 oral, 9 total communication. Matched on age at onset, age at implantation and duration of implant use

Demographics

Age at onset: total communication range 0:0–1:8 years, mean 0:5 years. Oral range 0:0–2:6 years, mean 0:7 years

Age at CI: total communication range 2:9–5:3 years, mean 4:4 years. Oral range 2:8–5:7 years, mean 4:0 years

CI use: total communication range 2:5–3:0 years, mean 3:6 years. Oral range 2:5–5:4 years, mean 3:4 years

CI device: Nucleus multichannel

Selection criteria

Oral children were sampled from the CID. The total communication group was sampled from the Indiana University School of Medicine. Selection criteria: implanted by age 5, at least 2 years of experience with CI

Dependent variables

Beginners' Intelligibility Test (BIT, developed at Indiana University School of Medicine). Uses object and pictures to convey target sentences; procedure similar to GAEL

Independent variables

Communication method: oral and total communication

Method

Chi-square test

Results

Mean intelligibility score on BIT 27% higher for the group using oral communication ($p <$ 0.05) (p.175). The average speech intelligibility score of the children who used oral communication was 48%, which was significantly higher than the average score of 21% of the children who used total communication.

Conclusions

The range of scores for the children who used oral communication was relatively large, with the scores of the children with the lowest intelligibility comparable to those of the children who used total communication.

'... results suggest that the children who demonstrated the most intelligible speech used oral communication. The fact that some of the children in the oral group still had poor speech intelligibility suggests that factors other than communicator mode influenced the acquisition of speech production skills in these children' (p.176).

Observations

The speech intelligibility of 18 children with prelingual deafness was examined after using multichannel cochlear implants for an average of three years. Half the children used oral communication and half used total communication. The nine children in each group were matched in terms of age at onset of deafness, age implanted and duration of implant use. Sentences were elicited from the children on an imitative basis and played to panels of listeners who were instructed to write down what they thought the children had said. Intelligibility was measured in terms of the percentage of words correctly understood in the sentences. Speech intelligibility was here measured in two groups of cochlear implant users ($n = 18$) implanted by age 5, with prelingual deafness, but separated by communication mode (effect of placement), oral and total communication. The study is of modest size, with only nine children in each group. The authors report that:

'The average speech intelligibility score of the children who used oral communication was 48%, which was significantly higher than the average score of 21% of the children who used total communication' (169).

These results, as the authors themselves suggest, will have been affected by the fact that the oral children were enrolled in CID education, an intensive auditory/oral rehabilitation programme; the oral children therefore will have received more training. Second, the authors suggest that the teachers in the total communication setting might 'not be adequately trained' (p.177). It may also be that teachers in different settings have differing sets of priorities as well as teaching to a varied ranges of abilities and needs.

Third, parents, and teachers in oral settings, might have higher expectations related to speech outcomes. And fourth, oral rather than total communication peer group is also likely to affect outcome.

Osberger MJ, McConkey Robbins AM, Todd SL, Riley AI, Miyamoto R (1994) Speech production skills of children with multichannel cochlear implants. In: Hochmair-Desoyer IJ, Hochmair ES (eds) Advances in Cochlear Implants. Vienna, Austria:, pp.503–508.

Population size
   29
Population comments
   Aged over 4 years. Comparison groups of HA users, in bronze (PTA > 110 dB HL), silver (PTA = 103 dB HL) and gold (PTA = 93 dB HL) categories
Demographics
   Age at onset of deafness: mean 0.9 years
   Age at CI: mean 5.7 years
   No further details given
   Control groups of HA users vary on both age and onset of deafness against CI group and across groups
Selection criteria
   No sampling criteria detailed
Dependent variables
   Ten-sentence elicitation task with speech production judged by inexperienced listeners
Independent variables
   CI versus HA
   Over-time improvement of speech intelligibility
   Placement (oral/total communication)
Method
   Plotting over time, using test percentage scores
Results
   The cochlear implant subjects showed a gradual improvement over time; after 2.5 years of implant use average performance exceeded that of 'silver' hearing aid users. However, speech intelligibility scores of 'gold' hearing aid users remained 30% above those of cochlear implant users across the period of study. Large individual differences in over-time outcome scores were noted (p.505).
   Overall higher performance was associated more with oral education than with total communication education.
Conclusions
   Substantial improvements in intelligibility occurred in the speech of children with cochlear implants with prelingual deafness over time. The largest changes in speech intelligibility occurred after two years of implant experience (p.506).
Observations
   This is an early study in the collection reviewed here to contrast the speech intelligibility of implanted children with that of bronze-, silver- and gold-standard hearing aid users.

Paganga S, Tucker E, Harrigan S, Lutman M (2001) Evaluating training courses for parents of children with cochlear implants. International Journal of Language and Communication Disorders 36: s517–s522.

Population size
   18

Population comments
Parents of cochlear-implanted children
Demographics
None detailed
Selection criteria
None detailed
Dependent variables
Interaction rating produced by naive raters of interaction between parent and cochlear-implanted child following a course aimed at improving parent–child interaction
Independent variables
Pre-course interaction rating
Method
Two-tailed t-test comparison of paired (pre- and post-course) rating samples ($n = 126$, p.520)
Results
Post-course ratings were significantly higher ($p < 0.05$) than the pre-course ratings (p.520).

> 'The most striking change noted was the reduction in parental directiveness when playing and communicating with their implanted child, immediately after the courses. This was probably due to the emphasis on allowing the child to lead the play/conversation during the course. [...] Parents used more "motherese" at the end of the courses, by increasing the use of repetition, good positioning and other strategies covered in the course' (p.521).

Conclusions
'The positive increase in effective communication skills is consistent with the therapists' views at the end of the courses' (p.520).
Observations
This is a study of a relatively simple and clearly effective design, in which naive raters judge the quality of parent–child interactions recorded before and after a course specifically targeted at improving parent–child interaction. The two recordings were presented to them in random order, so that the overall significantly higher ratings raters gave to post-intervention recordings offer clear, objective evidence for the effectiveness of the course – and this was exactly the point of the study.

The aim of the courses, run twice in Southampton and once in Nottingham (for 18 parents in total), was to: 'help parents gain information about language development and adopt interactive styles that promote their own child's communication' (p.518).

A clear problem in a course like this is measuring its effectiveness: parent questionnaires were used, reporting positive effects, as did therapists involved (p.519). The measure reported here provides additional evidence of a different order as to the effectiveness of the programme.

Parisier SC, Chute PM, Popp AL, Suh GD (2001) Outcome analysis of cochlear implant reimplantation in children. Laryngoscope 111(1): 26–32.

Population size
25
Population comments
Concerns a cohort of reimplanted children
Demographics
Age at initial implant: range 10 months–10 years (mean 3.9 years)
Gender: males (13), females (12)
Surgery interval: range 5 months–7 years (mean 32.5 months)

CI device: Nucleus 22 (14), Nucleus 24 (1), Clarion (10)
Aetiology: congenital (12), meningitis (13)
Number of electrodes: detailed
Ossification: detailed

Selection criteria

All child reimplantations carried out by the main author in Cochlear Implant Center of The Manhattan Eye, Ear and Throat Hospital up to 1998 and subsequently at Lenox Hill Hospital
No deselections (two children who were reimplanted in the other ear were excluded)

Dependent variables

Outcomes at six months, and where available, one month post reimplantation.
Test battery including GASP, PB-K, NU#6, CPT, LNT, BKB, with age-appropriate selections

Independent variables

Best prior speech perception results (achieved before reimplantation)

Method

Contrasting best results obtained with the first implant before failure to those obtained following reimplantation. Reports test battery outcome scores
No calculations of statistical significance performed on the data

Results

Overall, the speech-perception abilities of all of the children either remained the same or improved following reimplantation. Of the children (*n* = 5) who were already capable of reliable open-set speech recognition before implant failure, all were able to continue to perform at this level within six months of reimplantation. Three children were classified with no pattern perception (category I) abilities with their first implant system. Two of these children were capable of open-set speech recognition within one year of reimplantation. The other child was still classified as category I after one year. The remainder of the cohort either maintained their ability within the particular speech-perception category or achieved at a higher level, with five of these children being capable of open-set speech recognition within one year of reimplantation. No child had poorer performance in terms of pattern perception category after reimplantation.

Open-set speech recognition scores and speech-perception abilities remained stable or improved compared with results before reimplantation.

Conclusions

Cochlear implant reimplantation is technically feasible and allows for continued auditory development for the child who has a cochlear implant device failure. The length of electrode insertion may be slightly reduced.

Observations

This study is mainly of value for its reporting on a specific subgroup of children with implants, those who suffered device failure following initial implantation. The point of the article is to review experience gained technically and medically as well as reporting on outcomes; therefore this last element forms only a minor part of the overall reporting. The test battery included GASP and PB-K. The authors have measured outcome improvements mostly only at six months after reimplantation (with some data available for the one-year post-reimplantation interval), so that results must be considered tentative. However, the findings are encouraging, indicating improvements for most children very quickly, at the six-month interval.

Another comment can usefully be quoted regarding device failure rates reported more generally:

'Recent reports have shown a cumulative survival of 99.2% at four years and 97% at six years for the N-22 device. Recently, Kessler reported an electronic failure rate of less than 0.1% per year for the Clarion cochlear implant, including children and adults. Although no reported data exist for the N-24 device, the series of patients followed at Lenox Hill Hospital indicates an even lower failure rate for this device' (p.26).

Because of the range of ages of the children, their linguistic capacity and the variety of speech perception measures used, children were grouped using the standardized categories of speech-perception abilities for comparison. The five categories of speech perception range from the lowest level (no pattern perception, category I) to the highest (open-set speech recognition, category V).

Perrin E, Berger-Vachon C, Topouzkhanian A, Truy E, Morgon A (1999) Evaluation of cochlear implanted children's voices. International Journal of Pediatric Otorhinolaryngology 47(2):83–98.

Population size
4

Demographics
Gender: ratio 3/1
Age: range 9–14 years
Number of electrodes: range 18–22
CI experience: range 2–4 years
Age at onset: birth (3), at 4.5 years (1)
CI device: Nucleus 22
Encoding strategy: SPEAK
Age- and gender-matched hearing control group

Selection criteria
No criteria or sampling method detailed

Dependent variables
Story-telling. Scored subjectively by a listening jury (speech therapist) and 'objectively' by IT analysis using ILS software

Independent variables
CI

Method
No statistical evaluation due to low numbers. Each CI paired with a control child on outcome scores

Results
Score items varied between outcome pairs (no generalizations possible). Specific observations.

Subjective measures
'(1) intensity had a larger variation, but this was not seen with patient BA; (2) pauses were more numerous and their duration was longer' (p.184).

Objective measures
'(1) formant values for control children tended to be above the normal range (thus the normal range has to be seen again). They tended to be below the range for the implantees, and some kind of 'compensation' occurred on the total. (2) Speaking duration was much higher with the implantees' (p.184).

In summary, intensity variations were different between control and implanted children. Also voice formants were not situated in the same region regarding the normal ranges, but differences were difficult to assess. Globally, the main change was in the speaking duration.

Conclusions
'It produced four kinds of information: (1) the speaking duration was much higher with the implantees; (2) formant values tended to be lower with the implantees than with the control children; (3) the objective assessment pointed out differences, but they were not systematic; (4) pauses (subjective) and duration (objective) assessments should be correlated and it is worth seeing them more deeply' (p.186).

Observations

Compared to hearing children of the same age, so the authors claim, the voices of cochlear-implanted children are far from being similar. In this study, the voice of cochlear-implanted children has been compared with the voice of corresponding children (same age, same sex) included in the mainstream, with six girls and two boys participating in the experiment, although two are lost at the reporting stage. The phonetic material was a paragraph of the French standard text *La bise et le soleil* (The North Wind and the Sun). An objective and a subjective analysis of the voice were done and parameters were compared between both groups of people (children with implants and control). Studied parameters were voice pitch, intensity, fluency, pauses, articulation and pleasantness in the objective analysis, and voice pitch, formants and duration for the objective study.

Although the number of children reported on is low in this study – it presents a report on four case studies – the article is included here for a number of reasons. First, the authors report on a group of children implanted in France, hence the report contributes to the international data available on cochlear-implanted children. Second, the assessment procedure on speech intelligibility contains an exact reference to using both 'subjective' assessment through the use of individuals' scoring of the children's speech, and 'objective assessment' through the use of the standard ILS software. Third, the comparison is between deaf children with cochlear implants and the 'ideal target' of cochlear implantation outcome, an age- and gender-matched group of hearing children, a comparison that is obvious – arguably more so than comparisons with other, non-implanted deaf children – but rarely attempted. And fourth, although the results are not so different from those reported elsewhere for speech intelligibility (without the quantification, and given the wide individual variation reported between children), the authors arrive at a very distinctive conclusion:

> 'Is cochlear implantation an efficient means to improve the quality of the voice? Previous studies tended to answer "yes" to this question. No support to this answer could be given in our work. In the case of children the problem is more complicated as the total deafness also affects the acquisition of language. A hearing correction cannot change the past. Consequently, a child with a good auditory correction is bound to have more difficulties than a normal one to speak a sentence' (p.185).

It should be noted that the ages of the four children ranged from 9 to 14 years with experience of cochlear implant ranging from 2 to 4 years, so that none were implanted early, which is an important consideration.

Pisoni D, Geers A (2000) Working memory in deaf children with cochlear implants: correlations between digit span and measures of spoken language processing. Annals of Otology, Rhinology and Laryngology 109(12): s185.

Population size
43

Demographics
Age at onset: prelingual
Age: range 8–9:11 years
CI use: ≥ 4 years, mean 5.5 years
Communication mode: oral, total communication, 'approximately half' (p.92)
Total communication group received half the number of speech therapy hours per year (42 versus 81)

Selection criteria
No selection criteria detailed. Population the same as that reported in Geers et al. (2000)

Dependent variables
Speech perception
- VIDSPAC
- ESP
- WIPI
- LNT
- BKB
- CHIVE
- TACL

Speech intelligibility
- 32 McGarr sentences to three naive listeners

Reading
- Word Attack subtest of Woodcock Reading Mastery Test
- Two subtests of the Peabody Individual Achievement Test (Recognition and Comprehension)

Independent variables
  Working memory

Method
  Correlation

Results
  'Forward digit spans were correlated with the four sets of outcome measures obtained by Geers at al. [2000]: speech perception, speech intelligibility, language, and reading' (p.92).

Conclusions
  '... some component of working memory plays an important role in mediating performance across a range of different tasks. Moreover, this component of memory contributes a common underlying source of variance to tasks that measure speech perception, speech production, language comprehension, and reading. [...] The differences in performance among cochlear implant users on these four outcome measures may reflect fundamental differences in the speech and efficiency of elementary information processing operations that are used in the encoding, rehearsal, retrieval, and manipulation of the phonological representations of spoken words' (p.93).

  'The identification of working memory as the "locus" of the differences in performance between children with cochlear implants also suggests that what the child does centrally with the information received through a cochlear implant may be just as important as the nature of the sensory information and the initial neural representations of speech signals at the periphery' (p.93).

Observations
  The authors address the considerable individual differences in performance among children on many spoken-language outcome measures, suggesting that some findings point to an effect of working memory in spoken-language tasks. The authors obtained memory auditory digit spans from 43 8- and 9-year-old prelingually deaf children for a period of at least four years, and having used their implants for at least four years (p.92).

  The authors report that correlations exist between auditory digit span and the four sets of outcome measures obtained, but they fail to establish either a pattern of correlation, or a clear cause and effect.

  The result reported here is tentative, representing a single point-of-time measure (with individual variation) for a sample about which limited information is provided, especially so in relation to memory tasks. There is no account of language variation, prior language learning, or a histogram of placements to suggest differences in the use of working memory between individuals. It is not clear why working memory would account for individual variation in the light of the results reported, since no measures were taken to demonstrate differences in working memory in the first place. Indeed, working memory is simply demonstrated to correlate with performance; it is not demonstrated that working memory accounts for clearly significant variation in performance with other intervening variables factored out of the equation.

Preisler G, Ahlstrom M, Tvingstedt AL (1997) The development of communication and language in deaf preschool children with cochlear implants. International Journal of Pediatric Otorhinolaryngology 41(3): 263–272.

Population size
   19
Demographics
   Age: range 3.0–6.11 years
   Gender: males (9), females (10)
   Aetiology: meningitis (6), hereditary congenital (9), progressive (4)
   CI device: Nucleus 22 multichannel
   Age at CI: range 1.11–5.4 years
   CI experience: range 4 months–3 years (average 20 months)
   Parents' status: all hearing
   Educational setting: original: all preschool. Fifteen attended special preschool; for four
      there was no special preschool in the locality; current: range of special and mainstream
      pre- and primary schools. Mainstream placements have signing assistants
Selection criteria
   All children born between 1990 and 1994, receiving implants before the summer of 1996
   (n = 27).
   Deselection: one not using CI, one parental refusal, in remaining cases no contact
      established
Dependent variables
   Direct measures: video observation in home and school settings
   Indirect measures: teacher and parent interviews
   Average four video recordings of each child
Independent variables
   Not applicable
Method
   General descriptive reporting; no statistical analysis
Results
   The study is an ongoing longitudinal and qualitative psycho-social study of the
   communicative development in 19 preschool children with cochlear implants, using sign
   language. The children are video-recorded in natural interaction settings.
      Analysis of patterns of communication shows that 16 of the children use sign language
   in communication with adults and peers. With regard to oral communication, 13 children
   were observed to utter single words or speech-like sounds on an adult's request, but
   seldom used spoken words spontaneously. Six children used single spoken words in
   dialogues with adults if the content of the dialogue was about the here and now, and if
   the topic of reference was clear (these children had been using their implants for
   between one and almost three years, with a mean duration of 2.8 years). None of the
   children in the study was able to take part in age-adequate play activities with peers
   when speech was used in communication.
      Three children were still learning sign language because of late diagnosis of deafness, or
   because they had not had access to a signing environment. As a consequence they still had
   difficulties in participating in linguistic communication with adults and with other children.
      Generally, children were:

      '... observed to respond with sign language sentences mixed with one or two
      spoken words. One of the children used spoken sentences with adults, but
      depended on sign language in order to understand the meaning of the message.

As the adults had difficulties in understanding the child's spoken language, the child's articulation was poor, and as the child had just recently started learning sign language, there were considerable problems, both with respect to oral and signed dialogues' (p.268).

Parents and teachers reported that all of the children vocalized more since they started to use their implants (p.268).

'The majority of the parents were convinced that sign language was of utmost importance for their child's well-being, enabling them to communicate with peers, parents and teachers. But all of them nourished a hope that someday in the future, their children would be able to communicate with speech, at least to some extent. This would enable their children to take part both in the deaf society and also in the world of the hearing' (p.269).

Conclusions

Common traits are shared with international studies on cochlear implant outcomes:

'... all of the children perceive environmental sounds, and most of them perceive and produce a limited set of spoken words/sentences in well defined contexts. The children who use sign language and attend preschools with deaf children, command a language that enables them to take part in the world around them, to join in and interact with others, and share meanings and ideas with adults and peers' (p.270).

'The situation of the cochlear-implanted children in preschools/schools where speech is the main language, gives cause for apprehension. Their opportunities to take part in dialogues with peers are limited, they interact mostly with signing adults, and adults often take the role of interpreter for both other adults and children' (p.270).

Observations

This research is interesting because it is the only research in the studies reviewed here to draw on long-standing experience with sign bilingualism as targeted language development. Effects of cochlear implantation on communication are discussed with reference to early mother–infant interaction, the development of communication and language, and the significance of early close relationships for children's social and emotional development.

The authors take a radically different approach to investigating outcomes of pædiatric cochlear implantation, one that necessarily places outcomes in the context of a predominantly bilingual education environment.

The work is purely qualitative in nature, using no statistical analyses. Moreover, the article is an interim report based on only two years' post-implantation data. The authors report that progress made by the cochlear-implanted children in their sample is comparable (in terms of spoken language acquisition) to that of children elsewhere. As one of the findings of interest, the authors report that teachers tended to overestimate cochlear-implanted children's spoken-language skills, while at the same time tending to underestimate children's cognitive ability. It is clear that more research into sign bilingualism would be of very great value, and that this should draw on quantitative as well as qualitative assessment. As yet, little of this research has been published in English.

Purdy SC, Chard LL, Moran CA, Hodgson SA (1995) Outcomes of cochlear implants for New Zealand children and their families. Annals of Otology, Rhinology and Laryngology (Supplement) 166:102–105.

Population size

6

Demographics
CI device: Nucleus multichannel
Aetiology: congenital (3), meningitis (3)
Gender: males (4), females (2)
Communication mode: oral (1), total communication (5)
Age at onset: range 0–4:10 years, mean 2:0 years (SD = 2:1)
Duration of deafness: range 2:3–8:0 years, mean 4:10 years (SD = 2:1)
Age at CI: range 2:6–12:10 years, mean 6:3 years (SD = 3:2)

Selection criteria
No selection criteria detailed

Dependent variables
Speech perception:
- PLOTT subtest 1, 2-9
- Discrimination After Training (DAT)
- CID ESP
- NU-CHIPS
- PB-K words
- BKB/A sentences
- TACL-R
- GAEL-S
- PPVT-R

Parental stress – parents used a diary to record comments and rate changes in communication, interaction, discipline and behaviour using a five-point Lickert scale. Structured interactions between child and parents were videotaped and analysed

Parents of older children (n = 4) completed the Revised Behavior Problem Checklist (RBPC). Teachers rated child classroom behaviour using the Connor's Teacher Rating Scale

Parents completed the PSI, while their social support was assessed using the Norbeck Social Support Questionnaire (NSSQ)

Independent variables
Speech perception
Parental stress

Method
No statistical analysis, presumably due to low numbers

Results
'At 6 to 12 months, speech perception had improved to the level of good detection in one child and to good discrimination and closed-set word recognition in others' (p.103).

'Age equivalent scores for four children evaluated at 6 to 12 months after implantation indicate language delays of 1:6 to 4:7 years (mean 2:7, SD = 1:5)' (p.103).

For five out of six parental reports, 'the pattern of change was varied, with little change at times and big changes at others' (p.104).

'On average both parents and children signed about half as often as they vocalized. There was wide variation, but in general, communication between parent and child was very good and parents were effective at keeping the child on task' (p.104).

With regard to child behaviour: 'Some children had problems in specific areas, especially conduct and socialized aggression [...] but otherwise no significant problems were evident (p.104).

'The range of [parental stress] scores indicates extremely high parenting stress for some families. [...] PSI scores were generally consistent across time, but increased slightly in the three families studies at 12 months' (p.104).

Observations
Six children with multichannel cochlear implants and their families were evaluated by means of multiple measures to determine the impact of the cochlear implant on the child's speech perception, language, communication mode and behaviour, and on the

parents' stress levels.

Although this study reports on only six cochlear-implanted children, the results are included here because the data derive from New Zealand (where large datasets are unlikely, if only in light of population size), and because the study reports both spoken-language outcomes and stress levels among parents.

Results show high individual variation in outcome, and very high parenting stress in some families,

> 'but on average, stress was lower and social support networks were more extensive than those previously reported in studies of parents of deaf children in the United States' (p.102).

Results are drawn from a very wide range of measures focused on a narrow set of variables in relation to spoken language outcome and parental stress. Nevertheless, the results are not out of keeping with those reported elsewhere in this volume, with the exception of the comparatively milder levels of parental stress, which the authors note may be attributable to cultural variation (pp.104–5).

Pyman B, Blamey P, Lacy P, Clark G, Dowell R (2000) The development of speech perception in children using cochlear implants: effects of etiologic factors and delayed milestones. American Journal of Otology 21(1): 57–61.

Population size
75

Demographics
Age: up to 5 years
Age at CI: range 1.5–5.9 years, mean 3.2 years (SD = 1.2)
CI experience: 0.5–12 years, mean 4.1 years (SD = 2.8)
Encoding strategy: range F0F1F2 - SPEAK
CI device: Cochlear multichannel
Aetiology: detailed range
Other: delayed 'milestones'; cognitive and motor delays

Selection criteria
Consecutively implanted children at the Melbourne Royal Victorian Eye and Ear Hospital between 1985 and 1998. Two exclusions accounted for

Dependent variables
Speech perception scores. Different tests used with different children, therefore a five-scale classification of performance levels was used

Independent variables
Aetiology
Motor and cognitive delays

Method
Chi-square analysis; linear model analysis of variance (delayed/non-delayed co-varied with outcome scores over time)

Results
'The incidence of motor and cognitive delays were fairly evenly spread across etiologic factors, except for cytomegalovirus, which had a much higher than average incidence. Children with motor and/or cognitive delays were significantly slower than other children in the development of speech perception skills after implantation. Etiologic factors did not have a statistically significant effect on speech perception outcome' (p.57).

The proportion of variance accounted for in the analysis was 39% (p.59). There was a highly significant association between cause and the incidence of delays ($p < 0.001$); moreover, children who show evidence of cognitive delays are also likely to show evidence of motor delay, and vice versa. (p.59)

'The proportion of children in oral/aural [*n* delayed = 6/37] rather than in total communication and other manual communication educational settings [*n* delayed = 14/18] was the only one of the [non-central] variables that was significantly different for groups A [not delayed] and B [delayed]' (p.59).

Conclusions

'It is likely that central pathologic states account for a substantial part of the variance among children using cochlear implants. Specific indicators of central pathologic states should be used to assess a child's prognosis in preference to less specific information based on etiologic factors alone' (p.57).

Observations

This is an article of considerable significance in that the authors investigate the considerable individual variation in achievement between paediatric cochlear-implanted children. They focus on the notion of 'delayed milestones' in cognitive development as caused by motor and cognitive characteristics in cochlear implant candidates. However, an assessment of cognitive delay when this is based on speech-perception outcome scores suggests only a reductive operational definition of cognition; excluding linguistic, psycho-social and educational measures.

The authors found significant correlation between performance measures (speech perception scores only) and the pathological states of the children in the post hoc analysis. The research population of 75 is a subsample from the group of consecutive implanted children at the Melbourne Royal Victorian Eye and Ear Hospital between 1985 and 1998, and in terms of the characteristics for inclusion in the study this represents a considerable size population. The population derives from a longitudinal outcome assessment reported by Blamey et al. (2001), included elsewhere in this volume.

Research of this type should really be extended to cover a more longitudinal, and critically, a wider assessment of performance of this group of children over time and in various aspects of their lives.

As an aside, the article shows a clear link between placement and cognitive and motor ability that the authors found to be statistically significant (*p* = 0.004). Whereas 16% of the oral population (*n* = 43) were delayed on the basis of pathological and/or psychological diagnosis, 78% of those in total communication/manual settings were delayed (*n* = 32) (p.60). This can probably be explained by school-entry procedures and patterns of auto-selection among schools' candidature, since those least delayed are also those most likely to derive greater performance results from aural rehabilitation and mainstreaming/inclusion.

The relatively high incidence of underperformance among cochlear implant candidates is explained by a high correlation between cause of deafness and motor and cognitive delays.

Quittner AL, Smith LB, Osberger MJ, Mitchell TV et al. (1994) The impact of audition on the development of visual attention. Psychological Science 5(6): 347–353.

Population size

28

Population comments

Matched group of non-implanted deaf children; control group of age-matched hearing children (experiment 1)

Demographics

Experiment 1 (n = < 28)

Age: range 6–13 years in two groups, 6–8 (mean 7.4 years) and 9–13 (mean 10.5 years)

CI use: range 1–6 years

CI device: single channel and multichannel (numbers not detailed)

Communication mode: oral (14), total communication (13)

Educational setting: residential (5), self-contained classroom (7), mainstreamed (15)

Experiment 2 (n = 11)
  Age: range 6–14
  CI use: average 8.9 months (first test), 18.1 months (second test)
Selection criteria
  Recruited via the Indiana University School of Medicine
Dependent variables
  Visual attention:
Experiment 1
  Speeded selective response task using numbers (pushing a button whenever a nine
  appeared following a one); stream of 540 numbers
Experiment 2
  As experiment one, but twice, with an average 8.2-month test interval
Independent variables
  Audition
Method
Experiment 1
  3 (group) × 2 (age) analysis of variance (ANOVA)
Experiment 2
  3 (group) × 2 (time of test) analysis of variance (ANOVA)
Results
Experiment 1
  Data for one cochlear implant child was not analysed because the child made more than
  100 false alarms. Analyses indicated no differences between single- and multi-channel
  implants, so this difference was not entered as a variable (p.348).
    Significant effects were observed for both group ($p < 0.001$) and age ($p < 0.05$), with
  older children making more reliably correct responses, but did not differ in the number of
  correct responses. Among the younger children there was a difference between hearing and
  deaf groups, but this difference in performance was not observed in older children (p.349).
    Similar main effects were also observed for incorrect responses, with a significant
  decline in incorrect responses with age only observed in the cochlear implant group:
  older children with a cochlear implant made substantially fewer false alarms than
  younger deaf children with a cochlear implant (p.349).
    This effect of reliable performance increases between age groups was replicated using
  a statistical measure indexing the degree to which children's responses discriminated
  between the correct response signal and all other input (p.349).
    While younger deaf children employed different response strategies than same-age
  hearing children, all the older children utilized similar response strategies (p.349).
Experiment 2
  A main effect of time only was observed ($p < 0.05$), with both groups making more
  correct responses at the second test interval. Analysis of time revealed a significant
  group and time interaction ($p < 0.05$), with the cochlear-implanted group making half as
  many false alarms at the second test than at the first, while the non-implanted group
  made slightly more false alarms at the second test (p.351). Similar findings were also
  observed for the type of responding (impulsive or showing greater inhibitory control)
  (p.351).
Conclusions
Experiment 1
  '... deaf children have more difficulty in a visual task requiring selective responding than
  do hearing children [and] as indicated by the false alarms and the measure of d', older
  deaf children who have access to sound through cochlear implants have less difficulty in
  discriminating and responding selectively to relevant visual information than do older
  deaf children without implants. These results are consistent with the idea that access to
  sound through an implant accelerates the development of selective processing in deaf
  children' (p.349)

Experiment 2

'Individual deaf children using cochlear implants showed more rapid developmental gains in a visual task than did deaf children using hearing aids. [...] However, these changes did not occur immediately, but were measurable some time after a year's experience with the implant. Thus, a history of auditory experience promotes the ability to respond to some visual targets while not responding to others' (p.351).

Observations

The authors argue that there is compelling evidence for developmental dependencies between sensory modalities. In this study, they test the responses of children to visual cues; the children are divided into three groups, hearing children, deaf children without cochlear implants and deaf children with cochlear implants. They observe that deaf children perform much more poorly than do hearing children, but those deaf children with cochlear implants perform better than those without. The results, the authors conclude, suggest that a history of experience with sound matters in the development of visual attention (p.347).

'The idea that hearing might play an important role in the development of visual attention derives from clinical reports that deaf children are more distractible and impulsive than same-aged hearing children, and specifically, show deficits in visual matching tasks requiring selective attention...' (p.347).

Such clinical evidence would seem at odds with evidence collected from deaf education classrooms, for example the educational research by Erting (1987), Johnson and Erting (1989) and Erting et al. (1990).

As the authors suggest, rather than considering different abilities in different sensory modalities, their study seeks 'evidence for a specific role of hearing, by studying changes in deaf children's performance in this visual task after they have "been made to hear" via a cochlear implant' (p.347).

Experiment 1 is limited by a lack of description and the single point-in-time measure, while the significant difference of performance is measured for age (not a true over-time development measure), with older implanted subjects attaining higher performance than younger implanted subjects, relative to non-implanted subjects. In this first experiment, no details are reported for actual experience of cochlear implantation within the two age groups, so that the effect cannot be attributed unequivocally to the cochlear implant (or audition).

Anticipating these two objections, experiment 2 therefore replicates the exercise, but for a smaller group of subjects (*n* = 11) over an eight-month average test interval. Although the test interval covers only eight months of cochlear implant experience on average, results indicate significantly greater improvement in the visual task for cochlear-implanted subjects than for non-implanted subjects.

The authors conclude that:

'Because sound is part of the expected environment of epigenetic process, it is not surprising that development without sound in altered in some way. This changed developmental course need not be one of "deficits". For example, deaf adults are better than hearing adults at detecting motion in the periphery and show enhanced ability to pick up and remember complex visual signs [...] However, impoverished experiences with sound do appear to limit the development of attention, such that relative to their hearing peers, deaf children have difficulty responding only to target information' (p.352).

In line with the authors' observation, we would agree that it 'is not logically or intuitively obvious why access to sound via a cochlear implant should matter for success in the visual task' used in this study, even though the authors note that it does. They conclude that

'attention may best be viewed as a behaviour of the whole organism, one that emerges in and depends upon the developmental interplay of a variety of processes and experiences' (p.352).

Rose DE, Vernon M, Pool AF (1996) Cochlear implants in prelingually deaf children. American Annals of the Deaf 141(3): 158–261.

Population size
151

Demographics
No demographic data collated, but 3 were single-channel CI users (p.260)

Selection criteria
All public and private residential and day schools for the deaf with 100 or more students in the US were targeted. Response rate 70% (45 out of 64)

Dependent variables
Not applicable

Independent variables
Not applicable

Method
Not applicable

Results
'Of the 151 implanted children identified, 71 (47%) were no longer using the cochlear implant. Of the remaining 80 children (53%) still wearing the device, we could not specifically determine the percentage who derived significant benefit from the device and the percentage who did not' (p.258).

Eighty (53%) of the children are wearing their units on a regular basis (p.260). Sixty-five percent of those wearing their units were concentrated in three programmes, all running oral programmes.

Conclusions
'If this sample is representative, it would mean that of the over 1800 children who have been implanted in the United States, a large number (perhaps over half) may have ceased to wear the device or receive little benefit from it' (p.260).

Observations
All private and public residential and day schools for the deaf in the US that have 100 or more students were surveyed to see how many prelingually deafened students they had with cochlear implants and how many of these students were still using the device. Responses came from 70% (45 of 64) of those schools surveyed.

This often-quoted study is a particularly controversial one among those reviewed here, and it has been extensively reviewed and criticized. Nevertheless, it merits attention because of a number of key characteristics.

First, it targets a highly contested area of outcomes of paediatric cochlear implantation, namely the extent of non-use of the device by recipients. Generally statistics on non-use are being kept by implant centres, but since users may be inaccurate in the information they give about use of their implant to centre staff, these data are not necessarily a good source of information. By the same token, the questionnaire respondents in this study may not accurately state their use of the implant. Second, the number of children sampled in this study is considerable, with 151 children included by targeting residential and day schools for the deaf in the US.

According to Kluwin and Stewart (2000), the study is limited by the fact that only residential schools were sampled.

'Consequently, the negative results reported by Rose et al. (1996) are just as suspect as the positive results reported by other researchers' (Kluwin and Stuart 2000, p.27).

However, the sample did, according to Rose et al., include three oral programmes. These three schools (of the 45 responding, 7%) contributed 65% of the children wearing their implants. This observation suggests that a supportive educational environment can contribute to continued device use. However,

'Many other children were in oral-only programs after receiving the implant, but transferred to residential, total communication, or ASL oriented schools when the implant failed to enable them to understand speech after extended auditory rehabilitation. Often the transfer was made on the advice of the teachers and staff of the oral program' (pp.259–60).

It is clear that at least no children with implants in mainstream schools were included. With regard to the devices, it is noted that three of the 151 children wore single-channel devices. Rather than the focus on programmes being a weakness, it is likely that the research is affected by age at implantation. The research does not take into account the current move towards earlier implantation.

Schulze-Gattermann H, Illg A, Schoenermark M, Lenarz T, Lesinski-Schiedat A (2002) Cost-benefit analysis of pediatric cochlear implantation: German experience. Otology and Neurotology 23: 674–681.

Population size
Group 1: 34 children implanted between the ages of 0 and 1.9 years; group 2: 43 children implanted between the ages of 2 and 3.9 years; group 3: 48 children implanted between the ages of 4 and 6.9 years; and group 4: 33 children with hearing aids

Demographics
Current age: not reported
Age at onset: not reported
Age at CI: as stated under 'Population size' above
Duration of deafness: not reported
Life expectancy: study reports costs until the child is 16 years old

Setting The Medical University of Hanover, Germany

Method
Economic evaluation type: cost-benefit analysis
Study perspective: payers
Comparator intervention: hearing aids
Source of effectiveness data: none incorporated
Direct costs: charges
Indirect costs: educational expenses
Discount rate for costs and benefits: 6%
Outcome measure: cost savings to education
Currency and price year: €, 1999
Sensitivity analysis: two scenarios are used to vary costs. The first lowers costs for CI
    users and the second lowers costs for hearing aid users

Results
In the base case only cochlear implantation in the under-2-year-olds (group 1) produced a lower net present value for cumulated discounted costs of €138,000 (£99,479 or US$149,567) compared to €160,000 (£115,339 or US$173,412) for hearing aid users (group 4). Group 2 had a net present value of €170,000 (£122,548 or US$184,251) and group 3 of €177,000 (£127,594 or US$191,838). The same finding was found in scenario 1, although the net present values were €138,000 (£99,479 or US$149,567) for group 1, €170,000 (£122,548 or US$184,251) for group 2, €185,000 (£133,361 or US$200,508) for group 3 and €172,000 (£123,989 or US$186,417) for group 4. In sensitivity analysis 2 none of the implanted groups had a lower net present value than the hearing-aided children; group 1 €128,000 (£92,271 or US$138,729), group 2 €147,000 (£105,967 or US$159,321), group 3 €146,000 (£105,246 or US$158,237) and group 4 €123,000 (£88,667 or US$133,311). (All figures in brackets are £ or US$ for 2001/2).

Conclusions
'This study shows that pediatric cochlear implantation has positive cost-benefit ratios

compared with hearing aid users, depending on the age at implantation. From the payers' perspective, implantation of prelingually deafened children is strongly recommended if children receive implants before the age of two years because of costs savings of 13% ... compared with hearing aid users up to the age of 16 years. Implantation between the ages 2 and 3.9 years can be recommended from an educational perspective because of statistically significant differences of educational settings compared with hearing aid users. Those lead to 7% higher total costs. Implantation of children between ages 4 and 6.9 years must be seen more critically on the basis of cost-benefit results because of a negative cost-benefit ratio' (p.679).

Observations

This paper is not a true cost-benefit economic evaluation; it would be more appropriately described as a cost-minimization study. The study does not attempt to attach a value to benefits in monetary terms – this would require the use of methods such as contingent valuation or conjoint analysis. An analysis that only considers changes in costs is misleading for resource allocation decisions, since only programmes that are cost saving would be seen as worthwhile – this ignores the effectiveness of the intervention. In addition, educational placement is only an intermediate measure of outcome. That is it may be an indicator of what a child is likely to achieve but does not actually measure the end-point outcome of educational qualifications achieved or higher income earned as a result of improved educational opportunities.

Shea JJ, Domico EH, Lupfer M (1994) Speech perception after multichannel cochlear implantation in the pediatric patient. American Journal of Otology 15: 66–70.

Population size
30

Population comments
Subsample from total of 39 implanted at the Shea Clinic, Tennessee

Demographics
Demographics detailed in table by group, covering:
* gender
* aetiology
* communication mode

Selection criteria
Children who had at least 6 months' experience with their cochlear implant

Dependent variables
Speech perception test battery
Closed-set: Iowa, MTS, ESP, NU-CHIPS
Open-set: GASP, MAC, PB-K
Numbers of children participating fluctuates between tests and over time

Independent variables
Preimplantation scores
For group 2 (prelingual deafness) only:
* age at CI
* age at onset of deafness

Method
Binomial statistical measures at each test interval. ANOVA for group 2 (prelingual deafness)

Results
Group 1 (postlingually deafened children)
Results concern only four children, with open-set results being achieved by six months post-implantation. There were no statistically significant changes in test scores after the 18-month test interval; two children continued to improve at 36-month test interval (p.68).

Group 2 (prelingually deaf children)
Group performance tended to be poorer than that of group 1 subjects, although all subjects did improve over time. ANOVA analysis via Pearson Product Moment correlation revealed that older children, as indicated by their age at implantation, tended to perform better on the Iowa Male/Female ($p < 0.01$) and MTS ($p < 0.01$), while age at onset of deafness was significantly correlated with scores on GASP Words ($p < 0.01$), GASP Sentences ($p < 0.01$ and Monosyllabic Words ($p < 0.05$) (p.69).

Conclusions
Multichannel cochlear implantation is a safe and effective treatment for profound hearing loss in the paediatric population (p.69).

Prior experience of auditory input is thought to be a significant contributory factor to postimplantation test performance, with postlingually deaf children outperforming prelingually deaf children (p.70).

Observations
This research is an early report comparing postlingually implanted children with prelingually implanted children. The weakest element in the research is the serious migration in and out of tests and test intervals, while findings are reported for just four postlingually deafened children (ranging in age at onset of deafness between 5.3 and 15.0 years). Therefore the reported conclusions pertaining to age at implantation and onset of deafness are tentative.

Smith LB, Quittner AL, Osberger MJ, Miyamoto RT (1998) Audition and visual attention: the developmental trajectory in deaf and hearing populations. Developmental Psychology 34(5): 840–850.

Population size
51
Population comments
With age-matched controls: HAs ($n = 51$) and hearing ($n = 51$)
Demographics
Experiment 1 (n = 51)
Age at onset: prelingual
CI experience: 0.6–6.6 years
Educational setting, language mode (oral/total communication) and aetiology are detailed in Table 2 (p.843).
The group included both single-channel and multichannel users
Experiment 2 (n = 18)
Age at onset: prelingual
CI experience: 0.6–2 years
Age: mean 67 months, range 51–86 months
Selection criteria
All implanted at the Department of Otolaryngology at the Indiana University School of Medicine
Dependent variables
Visual attention
Experiment 1
Speeded selective response task using numbers (pushing a button whenever a 9 appeared following a 1); stream of 540 numbers
Experiment 2
Simplified speeded response task: pushing a button whenever a 0 appears
Independent variables
Audition

Method
Experiment 1
  3 (group) (2 (age) analysis of variance (ANOVA)
Experiment 2
  One-tailed t-test
Results
Experiment 1
  Analysis of variance demonstrated main effects of group ($p < 0.001$) and age ($p < 0.001$), and an interaction between group and age ($p = 0.05$). Post hoc comparisons indicated that at the youngest three age levels, both groups of deaf children performed reliably more poorly than did hearing children, and the two groups of deaf children did not differ from each other. In the other age groups, children in the cochlear implant group performed reliably better than did those in the deaf control group. In summary, the difference between the two groups of deaf children is more in the magnitude of the developmental gain than in the timing of the developmental shift (p.843).
  'The timing of major developmental change in this task occurred between 7 and 9 years of age, with deaf children just slightly delayed behind hearing children' (p.844).
Experiment 2
  Overall, the young deaf children subselected for this experiment did not perform particularly well on this task. Six of 18 children in the cochlear implant group and nine of 18 in the deaf control group scored at or below the 5th percentile of the (hearing) normative sample for this task. But although the group performance was weak, there was age-related incremental growth, more pronounced for the children in the cochlear implant group than in the deaf control group (p.845).
Conclusions
  Results suggest that sensitivity to environmental sounds is related to the beginning of developmental changes in the control of visual attention (p.846).
Observations
  This research continues the themes of earlier research by Quittner et al. (1994) concerning the contribution of sound to visual attention performance, as measured by a selective response task using numbers flashed on a CRT screen. It takes from that earlier study a notable issue in that some demographic variables are described (reported) but not controlled. In fact, the authors note that the cochlear-implanted children and deaf control children in this study were 'recruited from the same population, and thus population differences seem an unlikely source of the better task performance' (p.846) of cochlear-implanted children. But description does not equate with factoring out: in experiment 1, 10 out of 51 children with a cochlear implant were in fully mainstreamed setting, whereas only three in the deaf control group were. Twenty-seven (over 50%) used oral communication, whereas only 14 in the control group did. Since the authors are exploring a novel issue with no factors known to predict outcome – and are therefore not sure about the attribution of the effects measures, offering alternative explanatory theories to support findings at each step, in itself a good practice – it would seem a good idea to first control all the clearly identifiable factors known to account for variation in other measures.
  As a follow-up to the earlier research, these experiments are more targeted and better fitted to the explanatory theories proposed. Drawing on the patterning of the findings, the authors hypothesize on a multicomponent model of development and task performance, in which access to sound and performance on a task are related through an ability to visually select appropriate cues, an ability that 'kicks in' at a certain stage in child development. Borrowing from a 'division of labour hypothesis' they propose that deaf children may perform more poorly in laboratory tasks because:
  'in the larger attentional field of everyday life, distributed visual attention is more adaptive. Thus, access to sound may be an enabling condition because it frees up visual attention, allowing it to become task specific' (p.847).

This explanation is, however, not ultimately convincing, as the authors recognize in their reference to research on deaf children of deaf parents. Such research:

'suggests that deaf parents of deaf children are skilled in organizing their children's attention during social interaction and do so in ways that are not typical of hearing parents of deaf children [...] It is possible that these systematic cues may present an ecology in which highly selective visual attention can develop. In other words, although access to sound may play a critical role in the development of visual attention in typically developing children, there may be alternative routes – those that do not include access to sound – to the same end' (p.849).

This assessment leaves the very same query as at the end of the first set of results in 1994: 'is not logically or intuitively obvious why access to sound via a cochlear implant should matter for success in the visual task' (Quittner et al. 1994, p.325). More practically, perhaps, the question becomes: are there other factors that might explain the reported attention deficit behaviours which triggered the current investigative route?

Spencer LJ, Tye-Murray N, Tomblin JB (1998) The production of English inflectional morphology, speech production and listening performance in children with cochlear implants. Ear and Hearing 19(4): 310–318.

Population size
25
Demographics
Age: range 5–16 years (mean 5.7 years)
CI experience: ≥ 2 years
Age at onset: before 18 months, 2 after (26 and 30 months)
Processing strategy: F0F1F2 (3), MPEAK (22)
Communication mode: 'simultaneous communication' speech and Signed English
Educational placement: residential school for the deaf (1) others not detailed
Second group of 13 HA, age range 6–14 years (mean 10.2) – difference quoted as not significant
All HAs were candidates for CI, four were subsequently implanted
Selection criteria
Not detailed
Dependent variables
12-minute spontaneous conversation, transcribed and coded.
SALT (conversation); WIPI (speech intelligibility)
Independent variables
CI experience
Phoneme production
Closed-set speech recognition performance
Method
Between-group comparison
Results
Children who had cochlear implant experience produced significantly more English inflected morphemes than children in the hearing aid group. Cochlear implant participants also expressed the inflected endings by using voice-only mode 91% of the time, whereas hearing aid participants used voice-only mode 1% of the time. In the cochlear implant group, a strong relationship was found between number of morpheme endings used and speech-recognition scores, length of cochlear implant experience and accuracy of phoneme production.

Bound morphemes

The total number of morphemes used by individual members of the cochlear implant group ranged from 0 to 59, with a mean of 16 (SD = 17). Totals for the hearing aid group ranged from 0 to 12, with a mean of 3 (SD = 1). The difference in the use of bound morphemes between groups was statistically significant (p = 0.015).

Speech perception

There was a tendency for children who scored better on the WIPI to include more English inflected endings within conversation.

Speech production

Combined use of all five morpheme endings was also significantly related to accuracy of phoneme production (p = 0.0001) for cochlear implants. No statistically significant correlation for the hearing aid group observed.

Speech and language results + cochlear implant experience relationships were significant between cochlear implant experience and use of third person singular tense (p = 0.003). Length of experience with a cochlear implant was correlated with accuracy of words produced correctly on the imitative sentence task (p = 0.004). The relationship between age at testing, phoneme accuracy, use of plurals, possessives, present progressives, third person singular or regular past was not statistically significant.

Conclusions

The results of this study indicate that input from the cochlear implant facilitates children's ability to perceive and comprehend bound morphemes. The authors speculate that once the children in this study acquired a stable vocabulary base through sign and listening, they may have then extracted the significance of bound morphemes, perhaps through listening, and generalized their use to many contexts.

Observations

The study is a comparison between how children who use either cochlear implants or hearing aids express English inflectional morphemes during conversation, with voice, with sign or with both. A secondary objective was to investigate the relationship between morpheme use in paediatric cochlear implant users and their speech perception skills, length of experience with the device and accuracy of phoneme production. A 12-minute spontaneous conversation was elicited, transcribed and coded. This study compares the performance at a single point in time of a group of cochlear implant users with a group of hearing aid users. It is of particular interest because all children seemed to have been in a form of total communication programme using 'simultaneous communication'. Although it is noted that one child is enrolled in a deaf residential school, there is no account of other placements, but this may be accounted for by the fact that the tables were missing from the digital file reviewed. The study focused on the expression of English inflectional morphemes during conversation. The conversation was controlled by test administration parameters (i.e. it did not present real-life, natural incidents of conversation). The researchers observed that children in the cochlear implant group produced significantly more English inflected morphemes than children in the hearing aid group. It is surprising for a study published in 1998, that the authors report that few studies up to that point have reported on language skills in cochlear implant users. Of course their reference may be to detailed particular linguistic skills, such as morphemic inflections.

The reason for focusing on morphemic inflections (word endings in particular) here is that the authors hypothesize that deaf children, especially hearing-aided deaf children, may not have clear auditory access to detailed linguistic information, such as morpheme-level meaning discriminants, while cochlear implants may offer auditory improvements sufficient for accessing such information.

Two cochlear-implanted children were given a reduced set of WIPI (speech intelligibility), while one was not given the test; the reasons for this deviation are not detailed.

It is possible that the implanted children have increased accuracy in production of all phonemes in general as a result of cochlear implant experience and thus are better able to speak endings. Improvements in phonologic repertoire may give these children a means of marking a previously gained competence in morphology. However, there were some participants who did not use endings, or due to the nature of their productive language structure it was not possible to derive which ending would have been obligatory. In these cases it was not possible to assess the child's knowledge of an ending.

Spencer L, Tomblin JB, Gantz BJ (1997) Reading skills in children with multichannel cochlear-implant experience. Volta Review 99(4): 193–202.

Population size
40
Demographics
Age at onset: 'prelingual'
CI device: Nucleus multichannel
Age: range 6.9–17.5 years; mean 11.2 years (SD = 2.9)
CI use: range 24–108 months; mean 63.3 months (SD = 24)
Communication programme: range of public and private, oral and simultaneous communication placements. One child transferred to state school for the deaf 2 years prior to testing
Comparisons to earlier HA populations, but no clear replication structure or planning in place
Selection criteria
Not detailed. That students were nevertheless carefully selected is suggested by their performance
Dependent variables
Paragraphs comprehension subtest (form G) of the Woodcock Reading Mastery Test (Revised)
Independent variables
Reading achievement
Communication mode
Method
Reports scores, calculated on the basis of regression line function. Contrasted with earlier research on non-cochlear implant populations, not necessarily performing the same test
Results
'Results indicated that nearly one half of the children in this study were reading at or within eight months of their grade level. The reading grade quotient of 0.74 was calculated based on the slope of the regression line for the plot of years in school and reading grade level achieved' (p.193).
In greater detail, of the sample (in size of population):
- 32% read more than 30 months below grade level
- 23% read at or above grade level
- 18% read within eight months of grade level
- 15% read within 12–18 months of grade level
- 2% read between 18–30 months of grade level (p.194).
Conclusions
'This finding indicates that using a cochlear implant has a positive effect on reading achievement level' (p.193).
Observations
The study compared the reading-achievement level of 40 children with deafness who received the Nucleus multichannel cochlear implants between ages 2 and 13 with that of

children with deafness without cochlear implants. This research is of considerable importance, since it is one of very few studies reporting on a standard educational measure of achievement, reading. It is also important to note that the children were placed, according to the authors, in a range of public and private settings and across different programmes. The research population of 40 is not inconsiderable, but there are questions regarding their selection, as adequate details of the sampling criteria or strategy are not given. The wide age range should be noted, also especially significant because the research has not tracked performance over time, so that a number of outside variables may have affected results beyond the researchers' control.

The authors observe that all cochlear-implanted children were reading within eight months of their chronological age, with some reportedly performing at their chronological age. The quoted reading-grade quotient of 0.74 (nearly eight months within grade level on average) is very clearly affected by the top three performers, who, as can be seen in Figures 3 and 4, outperform the rest of the group by at least 50% of the total score range; especially given the relatively small size of the overall group, this clearly affects the overall regression line for the cochlear-implanted children.

In comparing and contrasting the cochlear-implanted children against earlier measures for non-cochlear-implanted populations, a number of other issues arise which make the comparisons extremely ambitious. The oldest quoted source dates back to Furth (1966), on research that included 5224 children, while some other research was conducted using different test batteries.

Summerfield AQ, Marshall DH (1999) Pediatric cochlear implantation and health-technology assessment. International Journal of Pediatric Otorhinolaryngology 47: 141–151.

Population size
Nil – data from published sources and tentative assumptions
Population comments
Educational placement of children on the Nottingham cochlear implant programme was observed
Demographics
Age at onset: not applicable
Age at CI: > 5 years (assumed)
Duration of deafness: not applicable
Life expectancy: 70 years (assumed)
Setting UK
Method
Economic evaluation type: tentative cost-benefit analysis
Study perspective: societal
Comparator intervention: no intervention
Source of effectiveness data: none
Direct costs: net cost to the NHS
Indirect costs: education and other (e.g. special equipment) cost savings
Discount rate for costs and benefits: 6%
Outcome measure: assumed cost savings to education and special equipment and
   improved productivity in adulthood
Currency and price year: £, 1996
Sensitivity analysis: none conducted
Results
Net societal costs ranged from £28,500 (£3,000 per year educational and £1,000 per year other savings assumed) (in 2001/2 prices – £34,497 or US$51,866) to £58,773 (no savings occur) (in 2001/2 prices – £71,141 or US$106,960). Average earnings would be

required to increase by 25–55% to offset these.

Conclusions

'It indicates that paediatric implantation would be cost-saving to society in the UK, provided that implantation saved £3,000/year in the cost of education, £1,000/year in other domains, and permitted an increase in personal income of 25% of the national median household income' (p.150).

Observations

The educational cost savings should have been reported in the numerator of the cost-benefit ratio. Otherwise it appears as if the costs with the programme are simply being compared to costs without the programme, without any attempt to value benefits in monetary terms. Such benefit valuation requires the use of methods such as contingent valuation or conjoint analysis, for example. An analysis that only considers changes in costs is misleading for resource allocation decisions, since only programmes that are cost saving would be seen as worthwhile – this ignores the effectiveness of the intervention.

Summerfield AQ, Marshall DH, Archbold SM (1997) Cost-effectiveness considerations in pediatric cochlear implantation. American Journal of Otology 18: s166–s168.

Population size

Nil – data from published sources (except that the educational placement of 67 children from Nottingham paediatric cochlear implant programme are incorporated)

Demographics

Current age: not reported
Age at onset: not reported
Age at CI: 3 years (assumed)
Duration of deafness: not reported
Life expectancy: 70 years

Setting Nottingham paediatric cochlear implant programme, UK

Method

Economic evaluation type: cost-utility analysis
Study perspective: societal (partial)
Comparator intervention: no intervention
Source of effectiveness data: published data
Direct costs: medical and rehabilitative care costs
Indirect costs: changes in education costs (cost estimates from Hutton et al. 1995).
Discount rate for costs and benefits: 6%
Outcome measure: utility (assumed from published adult literature)
Currency and price year: £, 1996
Sensitivity analysis: conducted by changing the HRQL gain between 0.15 and 0.30 (0.23 the base case value) and the length of device use between 20 and 70 years (70 years the base case).

Results

Cochlear implantation results in a cost per QALY of £12,100 (in 2001/2 prices – £14,646 or US$22,020) without including other special equipment and of £10,000 per QALY (in 2001/2 prices – £12,104 or US$18,198) including the cost savings associated with other special equipment. Cost per QALY estimates ranged from £5,200 (in 2001/2 prices – £6,294 or US$9,463) (HRQL gain of 0.30 and 70 years of use) to £36,000 (in 2001/2 prices – £43,576 or US$65,517) (HRQL gain of 0.15 and 20 years of use) depending on the HRQL and length of device use assumed.

Conclusions

'The present analysis extends the investigation of the cost-effectiveness of pediatric cochlear implantation described by Hutton and Politi by incorporating measurements of medical and educational assignments, in place of plausible estimates. The new evidence corroborates their conclusion that pediatric cochlear implantation *could* prove to be highly cost effective. However, as yet, the evidence is not conclusive' (p.s168).

Observations

This study, as with all cost-utility studies reported in this review, assumes that the gain in HRQL/utility resulting from implantation is achieved immediately and is constant over the implanted child's life. This may be an unrealistic assumption if, as one may expect, it takes time after implantation for a child to derive maximum benefit from implantation or if the gain varies over time, reflecting perhaps temporary problems with the device for example. The HRQL utility gain reported in this study is assumed from the published adult literature, which may not accurately reflect the benefits of cochlear implantation in children if their outcomes differ from those of adults.

Svirsky MA, Meyer TA (1999) Comparison of speech perception in pediatric CLARION® cochlear implant and hearing aid users. Annals of Otology, Rhinology and Laryngology (Supplement) 177: 104–109.

Population size

221

Population comments

Comparison group of 75 HAs, grouped by PTA, 90–100 dB HL ($n = 28$), and 101–110 dB HL ($n = 47$)

Demographics

Age: range < 6–12 years at implantation
CI device: Clarion
Encoding strategy: CIS
Communication mode: oral ($n = 111$) and total communication ($n = 111$)

Selection criteria

All Clarion implant users in the US as per early 1998, aged up to 12 years at implantation. One child excluded because communication mode was not available

Dependent variables

Speech perception: PB-K at 3-, 6-, 12- and 18-month intervals (auditory-only condition, p.106)

Independent variables

Age at CI
Communication mode
Comparison with HAs

Method

Linear regression on HA groups for age (maturation). Regression line used as benchmark comparison for CI children
Kruskal–Wallis one-way analysis of variance (ANOVA) for score against CI experience. This nonparametric test preferred over standard ANOVA because data were not normally distributed
95% and 99% confidence intervals determined for scores obtained by CI users at each test interval, and compared to the mean scores predicted for HAs matched for age at each interval (p.106)

Results

For hearing aid users, no correlation was observed between scores and either test intervals or communication mode, suggesting that no significant progress was made on the PB-K across the test intervals (p.106).

Cochlear implant users made improvements over time that were significant, across age (implanted < 6 and 6–12 years) and communication mode ($p < 0.001$).

For those implanted < 6 years of age, scores matched the HA101–110 dB PTA group by 112 months.

'By 18 months postimplantation, there was no significant difference between the cochlear implant group and the HA90–100 group' (p.106).

The cochlear implant group implanted between 6 and 12 years show similar patterns of improvement, scores being below those for hearing aid users preimplantation, 'but they matched the average levels of the group with more residual hearing (the HA90–100 group) in as little as 12 months postimplantation' (p.107).

No significant differences for communication mode were observed in the cochlear implant developments over time.

Conclusions

'These results clearly suggest that on average, children with hearing losses in the 101 to 110 dB HL range (HA101–110 group) would receive greater speech perception benefits from a cochlear implant than they do from their hearing aids, irrespective of the mode of communication they are currently using' (p.108).

Observations

In order to develop optimal criteria for implantation, the authors suggest it is crucial to test representative samples (or, if possible, full populations) of cochlear implant users and compare their results to those of hearing aid users of the same age and communication mode (oral or total communication), to determine which subgroups of hearing aid users may obtain more perceptual benefit from a cochlear implant than from a hearing aid. This concerns the thresholds of cochlear implant candidacy. In this study, the word- and phoneme-identification skills of deaf children who use either hearing aids or cochlear implants were evaluated and compared.

The authors measured a large population of implant users in speech-perception test intervals for up to 18 months post-implantation. However, as they note, the time interval of testing and the number of children evaluated at each test interval varied, with 'few data at the 18-month test interval' (p.106). It is also worth noting that the numbers of hearing aid users in the comparison groups were significantly smaller at outset.

The findings suggest that by 18 months post implantation, the PB-K scores of cochlear implant users are roughly similar to those of 90–101 dB HL hearing aid users.

This research is significant for the number of children participating (221), but the measure is limited to one single speech-perception task (PB-K). The appropriateness of the PB-K for younger children in particular is in doubt. The authors only report on group results, which can hide the often reported wide distribution of individual performance. The method's disaggregation of children with implants into two groups of age at implantation (< 6 years and 6–12 years) does not result in any differences in findings. Nevertheless, these results are of particular interest in debates on cochlear implant candidacy and the notion of equivalent hearing loss.

Szagun G (2001) Language acquisition in young German-speaking children with cochlear implants: individual differences and implications for conceptions of a 'sensitive phase'. Audiology and Neuro-Otology 6(5): 288–297.

Population size

22

Population comments

Control group of 22 age-matched hearing children

Demographics

Gender: male (10), female (12)

Age at CI: range 14–46 months, mean 29 months

Age at onset: prelingual

Selection criteria

All children attended Cochlear Implant Center Hanover for aural rehabilitation. Only children from monolingual, spoken-language backgrounds (no sign language) and with no additional disabilities were included. The sample was controlled for intelligence on the basis of IQ test scores falling within the normal range

Dependent variables

Grammar and vocabulary measures, collected over 36-month post-implantation period at regular intervals

Vocabulary assessed using parental report

Grammar assessed as mean length of utterance (MLU)

Free play-triggered conversation was video-recorded, transcribed using CHILDES and scored by three researchers

Independent variables

Age

Preoperative residual hearing

Method

2-way ANOVA

Results

There was a significant effect of age ($p < 0.001$), a significant effect of group ($p < 0.001$), and this combined into a significant age and group interaction ($p < 0.001$). Post hoc comparisons revealed that the hearing children increased their MLU significantly between adjacent age points, but for the cochlear-implanted children only the increase between the last two age points was significant (p.292).

Disaggregating the group data to compare individual developmental patterns revealed that three cochlear-implanted children progressed as rapidly as 13 hearing children. Seven cochlear-implanted children had MLU curves similar to nine more slowly progressing hearing children. Six cochlear-implanted children remained at the two-word stage, while slow cochlear-implanted children remained at low MLU levels right up to the 36-month data-collection point. Overall, therefore, the differences between cochlear-implanted children and hearing children became more and more pronounced over time (pp.292–3).

Vocabulary development confirmed the above trends. There was significant correlation between MLU (grammar) and vocabulary development (p.293).

Preoperative residual hearing correlated significantly with linear growth in MLU at all data points, accounting for 53% of variance. Age at implantation correlated significantly with linear growth in MLU at three data points but less strongly, accounting for 25% of variability. Preoperative residual hearing correlated significantly with vocabulary growth, accounting for 42% of variance, but age at implantation did not (p.295).

Conclusions

Young cochlear-implanted children (when considered as a group) acquire spoken language more slowly than do hearing children – but there is significant variation in performance between individuals (p.295).

'The fact that 10 cochlear-implanted children developed at a pace with normally hearing children argues against a "critical period" viewpoint with its narrow age range for setting off grammar...' (p.296).

But the 'sensitive period' view can accommodate slower grammatical development and vocabulary growth as well as typical development because it does not specify a 'trigger age' and extends the sensitive period up to puberty (p.296).

'The fact that implantation age predicted growth in grammar but not in vocabulary lends support to the view that the acquisition of grammar is more strongly determined by age-related maturational processes than the acquisition of vocabulary...' (p.296).

'The present study allows for the conclusion that, for children who undergo cochlear implantation before 4 years of age, it becomes evident around 2–2.6 years after the operation whether a child develops language near normal or not. [...] It is conceivable that a programme of total communication – as is practised in countries such as the USA, Great Britain, or Israel – would be of benefit. Using gestures or sign language would promote the use of symbols, which is an essential component of cognitive development, and could prevent a possible negative influence of insufficient symbol use on cognitive development' (p.297).

Observations

The author notes that, to date, no study has focused on the acquisition of grammar by children implanted before the age of 4, comparing their development to that of hearing children. This study takes a developmental psycholinguistic viewpoint, focusing on the acquisition of grammar and vocabulary (p.289). Two views on language development are pertinent to the study: the notion of a 'critical period', according to which triggers for the development of specific language functions are closely matched to age-points; and separately the notion of a 'sensitive period', a period in which humans have an enhanced capacity for language learning early in life, decreasing gradually up to puberty (p.289). Both views take age as a determining factor in language development. However, for cochlear-implanted children another factor may be the quality of preoperative hearing, and this possibility is included as a factor in the research.

The study focuses on 'mean length of utterance' (MLU) and vocabulary growth as two core measures of language development performance (p.290).

The study reports delays in both grammar and vocabulary development for the cochlear-implanted children as a group, although the performance is characterized by wide individual variation in performance, persistent over time (i.e. those who progress most at first also progress most over time). This delay in spoken language development occurs in young-implanted children (aged below 4), despite the implant being in situ at the time of both 'critical period' and 'sensitive period' of language development. Hence the authors hypothesize that a programme of total communication may be beneficial in preventing a possible negative influence of insufficient symbol use on cognitive development in totally oral/aural programmes (p.297).

Tait DM, Lutman ME (1994) Comparison of early communicative behaviour in young children with cochlear implants and with hearing aids. Ear and Hearing 15: 352–361.

Population size
9

Population comments
n = 27 in total, in three groups of 9: CIs, proficient 'gold/silver' hearing aid users, and in 'bronze' users, not using hearing aids proficiently

Demographics
CI: Nucleus multichannel
Age: < 5 years, detailed per child, range 2:6–4:5 years
Age at onset: detailed per child, range 0:0–2:8 years
Length of hearing aid use: detailed per child, range 0:8–3:9 years
Hearing loss: detailed per child, range 116–120 dB HL better ear
Number of electrodes: detailed per child, range 10–22
Aetiology: CIs early acquired, hearing aid users congenital

Selection criteria
Age-matched, range 2–5 years
No other disability

Dependent variables

Scores of communicative behaviour, including:
- vocal auditory turn-taking
- development of autonomy
- eye contact
- auditory awareness

Independent variables

Hearing technology status

Method

Quantitative video analysis at 6- and 12-month intervals

Pearson correlation coefficients relating first and second replications of each measure

Subsequent pattern correlation analysis

Results

Vocal auditory turn-taking increased steadily for the cochlear-implanted children and gold/silver groups (not for the bronze group where it decreased), while they are more likely to vocalize. This outcome is statistically significant. The cochlear-implanted children outperformed the gold/silver group after 12 months. For eye contact there was a significant linear increase for all groups, but no differences of significance were revealed until one case (with high signed communication skills) was removed.

Conclusions

Over the 12-month assessment period, cochlear-implanted children and proficient hearing aid users developed a strongly vocal/auditory style of communicative behaviour, especially the cochlear-implanted children. This contrasted with a strongly visual/gestural style developed by the poor hearing aid users (in fact, there was no overlap between the scores). It is concluded that children with implants develop their early communicative behaviour along lines that are similar to proficient hearing aid users, but more rapidly and more strongly in the vocal/auditory direction.

Observations

This is a valuable study in that it monitors early communicative behaviour over time (although only two intervals are being reported here) in a comparison between cochlear implant children and 'gold' and 'bronze' hearing aid users, broadly matched on age and hearing loss. The research shares with other research in this series that there is an implied focus in the categories of assessment on eventual spoken-language development and outcome. The research is included in this review despite its low number of nine children in the cochlear implant group because of its relevant data on communicative behaviour patterns (including turn-taking and eye-gaze) in very young cochlear implant children. Given the predominant move towards early implantation, research in this area of outcome is an extremely valuable precursor to tracking a broader set of outcomes over time; the data reported here might suggest means to develop some form of 'baseline assessment' to assist in predicting later results. In these results the data suggest a possible future bifurcation among children's placements along spoken-language and sign bilingual lines.

The authors conclude that children with cochlear implants and proficient hearing aid users developed a strongly auditory/vocal style of communicative behaviour, contrasted with a strongly visual/gestural style developed by the poor hearing aid users.

As an aside: among outcomes for cochlear-implanted children, it was noted that

'one outlying child on the "eye contact measure" had been remarkably proficient at signed communication and retained strong eye contact for over 1 year after implantation' (p.358).

This raises a prior issue about early communication preferences and/or strengths. After removing this case, 'the difference between the two groups [cochlear-implanted children and proficient hearing aid users] became highly significant' ($p = 0.002$), but this also indicated the strong effect of a single case on the low numbers involved.

No details were available on the conditions and contexts of the recordings (i.e. the skills of the interlocutors involved) so that the slightly depressed scores on eye contact among the bronze group cannot be analysed without referring back to previous publications on the methodology.

Tait DM, Lutman ME (1997) The predictive value of measures of pre-verbal communication behaviours in young deaf children with cochlear implants. Ear and Hearing 18(6): 472–478.

Population size
17

Demographics
Age at CI: < 5 years (range 2.7–4.6 years, mean 3.74 years)
Experience of deafness: range 0.7–4.4 years (mean 2.54 years)
Prior experience of hearing: range 0–2.8 (mean 1.14 years)
Education programme: oral (7), total communication (10)
CI device: Nucleus 22
Aetiology: congenital (4), encephalitis (1), meningitis (12)

Selection criteria
'Unselected' range of consecutively implanted children at Nottingham Cochlear Implant Centre
However, one child excluded for 'sporadic use' of CI

Dependent variables
Speech perception measures after 3 years CI:
• Iowa closed-set sentence test
• continuous discourse tracking
• rating of ability to use telephone
• categories of auditory performance (CAP)

Independent variables
Age at CI
Prior performance on video analysis measures taken within one year post-CI

Method
Test percentage scores. Some ceiling effect for Iowa. Battery composite measure (normalized) correlated with video analysis measures using linear regression

Results
There was a significant correlation (p = 0.006) between the video analysis measure taken at the 12-month interval, specifically the extent of auditory and vocal behaviours, and three of the outcomes obtained at the three-year interval: both performance-based measures and the telephone rating. When the four outcomes were aggregated to form a composite measure, the correlation was highly significant (n = 14; not all completed all four tests). There was no significant correlation between the composite measure and the video analysis measures obtained earlier than the 12-month interval.
Outcome measures were highly correlated among each other, indicating statistical redundancy between them (hence composited).

Conclusions
Development of a predominantly auditory and vocal style of early communicative behaviour is predictive of relatively high levels of skill on speech and language tasks measured two years later. Hypothesis that early communicative behaviour can help predict future auditory development is upheld, but confirmation by larger populations is needed.

Observations
This study concerns an analysis of preimplant measures of preverbal communicative behaviour as a predictor of post-implantation speech perception and speech-production tasks. The design used video recordings of preverbal communicative behaviour at the

preimplant stage and the Iowa closed-set sentence test, continuous discourse tracking and a telephone use measure at up to three years post implantation.

There appear to be some ceiling effects at level A of Iowa in the study reported. The wide range of outcomes suggests intervening variables (individuals discussed, see below). Although no such correspondence between intervening variables and outcomes was found, the low sample does not put interventions by other measures beyond doubt; otherwise results such as the ones quoted below are difficult to explain.

> 'The range of performance is best illustrated by two examples. Child A was implanted at the age of 4 years 0 months, having become profoundly deaf as a result of meningitis at 7 months of age. She had a full insertion of 22 electrodes. Her mode of communication was primarily based on signing and she remains in a total communication environment. Twelve months after implantation, her auditory/vocal score was 165, towards the lower end of the range of this sample of children. At the three-year interval she was unable to perform CDT. She achieved 97% in the Iowa test at Level A, but was unable to cope with Level B. She achieved 53% on the Telephone Profile and was one of the four children rated at Category 5 on CAP, being able to understand common phrases without lip-reading, but not to carry out a simple conversation without lip-reading. Child B was implanted at the age of 2 years 8 months, having become profoundly deaf at the age of 1 year 2 months (aetiology uncertain). She also had a full insertion of 22 electrodes. Her mode of communication was primarily based on signing but has become oral/aural. Twelve months after implantation her auditory/vocal score was 267, the highest in this sample. At the three-year interval she was able to perform CDT at 59 words per minute without prior exposure to the material, scored 100% on the Iowa test at both Levels A and B, scored 97% on the Telephone Profile and was consequently the only child in the sample rated Category 7 on CAP.'

Tait DM, Lutman ME, Robinson K (2000) Preimplant measures of preverbal communicative behaviour as predictors of cochlear implant outcomes in children. Ear and Hearing 21(1): 18–24.

Population size
   33
Demographics
   CI device: Nucleus 22 multichannel
   Age at CI: ≤ 5 years (median 45 months (range 30–69 months))
   Aetiology: 13 congenital, 19 meningitis, 1 encephalitis
   Age at onset: median 7 months (IQR 0–20 months)
Selection criteria
   Consecutive selection of all CIs (Nottingham) – no deselections
Dependent variables
   Pre-CI: video analysis measures of vocalizations and gestures
   Post-CI: speech perception: Iowa closed-set speech perception sentence test (both levels), Connected Discourse Tracking (CDT) and an observational measure of telephone use
      Speech production: Edinburgh Articulation Test (EAT)
Independent variables
   Not specified
Method
   Associations between preimplant measures and three-year outcomes were assessed by correlation analysis
   Regression analysis to examine covariation

Results

Three-year post-implantation performance measures of speech identification were correlated with the preimplant measure of autonomy. Telephone use and speech production ability were not significantly associated with preimplant measures. For seven cochlear-implanted children EAT results were unavailable (unexplained). Outcome measures are significantly dependent on age at implantation, but not on age at onset.

Conclusions

Up to 25% of variance (16% Iowa, 27% CDT) in speech identification at three-years post-cochlear implantation may be predicted from pre-cochlear implant communication characteristics — mainly demonstrations of autonomy in preverbal communicative interactions (vocalizations or gesture).

> 'It is likely that a child who is a good communicator before implantation, whether silently or vocally, is likely to have good speech discrimination and intelligibility in later years [of CI]'.

Observations

This study continues the work reported in 1997 into the analysis of preimplant measures of preverbal communicative behaviour as a predictor of post-implantation speech perception and speech production tasks. The design used video recordings of preverbal communicative behaviour at the preimplant stage and the Iowa test, continuous discourse tracking and a telephone use measure at up to three years post-implant. Although the number of children in 1997 (14) was insufficient for a clear assessment of the predictive value of the test of preverbal communicative behaviour, this time the authors concluded, on the basis of an assessment of 33 children, that up to one-third of variance in speech identification performance three years post-implant can be predicted from communicative characteristics inherent to the child prior to implantation.

Tobey EA, Geers AE, Douek BM, Perrin J, Skellet R, Brenner C, Toretta G (2000) Factors associated with speech intelligibility in children with cochlear implants. Annals of Otology, Rhinology and Laryngology 109(12): 28–30.

Population size

46

Demographics

Age: 8–9 years
CI use: 4–6 years
CI device: Nucleus
Communication mode: oral, total communication, 'half' (p.29)

Selection criteria

None detailed, but authors include those responsible for CID studies, also focusing on 8- to 9-year-olds with Nucleus implants

Dependent variables

Speech production
Reading sentences to 'three hearing judges' (p.29)
Speech perception
LNT
No details on test administration or listening experience of judges

Independent variables

Communication mode

Method

Direct linear correlation

Results

> 'Significantly higher open-set speech perception performance was observed for the children using auditory-oral communication as compared to the children

using simultaneous communication on the LNT', scoring 50% versus 30% correct (p < 0.05)' (p.29).

Analysis of variance revealed that the auditory-oral group was significantly more intelligible than the total communication group ($p < 0.01$) (p.29), with scores averaging 81% versus 51% for total communication children.

Higher speech intelligibility was found in individuals who had higher speech perception scores, as a 'moderately strong relationship' (p.30).

Conclusions

'... the overall speech intelligibility appears to be better in children using an auditory-oral mode of communication than in children using simultaneous communication. The variability across children on speech intelligibility measures also appears to be greater in the simultaneous communication group of children. Positive relationships appear between speech perception and overall speech intelligibility in both groups of children' (p.30).

Observations

The authors claim that this research is of significance because it concerns a population of relatively comparable age (8–9 years) who have similar (4–6 years) experience of cochlear implants. However, the study concerns not the analysis of factors associated with speech intelligibility, as suggested by the title, but rather an assessment of communication mode measured at a single point in time.

Comparison of a number of demographic and socio-economic status variables revealed significant differences in the mother's education between oral and total communication children in favour of the oral children, and the fact that the oral children received nearly double the amount of hours of therapy (p.29). This was also detailed for other related research (Geers et al. 2000).

The results demonstrate higher outcome scores for auditory-oral children, but unfortunately the study lacks descriptive detail. There are no details about test administration (for example auditory-only or auditory plus visual modes), no factoring out of intensive oral rehabilitation or significant differences on socio-economic status measures and no account of prior achievement or over-time development.

Tomblin JB, Spencer L, Flock S, Tyler R, Gantz B (1999) A comparison of language achievement in children with cochlear implants and children using hearing aids. Journal of Speech, Language and Hearing Research 42: 497–511.

Population size
29

Demographics
CI device: Nucleus 22 multichannel
CI use ≥ 3 years (2 non-users, 6 minimal users)
Age at CI: range 2.6–13.2 years (mean 4.7 years)
Age: average 10 years.
Audiology: mean R111.9/L114.8 dB
Aetiology: 18 (62%) are 'unknown''
Educational programme: 25 mainstream with interpreter (3 part-time mainstream); 1 oral school for the deaf, 2 state schools for the deaf; 1 category not detailed
(Comparison group n = 29 of non-CI)
No additional complications (normal cognitive ability)

Selection criteria
Not detailed

Dependent variables
English comprehension
1 Rhode Island Test of Language Structure (RITLS)
2 Index of Productive Syntax (IPSyn) – signed and spoken English grammar

Language production
Story retell protocol, 'measure of signed and spoken [English] sentence comprehension'
Independent variables
CI/non-CI
Length of CI use
Prior achievement 6 years before assessment
Method
Percentile rank plotted against age. Confidence interval calculated and used to predict outcomes for age
Results
A mean percentile rank of 92.2 was obtained for cochlear-implanted children on RITLS, with clear overall ceiling effect (one exception); 'age-equivalent' scores; results for HA group not given. Cochlear implant users outperformed hearing aid users on IPSyn (differences in story length not found to be statistically significant). Based on prediction of gains derived from chronological age measures in the hearing aid group, the cochlear implant group consistently performed above predictions for hearing aid users.

In the story retell task the cochlear-implanted children showed opposite use of voice (23%) versus sign (6%) relative to children using hearing aids.
Conclusions
Cochlear implant users achieved significantly better scores (RITLS, IPSyn) than hearing aid users. Chronological age correlates highly with IPSyn levels only among cochlear-implanted children; length of cochlear implant use significantly correlated with IPSyn scores. Clear differences between cochlear implant users and hearing aid users were found after two years of post-implant experience. Length of cochlear implant use rather than age was the principal factor in accounting for IPSyn achievement levels. Children who receive cochlear implants benefit in the form of improved English language comprehension and production.
Observations
In this study the English language achievement of 29 prelingually deaf children with three years or more of cochlear implant experience was compared to matched children without cochlear implants using the Rhode Island Test of Language Structure (RITLS), a measure of signed and spoken sentence comprehension, and the Index of Productive Syntax (IPSyn), a measure of expressive (signed and spoken) English grammar. There are no details on sampling methods or selection criteria detailed in the article.

Children entered the study at different intervals and different ages, while some in the hearing aid group became part of the cochlear implant group during the study, and all were candidates for cochlear implantation. This does mean that the relevance of the prior achievement measure has to be judged against the changing population over time (i.e. the 95% confidence interval may not be an accurate measure).

The authors observed that test scores correlated with length of cochlear implant experience in the cochlear-implanted children, whereas chronological age correlated with non-cochlear implant children, suggesting increased rates of improvements for the cochlear-implanted children.

The hearing aid group age range was slightly higher (3.6–14.3 years) and the hearing losses slightly lower. Home and education situation were comparable.

Correlation of test results with chronological age for hearing aid users suggest a language development curve; the authors comment that the lack of correlation for cochlear implant users suggests that gains resulting from cochlear implant experience overwhelm the correlation. Despite this, the cochlear implant group continued to rely on a combination of speech production and signed English to communicate.

The authors reference research into sign language acquisition patterns (Bellugi 1988) to inverse the claims for natural language acquisition. Bellugi's work aimed to show that deaf children acquire sign language in a pattern in keeping with normal language acquisition in children generally. Their research was an early example to conclude that naturally occurring forms of sign language were a legitimate target for first language acquisition in deaf children. Tomblin et al. here suggest that:

'Thus, most children with prelingual deafness should be fully capable of acquiring any lexical and grammatical aspects of a language regardless of its modality, so long as the sensory system provides appropriate input and there are mature language users providing adequate communication experiences' (p.498).

Truy E, Lina-Granade G, Jonas AM, Martinon G, Maison S, Girard J, Porot M, Morgon A (1998) Comprehension of language in congenitally deaf children with and without cochlear implants. International Journal of Pediatric Otorhinolaryngology 45(1): 83–89.

Population size

13

Demographics

Age at CI: range 1.10–6.6 years (mean 2.8 years)
Age at end of follow-up: 3.9–11.3 years (mean 6.2 years)
HL: profound (mean PTA 113.4 dB)
Aetiology: congenital
CI device: Nucleus (11), Digisonic (2)
Control population of age-matched non-CI deaf children

Selection criteria

No multiple handicaps

Dependent variables

Speech perception battery:
- 'Nelly Carole' test (< age 3 years), 'Vocim' test (≥ age 3 years), validated French translation of IPTA
- single point-in-time measure; test administration adapted to children's preference

Independent variables

Prior achievement pre-CI
Non-CI

Method

Pearson's correlation and 2-way ANOVA to test significance; for each child the age-equivalent score was plotted against age, on tests pre- and post-CI, resulting in three regression curves. No multivariate analysis attempted due to low numbers

Results

The pre-operative receptive language development curve suggests a possible growth over time with the maturation and the speech therapy. Comparison showed the slope for post-operative cochlear-implanted children to be greater than for non-cochlear-implanted children, and that this difference is statistically significant ($p < 0.05$), and that the slope for cochlear-implanted children is greater post- than pre-operatively ($p < 0.05$).

Receptive language level is significantly improved by implantation: scores were better in cochlear-implanted children post-operatively than in non-cochlear-implanted children, and in cochlear-implanted children post-operatively than in cochlear-implanted children pre-operatively. Scores were better in non-cochlear-implanted children than in cochlear-implanted children pre-operatively.

Conclusions

The main conclusion is that receptive language scores grow significantly more rapidly over time after surgery in cochlear-implanted than in matched non-cochlear-implanted children, despite better hearing thresholds of the latter.

Observations

This is a small study carried out by a team at the Hôpital Edouard Herriot (Lyon) on cochlear-implanted children, comparing a cochlear implant population of 13 with an age- and hearing loss-matched population of non-cochlear-implanted children at two point-in-time test assessments: pre- and post-implantation. The design uses two different tests for age groups below 3 years and aged 3 years and above. The findings report accelerated receptive spoken language development for children with cochlear implants. The authors factored out the effect of maturation and rehabilitation in the statistical analysis. But most significantly, the authors go beyond only spoken language as an outcome measure. The test design and administration include cross-modal preferences for all children. Hence also the conscious exclusion of speech production measures:

> 'Speech production skills [...] are known not to be a reliable reflection of oral language competence as a whole. Oral language is an acquired common code in a specific group, enabling exchange of ideas, feelings and knowledge. In humans, speech is one of the channels conveying language' (p.83).

The authors are in agreement with other findings that early implantation is a topic for further investigation.

> 'Another major aim will be to see whether the gap persists between normal-hearing children and cochlear implant users over time. The younger a patient at implantation, the better cortical connectivity and plasticity is able to lead to a good result, but also the smaller the initial gap is. Our study did not distinguish the patients, and our sample was too small to compare subgroups according to the age at implantation. The impression we get, however, is that the earlier the implantation the better the results, with, in some cases, a nearly normal development' (p.88).

Tye-Murray N, Spencer L, Gilbert Bedia E (1995) Relationships between speech production and speech perception skills in young cochlear-implant users. Journal of the Acoustical Society of America 98(5/1): 2454–2460.

Population size
23

Demographics
CI device: Nucleus multichannel
Age at CI: range 2.7–14.2 years, avg. 7.3 years (SD = 3.6)
CI experience: ≥ 24 months, average 34 months (SD = 13)
Age at onset: 0–30 months
Aetiology, processing strategy (MPEAK or FOF1F2) and age at onset detailed in Table 1 (p.2456)

Selection criteria
None detailed. At least 24 months' implant experience

Dependent variables
Speech production:
• Children's Audio-visual Feature Test (consonant-vowel syllable test)

Independent variables
Speech features:
• voicing
• nasality
• duration
• frication
• place of articulation
Recognition mode:
• audition only
• vision only
• audition plus vision

Method
Paired comparison t-tests of individual performance scores

Results

Consonant production
Scores range from 12 to 78% correct (average 37%). With the exception of /v/, consonants associated with visible facial movement were produced with the highest accuracy, while the fricatives were mispronounced most often (p.2457).

Consonant perception
On average, subjects scored 25% consonants correct (SD = 16) in audition-only condition, 44% (SD = 7) in visual condition and 59% (SD = 21) in the combinatory condition, with performance exceeding chance for all conditions (p.2458).

Relationship between perception and production
Relationships between production and audition-only perception were significant for the features place of articulation (p = 0.01), nasality (p = 0.01) and voicing (p = 0.001). In audition plus vision condition, both nasality (p = 0.001) and voicing (p = 0.001) were significant. No significant relationships emerged in the vision only condition (p.2458).

Conclusions
Prelingually deafened children who had used their cochlear implants for at least two years spoke the consonant-vowel syllables with above-chance accuracy, scoring 37% of consonants correct on average. In many ways, the subjects' error patterns resemble those of profoundly deaf children who use hearing aids (p.2459).

However, information received from cochlear implants might influence young cochlear-implanted children's speaking behaviours after an average of 34 months of experience (p.2459).

The numerous consonantal errors spoken by the children in this study underscore the difficulties involved in learning to talk when minimal auditory information is available; however, the degraded signal of the cochlear implant can fulfil some of the roles of an intact auditory signal (p.2460).

Observations
The purpose of the study reported was to examine the relationships between young cochlear-implanted deaf children's abilities to produce the speech features of nasality, voicing, duration, frication and place of articulation in three different perceptual conditions (audition only, vision only and the combination). The central question was how the children's speech recognition and production skills correspond with each other, with the suggestion that speech recognition entails attending to both auditory and visual cues (p.2454).

Tye-Murray N, Spencer L, Gilbert Bedia E, Woodworth G (1996) Differences in children's sound production when speaking with a cochlear implant turned on and turned off. Journal of Speech and Hearing Research 39(3) :604–610.

Population size
20

Demographics
CI device: Nucleus 22
Age at CI: range 2.7–15.3 years, average 5.8 years (SD = 2 .9)
Age: average 9 years
CI use: ≥ 24 months, average 34 months (SD = 8)
Situation: all participants lived at home and attended public school
Communication mode: total communication

Selection criteria
Subpopulation from sample described in other Tye-Murray research

Dependent variables
Speech stimulus items of 14 words produced within target sentence

Independent variables
Speech intelligibility: story-retell activity
Speech perception: Audiovisual Feature Test; Children's Vowel Perception Test
Cochlear implant on and off situations
Speech intelligibility and speech perception test score

Method
Paired comparison t-test; Pearson calculation of significance

Results
'On average, participants were as likely to produce the sounds and features correctly when they spoke with their cochlear implants turned on as when they spoke with them turned off. For example, the average total vowels correct spoken during the device-on condition was 71%, and 70% in the device-off condition. [...] On average, no phoneme of feature of articulation was spoken more accurately in one condition that the other' (p.607).

Comparison with speech intelligibility scores
'On average, children spoke 47% of the phonemes correctly during the story-retell procedure, with scores ranging from 4% to 83%. [...] No significant relationships were revealed between performance on the story retell activity and any of the difference scores' (p.608).

Comparison with speech perception scores
'Two comparisons were significant. Participants who scored better on the Children's Vowel Test also were significantly more likely to show a greater decrement in their vowel production score (r = 0.64, p = 0.01) and their production of the vowel place of articulation feature (r = 0.61, p = 0.01) when speaking with their cochlear implants turned off as opposed to on. [...] Additional data are needed to evaluate whether this relationship is robust' (p.608).

In summary, on average no difference between speaking conditions on indices of vowel height, vowel place, initial consonant place, initial consonant voicing or final consonant voicing was found. Comparisons based on a narrow transcription of the speech samples revealed no difference between the two speaking conditions. Children who were more intelligible were no more likely to show a degradation in their speech production in the device-off condition than children who were less intelligible. In the device-on condition, children sometimes nasalized their vowels and inappropriately aspirated their consonants. Their tendency to nasalize vowels and aspirate initial consonants might reflect an attempt to increase proprioceptive feedback, which would provide them with a greater awareness of their speaking behaviour.

Conclusions
'Children with prelinguistic deafness who have prolonged cochlear implant experience do not change their speech output when speaking with their cochlear implants turned off (for a relatively short period [approximately overnight + 4 hours]) rather than on, in a way that is detectable by a trained listener [Speech and language pathologist...] These results suggest that any degradations that occur when children talk with their cochlear implants turned on are probably subtle' (p.608).

'The fact that children sometimes nasalised their vowels and added aspiration to their initial consonants suggests that they may be attempting to maximize proprioceptive information, even though they receive some auditory feedback via their cochlear implants' (p.609).

Observations
This report is interesting because it takes a higher face-value tack on speech intelligibility impact of cochlear-implanted children. This study reports on 20 children who have worn a Nucleus multichannel device for an average of 33.6 months, and who participated in a device on/off experiment measuring speech production in both conditions. The results of the experiment are modest, with the authors concluding that children with better speech-perception skills with the cochlear implant turned on were no more likely to demonstrate a degradation in performance in the cochlear implant turned-off condition than were the

other children. They shared with other children a tendency to nasalize and aspirate initial consonants, which the authors propose results from attempts to increase proprioceptive feedback during speech articulation.

To some extent, this may also reflect shared speech training, although this possibility is not discussed.

The significance of the study lies mostly in its comparison of outcome scores using two modes, the cochlear implant switched on and turned off. In so doing the authors aim to capture the actual contribution of the implant to test performance. However, this approach has the drawback that the implant-off condition is unfamiliar to the child, which may artificially reduce performance in that condition.

Conclusions seem to suggest that the benefits of cochlear implants on pure audiological perception may be modestly significant rather than spectacularly significant; perhaps analogous to the distinction between HA and HA+, or profound and severe hearing loss. However, note the methodological drawback indicated above.

Tye-Murray N, Spencer L, Woodworth GG (1995) Acquisition of speech by children who have prolonged cochlear implant experience. Journal of Speech and Hearing Research 38(2): 327–337.

Population size
28
Population comments
Divided into three age groups, 2–5 years, 5–8 years and 8–15 years
Demographics
Age at onset: prelingual ≤ 18 months
CI device: Nucleus 22
Age at CI: range 31–170 months, average 85 months (SD = 47)
Residence: all children lived at home
Mode of communication: total communication at home and at school
Placement: 25 were mainstreamed part of the time; 1 attended deaf school
Across the last three measures, the sample is claimed to be representative of the US
   deaf school population
Selection criteria
Children had to have at least 24 months of CI experience to participate. No sampling technique detailed
Dependent variables
Speech production and perception test battery, including:
 • long sentence test
 • story-retell task
 • CID Speech Intelligibility Evaluation (SPINE)
 • audio-visual feature test
 • fundamental speech skills test
 • parent questionnaire
Independent variables
Age
Prior achievement
CI
Method
Percentage scores (some aggregated across tests). Pearson correlation between composite scores and age groups
Results
Speech intelligibility
On average, the entire group of children produced 53% of the phonemes correctly and

22% of the words correctly. Performance within age groups varied widely, as indicated by the large standard deviation bars (p.330).

> 'Ratings of intelligibility were low, corresponding with the relatively poor word production revealed by the transcription procedure. The mean rating of the 10 raters, averaged over all children, was 2.5, on a scale of 1 to 10. Scores ranged from 1 to 9. [...] The 10 listeners who were assigned to the identification task identified which stories the children were describing in 51% of the samples...' (p.330).

Speech production and age at implantation
Older children tend to achieve higher scores than younger children prior to receiving a cochlear implant, but after at least two years of experience with a cochlear implant, older children no longer performed better than the younger group (p.333).

Relationship between speech perception and speech production
> 'Children's abilities to produce speech corresponded well with their abilities to perceive it, as all relationships were significant' (pp.334–5).

Use of sign language
> 'Children used both sign and speech for an average of 83 words (SD = 29) within their 100-word samples. Children used speech-only for an average of nine words (SD = 26) and sign without speech for an average of seven words (SD = 16). Parents assigned an average agreement score of 4.8 (SD = 2.7) to the questionnaire statement, "My child communicates without sign, using speech only." Thus, the questionnaire results indicate a lower incidence of signing than in the story-retell procedure' (p.335).

Conclusions
Conclusion on error analysis
> 'In some ways, their errors resemble those produced by children who have severe or profound hearing loss and use hearing aids' (p.335).

Speech production
Children who are deaf and who receive a Nucleus cochlear implant before the age of 5 years may show greater benefit in terms of speech production measures than children who receive a cochlear implant after the age of 5 years (p.336), while children's speech-production skills were significantly correlated with their speech-recognition skills. Children with better speech-production skills were more likely to have better speech-recognition skills (p.336).

Other outcomes
> 'Results from the story-retell procedure suggest that children who used manual communication or simultaneous communication prior to receiving a cochlear implant do not discontinue signing after receiving a cochlear implant. Use of simultaneous communication increases. The results from the parent questionnaire indicate a somewhat lower incidence of signing. [Yet we] have noted clinically that some children have sign skills that surpass those of their parents' (p.336).

Observations
The study reported has an ambitious range of aims,

> 'to assess whether children acquire intelligible speech following prolonged cochlear implant experience and examine their speech error patterns, to examine how age at implantation influences speech acquisition, to assess how speech production and speech perception relate, and to determine whether cochlear implant recipients who formerly used simultaneous communication (speech and manually coded English) begin to use speech without sign to communicate' (p.327).

The latter form of phrasing is slightly at odds with that reported in the background details, where it is said instead that,

'The final purpose of this investigation was to examine whether children who relied on simultaneous communication [...] prior to receiving an implant continue to integrate sign into their communication mode following implantation... (p.328).

The suggestion is that cochlear implantation does not necessarily lead to a decrease in the use of sign. The two aims are actually subtly different, while the authors conclude, based on their findings, that signing does not disappear from communication mode (p.327). In the former aim this is a negative response, in the second phrasing it is a positive one. The children reported here all used total communication at the time of implantation. The outcomes of the study, despite the ambitious aims, are more modest. There is also the consideration that the use of sign may depend on factors external to the child, such as local policy.

It is concluded that the children acquire some intelligible speech, that implantation before age 5 produces comparatively greater benefits and that children who recognize more speech are likely to speak more intelligibly.

The research population (n = 28), like others included in this review, is comparatively modest. As a criterion they had worn implants for at least 2 years (average 36 months); it is debatable whether this constitutes prolonged experience, although it is clear that studies reporting over very long time periods, such as five or seven years, also face issues about the direct effect of implantation on longitudinal outcomes, relative to those of, for example, rehabilitation services, schooling and maturation.

In relation to comparisons between cochlear implant users and hearing aid users, it is relevant to note the comment that in the error patterns analysed the cochlear implant children resembling hearing aid users (p.335).

Tyler RS, Fryauf H, Gantz BJ, Kelsay DMR, Woodworth GG (1997) Speech perception in prelingually implanted children after four years. In: Honjo I, Takahashi H (eds) Cochlear implant and related sciences update. Advances in Oto-Rhino-Laryngology 52: 187–192.

Population size

23

Demographics

No demography details, reference made to earlier research (Fryauf-Bertschy et al. 1997)
Generally children were deaf at birth or before 2 years of age

Selection criteria

Not detailed, reference made to earlier research (Fryauf-Bertschy et al. 1997)

Dependent variables

Speech perception test battery at age 4:
• MTS
• WIPI
• PB-K

Independent variables

Preimplant performance

Method

Percentages, no analysis of statistical significance

Results

Ceiling effects on MTS after two years of cochlear implant use. BP-K tests show limited improvement over first 12 months, increased performance gain between 36 and 48 months.

Conclusions

Average performance continues to improve as a function of time; asymptomic performance not observed after four years. Large individual performance differences. Preliminary measures suggest that preimplant hearing thresholds at 250 or 1000 Hz are not good predictors of postoperative speech perception performance at 36 months.

Observations

This research is of limited value because of lack of information on demographics, sampling criteria and analysis of results. The authors suggest that the report builds on earlier work, extending that research to outcome measures over four years post implantation. They also examine the relationship between pre-implant and post-implant performance. The authors report that the children continue to show improvements over time, but large variations across individuals in performance is noted (although not shown in the data).

Tyler RS, Fryauf-Bertschy H, Kelsay DMR, Gantz BJ, Woodworth GP, Parkinson A (1997) Speech perception by prelingually deaf children using cochlear implants. Otolaryngology – Head and Neck Surgery 117(3/1): 180–187.

Note

Same group as Fryauf-Bertschy H, Tyler RT, Kelsay DM et al. (1997) Cochlear implant use by prelingually deafened children: the influences of age at implant and length of device use. Journal of Speech, Language and Hearing Research 40(Feb): 183–199.

Population size

44

Demographics

Age: 2–15 years
CI use: ≤ 5 years
CI device: Cochlear Nucleus 22 multichannel
Mode of communication: total communication

Selection criteria

University of Iowa Implant Center
Grouped by age
16 children excluded: 6 (no detail); 2 for medical complications; 8 for non-use
Judged by clinical psychologist

Dependent variables

Speech perception test battery:
• range of MST to PB-K

Independent variables

Pre-implantation scores

Method

Reporting of scores

Results

Gains in speech perception within one year of cochlear implantation. Open-set perception gains slower than closed-set. Large differences exist between individual scores. Age at cochlear implantation ≤ 4 years higher gains than post-4 years. Perception of vowel and consonant features shows increased performance gains after two years of cochlear implant use. Minimal users score more poorly than full-time users. Outcomes repeat those of earlier studies.

Conclusions

Most children demonstrated some improvement; some children obtained limited benefits, and some of these discontinued use of their cochlear implant. Possible reasons for poor outcomes include inadequate fitting, insufficient cognitive skills, poor motivation, educational and social environment emphasizing manual communication, and limited parental support. Congenitally deaf children obtained higher scores than did children with acquired deafness; these observations are tentative. It is not obvious why children with no exposure to sound should lead to better word understanding than having limited exposure. The possible effects of meningitis are not mentioned.

Observations

In this study the researchers investigated the speech perception performance of a population of 50 prelingually deaf children, over a period extending to five years post-implantation. All were implanted at the University of Iowa. As with the 1997 study reporting on outcomes over four years, the study is limited by lack of demographic description, making it difficult to place the results into the context of other studies.

The sampling is accounted for as follows: the children formed part of a 73 consecutively implanted sample at the Iowa centre subsampled by experience of their implant for two or more years; two children with Goldenberg syndrome were excluded because only a limited number of electrodes were inserted. Eight other children were excluded because they stopped using their implants for a number of reasons. All children in the study used total communication.

The test battery was a combination of closed- and open-set word-recognition tests, including the Monosyllable Trochee Spondee (MTS) test, the Iowa Vowel Perception Test, the Word Intelligibility by Picture Identification (WIPI) and the PB-K test.

Open-set performance increases were slower than closed-set performances over time, while large individual differences were observed. The large individual differences might well point to the lack of population characteristics on record, including such elements as socio-economic status, ethnicity, additional handicap, variation in intelligence, prior performance, language preference, gender and educational measures.

Greater performance of prelingual deaf children might be attributable to a number of factors, including the effect of meningitis on children with acquired deafness, higher prior achievement in total communication programmes and longer/more pronounced parental and specialist support.

**Tyler RS, Gantz BJ, Woodworth GG, Fryauf-Bertschy H, Kelsay DMR (1997)
Performance of 2- and 3-year-old children and predictions of 4-year from 1-year performance. American Journal of Otology 18: s157–s159.**

Population size
Not specified
Demographics
Not detailed, reference back to earlier research (Tyler et al 1997, Fryauf-Bertschy et al. 1997)
Two age groups of CIs, 2–4 years, and 4–9 years.
CI use duration same for both groups
Selection criteria
Sampling criteria same as Fryauf-Bertschy et al. 1997
Dependent variables
Speech perception test battery:
- MTS
- PB-K
- Central Institute for the Deaf (CID) low-verbal test
Independent variables
Age at CI
Prior on speech perception tests
Method
Percentages of correct scores
Results
'Implanted young' group (2–4 years) outperformed 'implanted old' (4–9 years) after 36 months; one-year performance data are 'helpful' in predicting four-year performance. Ceiling effects reported on MTS and CID low-verbal tests; others scored below chance

levels. Prelingually deaf children implanted at age 2–4 years outperform 4–9 year age group. No test of statistical significance detailed.

Conclusions
It may be desirable for children to undergo implantation when under 2 years of age. Prediction conclusion: children who score less than 85% correct on CID low-verbal test or less than about 70% on MTS test at one year will likely perform more poorly after four years of implant use than children who score above these levels after one year of use.

Observations
Continuation of research based on single population (University of Iowa Implant Center). This study shares the characteristics of other research based on the same population published in the same year, including summary reporting and lack of population description. No assessment of significance is undertaken, the group is small and is underdescribed, the rationale for the age range division among the two groups is not given, and other variables may have affected the outcomes. As the conclusion to the study the authors report that it may be desirable for children to undergo implantation under age 2.

Tyler RS, Kelsay DMR, Teagle HFB, Rubinstein JT, Gantz BJ, Christ AM (2000) 7-year speech perception results and the effects of age, residual hearing and preimplant speech perception in prelingually deaf children using the Nucleus and Clarion cochlear implants. In: Kim CS, Chang SO, Lim D (2000) Updates in cochlear implantation. Advances in Oto-Rhino-Laryngology 57: 305–310.

Note
Seven-year outcomes of the Iowa CI group described by Fryauf-Bertschy (1997)

Population size
34

Demographics
Nucleus 22 population based on population detailed in Fryauf-Bertschy (1997)
Clarion population based on population details in Osberger et al. (1999)
No further details of overall population size

Selection criteria
Based on population detailed in Fryauf-Bertschy (1997)
Clarion population based on population details in Osberger et al. (1999)
No further details of sampling method

Dependent variables
Speech perception test battery (undetailed, but based on Fryauf-Bertschy 1997)

Independent variables
Duration of CI use (7 years)

Method
Outcome score percentage graphs per year of CI

Results
Three years of implant use needed for observation that younger age at cochlear implantation improves outcomes. Children implanted before 3.5 years generally obtain higher post-implant speech perception scores. Trend continues over six-year period. Easier tests are marred by ceiling effects. Results similar for two devices.

Conclusions
Children implanted ≤ 3 years appear to have an advantage over other children in speech reception skills gains.

Observations
This is a necessary longitudinal extension of earlier reported outcomes. Direct comparison is limited by the inclusion of a different population group. The population is insufficiently described while data are underanalysed, perhaps due to the limited size of the remaining population.

Tyler RS, Rubinstein JT, Teagle H, Kelsay DMR, Gantz BJ (2000) Pre-lingually deaf children can perform as well as post-lingually deaf adults using cochlear implants. Cochlear Implants International 1(1): 39–44.

Population size
   21
Population comments
   Sample concerns prelingually deaf CI children and in addition 81 postlingually deaf CI adults
Demographics
Prelingually deaf children
   Age at CI: range 2.5–16 years
   Duration of CI use: range 1–11 years
   CI device: Nucleus multichannel
Adults
   CI device: Clarion 34, Ineraid 24, Nucleus 22
   No further details.
Selection criteria
   Children selected to have vocabulary and language sufficient to complete the test (not noted for the adults): ≥ 95% on RITLS
Dependent variables
   Iowa Sentence test (IST)
Independent variables
   Age at CI: child versus adult
Method
   Test scores in percentages graphed for individual children
Results
   Scores for children ranged from 0 to 79% correct; 50% scored above 70% correct. Adults score range 0–100% correct; 50% scored above 60% correct. Large individual differences
Conclusions
   Many of the children scored as well or better than adults. The auditory system of prelingually deaf children is sufficient to obtain levels of speech recognition similar to postlingually deaf adults.
      Prelingually deaf children and postlingually deaf adults represent rather diverse biological systems. If they share similar upper bounds on performance with a cochlear implant, then these limits may be device-related rather than of biological origin (p.43).
Observations
   This study is limited by a lack of detail for the adult population, for example no detail on duration of cochlear implant use. The adult population administered IST over a range of years several years earlier. The children may have been familiar with IST since this population has been continually assessed since implantation (no details given).

Tyler RS, Teagle HFB, Kelsay DMR, Gantz BJ, Woodworth GG, Parkinson AJ (2000) Speech perception by prelingually deaf children after six years of cochlear implant use: effects of age at implantation. Annals of Otology, Rhinology and Laryngology (Supplement) 185: s82–s84.

Note Study continues tracking population described by Fryauf-Bertschy 1997, from Iowa Implant Center
Population size
   26

Demographics

Demographic details not given, but reference made to Fryauf-Bertschy et al. 1997

Selection criteria

As in Fryauf-Bertschy et al. 1997

Dependent variables

Speech perception battery detailed in Fryauf-Bertschy et al. 1997

Independent variables

Length of CI use (6 years)

Method

Percentage scores

Results

MTS test overall clear ceiling effects. PB-K scores averaging 27%; 20 scored 10% or above. Test ceiling effects restrict ability to observe changes beyond three years of cochlear implant use. Gains on PB-K continue to five years (but appear overinterpreted).

Conclusions

Overall continuing wide range of performance; some children require several years of implant use before showing improvements in open-set word recognition; 'small but consistent' gains observed four to six years post-implantation; cochlear-implanted children implanted at younger age show more rapid learning curves.

Observations

Detail in introduction: after six years of experience with a cochlear implant, two children are now enrolled in oral education; 24 are continuing in total communication programmes. Because of the overall clear ceiling effects, this research is hard to interpret and demonstrates the clear need for a battery of age-appropriate language skills tests stretching from pre-implantation (early communicative behaviour) to adult-equivalent language skills.

Despite the detailed testing, the fact that 24 out of 26 cochlear-implanted children continue in total communication settings is perhaps the most significant and 'real-life' outcome of this set of research articles so far. It also points to the clear need to develop a longitudinal system to track the use of cochlear implants in education itself (including actual education results). However, the preponderance of total communication may reflect local policy rather than benefit from the implant or children's intrinsic capabilities.

Uziel AS, Reuillard-Artieres F, Sillon M. et al. (1995) Speech perception performances in prelingual deafened children with the Nucleus multichannel cochlear implant. Advances in Oto-Rhino-Laryngology 50: 114–118.

Population size

37

Population comments

Divided into two groups for age at onset

Demographics

Age at onset: congenital (before age 1, n = 24), and prelingual (before age 2, n = 13)
Aetiology: mostly meningitis
CI device: Nucleus multichannel
Experience of deafness: shorter (range 2–3 years, n = 18) and longer (> 3 years, n = 19)
Age: range 2.2–9 years, mean 4.4 years

Selection criteria

Implanted by the Montpellier Paediatric Cochlear Implant Programme, age at onset occurring before age 2

Dependent variables

Speech perception test battery selected from the European Children Implant Programme battery:

- phoneme detection test
- closed-set word identification test
- closed-set sentence identification test
- open-set speech recognition test (audition only)

Independent variables

Age at onset

Over-time progress

Method

Group mean percentage scores

Results

Phoneme detection was achieved by all subjects three months post-implantation, with a mean group score of 85%; a ceiling effect is evident at one year post-implantation (p.115).

Closed-set word identification averages approximately 20% at three months post-implantation, reaching a plateau by 24 months post-implantation. Congenitally deafened children tended to achieve lower scores than prelingually deafened children; this effect was not significant, and the performance gap was closed two years post-implantation (pp.116–17).

Open-set speech recognition was not achieved until 12 months post-implantation. Performance increases were gradual, with no plateau even after 36 months post-implantation (p.117).

Conclusions

'Data from this study clearly indicated that profoundly hearing-impaired children with cochlear implants achieved significant improvement in their abilities to perceive speech during the first three years postimplantation' (p.117).

'... the prelinguistically [sic] deafened children tend to outperform the congenital children between 6 and 18 months postimplantation. This difference may be accounted for by the short linguistic-auditory experience of the prelinguistically [sic] deafened children' (p.117).

Observations

This research was designed to control for device and age at implantation, while collecting longer-term (36 month post-implantation) improvement data. The authors note that large individual variation in performance was typically reported, and suggest this may be partly accounted for by different devices, and the inclusion of single-channel devices in past research.

However, in reporting their findings the authors do not disaggregate their data into individual performance patterns, and no detail is provided on individual performance variation in this article.

The authors' finding that the better performance of prelingually deaf children relative to congenitally deaf children was a temporary one is not further analysed, yet makes an intriguing contribution to comparative findings reported elsewhere.

Vermeulen A, Hoekstra C, Brokx J, van den Broek P (1999) Oral language acquisition in children assessed with the Reynell Developmental Language Scales. International Journal of Pediatric Otorhinolaryngology 47(2): 153–155.

Population size

12

Demographics

Age at onset: around 3 years (graphed), average 2.4 years

Age at CI: range +3–6 years (graphed)

HA experience: average 3.4 years.

CI experience: range 1 to about 5 years (graphed), average 3.4 years

CI device: Nucleus 22

Aetiology: meningitis

Educational placement: oral (7), total communication (5)

Selection criteria

None detailed

Dependent variables

Reynell Developmental Language Scales (RDLS) Dutch version at 6, 12 and 24 months post-CI

Independent variables

CI; Reynell score pre-CI

Method

Score graph. No statistical analysis attempted

Results

The rate of receptive language development showed a gradual increase. In the interval between 12 and 24 months of implant use the ratio was 0.9 (normal development rate = 1). The rate of expressive language development showed a rapid improvement in the period between six and 12 months after implantation, up to 1.4.

'Although the rate of receptive language acquisition during implant use increased, the language retardation still increased as well. But, as said before, not at the same rate as in the period of conventional hearing aid use' (p.155).

'The average rate of expressive language acquisition with the use of conventional hearing aids was 0.1. After implantation the rate of language acquisition increased and became 1.3 and remained slightly above 1. Six months after implantation the rate of expressive language acquisition was higher than that of the hearing children. If this trend continues the children will catch up with their normal hearing peers' (p.155).

Conclusions

After implantation the language began to develop again, the results showing that the rate of receptive and expressive language acquisition increased.

'The receptive language retardation did not continue to increase at the same rate as in the period of conventional hearing aid use. The expressive language retardation commenced to decrease, implying a catching up with the language level of normal hearing children' (p.155).

Observations

This study is of interest because it reports on a Dutch population of cochlear-implanted deaf children with apparently excellent test outcomes. All were deafened by meningitis. The oral language development of the ten children was assessed with a Dutch version of the Reynell Developmental Language Scales. The test was administered preoperatively and at regular intervals after implantation and the average rate of spoken language development between two consecutive evaluations was computed. This rate was defined as the quotient of the increase of the spoken-language age and the increase of the chronological age between the evaluations, given a value of 1; this means 12 months' spoken language development in 12 months' time. In the case of language deemed retarded the rate of spoken language development is therefore less than 1.

After merely two years of implantation the deaf children demonstrate a developmental ratio of 0.9 – 1 constituting normal language development. Since some children demonstrated a ratio of 1.4 in the six- to 12-month period following implantation, the authors conclude that the cochlear-implanted children may likely catch up with their hearing peers in normal language development. This is notable, as there is, in fact, not much evidence of 'catching up' in the literature (other than for modest numbers), although there is other evidence supporting the notion of a period of accelerated speech reception and production development across the age-range.

There is no discussion of the Reynell test content or administration. Neither is there any detail on demographics other than periods of hearing loss and use of conventional aids prior to implantation, so that a comparison between this population and those reported is difficult. With regard to sampling, it is noted that all children demonstrated absence of psychological or developmental disorders.

Wald RL, Knutson JF (2000) Deaf cultural identity of adolescents with and without cochlear implants. Annals of Otology, Rhinology and Laryngology 185: s87–s89.

Population size
8

Population comments
With an additional non-implanted group of 37 deaf adolescents

Demographics
Age: mean 14.5 years, range 12–18 years
No further demographic detail provided

Selection criteria
Recruited from four different sources; no sampling criteria detailed, nor is it clear how or where the CI children in particular were recruited

Dependent variables
Self-assessment
Deaf Identity Development Scale (DIDS), five-point Lickert scale closed-response questionnaire
Teacher assessment
Teacher Rating Form (TRF)

Independent variables
Cultural identity

Method
T-tests

Results
'Both groups gave the most favorable ratings to items on the Bicultural scale. The cochlear-implant users rated hearing identity items significantly more favorably than did the adolescents without cochlear implants (p < 0.05)' (p.88).
Cochlear implant users rated immersion identity less favorably than did non-implanted deaf adolescents, but this difference was not significant; there were no great differences for Marginal and Bicultural scales (p.88).
No statistical differences between cochlear-implanted children and non-implanted children were found for social competence (teacher assessment), no matter which identity they favoured (p.89).

Conclusions
'... deaf adolescents with cochlear implants endorse beliefs about deafness and deaf culture that are similar to those of adolescents without cochlear implants' (p.89).

Observations
This study is of interest despite its small number of cochlear-implanted children (n = 8) because of its focus on cultural association in adolescent cochlear implant users, a hitherto neglected aspect of cochlear implantation outcome. The authors place the study in the context of a binary distinction, of whether deafness is to be considered a target for medical intervention or cultural identity. The authors note that the impact of cochlear implantation on identity choice among adolescents is unknown, an observation confirmed by the lack of evidence available for review here. They suggest that:
'In many ways, cochlear implant users may be described as poised between the deaf and hearing worlds. It is possible that such a position will facilitate the adoption of a bicultural identity in which individuals are able to negotiate social interactions within both communities' (p.88).

It is important to note that the measures reported here concern the beliefs of those responding, rather than actual outcomes. The findings suggest that the cultural identity ideal-targets are similarly distributed for both implanted and non-implanted deaf adolescents reported here, with a stronger preference for hearing identity expressed by the implanted children. The authors' comment on this reflects the overall trend in the research reviewed here:

'Because many implant users receive audiological benefit, it is not surprising that they describe emulating the hearing majority as a desirable goal' (p.89).

Waltzman SB, Cohen NL, Gomolin RH, Green J, Shapiro W, Brackett D, Zara C (1997) Perception and production results in children implanted between 2 and 5 years of age. Advances in Oto-Rhino-Laryngology 52: 177–180.

Population 38
Population comments
Sample dropping to n = 3 at 5-year postoperative test interval
Demographics
None detailed
Selection criteria
None detailed
Dependent variables
Speech perception: GASP and PB-K
Speech production: PPVT and Expressive One Word Picture Vocabulary test
Independent variables
Preimplantation scores
Method
Percentage reporting
Results
After using the device for one or more years the children had varying degrees of open-set speech perception (p.178).
Overall the mean growth was 33 months for receptive vocabulary and 48 months for expressive vocabulary (p.179).
Conclusions
The results demonstrate significant improvement in open-set speech perception, language acquisition and speech production in congenitally deaf children implanted below the age of 5 (p.179).
Observations
The authors set out to report long-term findings for a 'large' (p.177) group of congenitally deaf children implanted below the age of 5. Reported here are speech production and speech perception findings up to four years post-implantation.
The reporting on this study is summary, reflecting in particular the lack of demographic detail and the complex reporting of findings. There is no clear pattern of reporting, with test results quoted for different years and different subgroups and different tests on an apparently arbitrary basis. Results on the GASP Word test after one year of implant experience are reported for 23 children, while only six children completed the Sentence test. If there is an overall pattern of performance in the results, then the reporting does not reveal it. Otherwise, results quoted are not contradictory to findings reported elsewhere.

Waltzman SB, Cohen NL, Gomolin RH, Green JE, Shapiro WH, Hoffman RA, Roland JT (1997) Open-set speech perception in congenitally deaf children using cochlear implants. American Journal of Otology 18(3): 342–349.

Population size
   38
Population comments
   Sample size decreases rapidly to ≤ 5 over time, while most tests anyway concern subsamples
Demographics
   Age at CI: < 3 years (15), 3–5 years (23)
   Age at onset: congenital
   No further demographics
Selection criteria
   Implanted at the NYU Medical Center; no known additional disabilities
Dependent variables
   Speech perception test battery:
   • GASP
   • PB-K
   • Common Phrases Test
   • Multisyllabic Lexical Neighborhood Test
   • Lexical Neighborhood Test
   Divided into two groups, 'across all children for each yearly evaluation [and] across children who were administered the test at each yearly evaluation' (pp.343–4)
Independent variables
   Preoperative performance
Method
   Percentage scores over time. Correlation coefficients were calculated between scores at each interval and age at implantation; one-way analyses of variance were performed independently
Results
   In summary, all test scores improved steadily over time after first rapid improvement postoperatively.
      '... all children had significant open-set speech recognition at the time of the last postoperative evaluation. Thirty-seven of the children use oral language as their sole means of communication' (p.342).
Conclusions
   'Multichannel cochlear implants provide significant and usable open-set speech perception in congenitally deaf children given implants at < 5 years of age' (p.342).
Observations
   With this study the authors aimed to assess the development of open-set speech perception in congenitally deaf children, all implanted with the Nucleus multichannel device at < 5 years of age. Children formed a population of 38 consecutively implanted at the NYU Medical Center, and had been followed for up to five years at the time of reporting.
   All children are reported to achieve significant speech perception outcomes, while 37 of the 38 children use oral language as their sole means of communication.
   The study sample is a homogeneous group but the authors did observe wide variation between individuals. The population ranged from 38 (at one year post-implantation) to three (at five years post-implantation).
   The authors observed wide variation between individuals largely because of problems with the tests (none are age-appropriate) and because of extremely high population migration over time and between measures. A few remarks must be made about both the population and the outcomes reported.

First, increases in test outcomes are very large; the number of children at the three- and five-year intervals extremely low ($n \leq 5$).

It is relevant to note the absence of any demographic description of the sample. It is only in reading the discussion that it emerges that:

'... the commitment of the parents of the children in this study to oral education and mainstreaming as well as their willingness to expend the time and energy necessary to reach their goals were total. The influence and effects of these factors on the eventual outcome in congenitally deaf children with cochlear prostheses cannot and should not be underestimated' (p.247).

Interestingly, the authors conclude this without making reference to this fact in their demographic description, while attributing all outcome reported to the effect of the cochlear implant itself.

Furthermore,

'The children, with one exception, all use oral language as their only mode of communication. The only exception is a child who used total communication before implantation and who was the only one to consistently score 0% on PB-K words' (p.345).

'All children, with one exception, are mainstreamed with no assistance in the classroom, although preview/review sessions are held for the children when necessary' (p.345).

It must by concluded that the sampling and sample characteristics are insufficiently detailed; that the population size − as others reported here − is comparatively modest for these particular measures; that the sample became extremely small over time; and that the results reported are therefore limited and difficult to contrast with other outcome reports.

Wang HL, Toe D (1998) The development of communicative competence in adolescents with cochlear implants. Caedhh Journal/La Revue Acesm 24(1): 27–45.

Population size
4
Demographics
Age at CI: range 13.11–17.6 years
Aetiology: Mondini's ($n = 2$), Usher's ($n = 1$), congenital, unknown ($n = 1$)
CI device: Nucleus multichannel
Selection criteria
Selected due to data availability at the Victorian Eye and Ear Hospital, Melbourne
Dependent variables
Discourse sample recording over a 2-year period with a conversation partner (CP)
Independent variables
Late implantation (in adolescence)
Over-time development (2 years post-implantation)
Method
Percentage scores, Spearman's ranking correlation for over-time score differences
Results
Results reveals an increase over time in the three out of four adolescents in talk time, significant for all three ($p < 0.05$, p.37).

'There was an overall increase in the frequency of appropriate responses over time by all four participants [...] For all participants the post-implant samples had a greater proportion of appropriate responses than preimplant samples' (p.39).

Seeking clarification from the CP was also measured over time, and is discussed qualitatively per subject, suggesting some over-time improvement (pp.39–40).

Conclusions

In the study, a longitudinal increase in the communicative skills and competence is reported for the four adolescents of the sample. Aspects that showed improvement were:

'... (a) an increase in the ability to resolve questions, (b) increased talk time for three participants, and (c) a greater range and sophistication in the use of repair strategies' (p.43).

Observations

This study focuses on four deaf adolescents, who were implanted during their adolescence. Since data from this age group are rare (whether young-implanted or, as here, late-implanted), the article is therefore included in this review despite its small sample size. Indeed, a more qualitative-oriented study might have suited the subjects better, and allowed for more conscious participation by the adolescents themselves, perhaps incorporating a wider range of outcome measures than are being reported here. Nevertheless, the authors report clearly useful data, and there is no attempt to overinterpret or overgeneralize the findings reported.

The authors note that prelingually deaf teenagers who have been implanted in their adolescence comprise a small group in the overall population with cochlear implants (p.28). Indeed, all the evidence to date suggests that the group will become smaller in size, given that more and more deaf children are implanted at a very early age. The authors note that for this age group it is more useful to measure communicative competence rather than e.g. speech perception or speech production, noting in particular that speech intelligibility, due to the long experience of deafness, is unlikely to reach much higher levels of competence. On the other hand,

'... the extraneous variable of maturation, often considered an issue in research with young children, should have less influence on the results of developmental studies in teenagers' (p.29).

Communicative competence is defined operationally as the communicative knowledge that individual members of cultural groups need to possess to be able to interact with one another in ways that are both socially appropriate and strategically effective (p.28).

The study focuses on changes in communicative behaviour over time in samples derived from spontaneous conversational interaction between the participants and a conversational partner in a clinical context, focusing in particular on query–response sequences.

Results reported demonstrate some valuable improvement over time, but as in studies concerning younger children, the results also demonstrate considerable individual difference, which fails to demonstrate any patterning due to the small number of adolescents included in the study.

Young NM, Gorhne KM, Carrasco VN, Brown C (1999) Speech perception of young children using nucleus 22-channel or CLARION® cochlear implants. Annals of Otology, Rhinology and Laryngology 108(4): 99–103.

Population size

43

Population comments

Disaggregated for device, Nucleus (*n* = 23) and Clarion (*n* = 20)

Demographics

Age at CI: mean Nucleus (3.1 years, SD = 1.0), Clarion (3.3 years, SD = 0.9)
HA use: mean Nucleus (19.3 months, SD = 11.1), Clarion (22.8 months, SD = 10.6)
Education: oral (Nucleus 11, Clarion 12), total communication (Nucleus 12, Clarion 8)
Encoding strategy: SPEAK (Nucleus), CIS (Clarion)

Selection criteria

Children implanted at the Children's Memorial Medical Center in Chicago or the

University of North Carolina in Chapel Hill. Inclusion criteria: under age 5 years at time of CI, congenitally deaf, normal cochleas (computed tomography), English as primary language in family, absence of confounding medical conditions

Dependent variables

Speech perception at 6 and 12 months post-implantation
ESP, PB-K, GASP

Independent variables

Device: Nucleus, Clarion

Method

Parametric and non-parametric tests used as appropriate: Levene's tests for equality of variances, and Mann-Whitney U test (p.101)

Results

'Generally, the mean scores [post-implantation] were higher for the Clarion group. These differences reached statistical significance for ESP Pattern Perception and ESP Monosyllables at six months, and for the GASP Word scores at 12 months' (p.101).

Conclusions

'This study demonstrates that children implanted with the Clarion device and who use the CIS strategy may develop better auditory perceptual skills during the first year post-implantation than children implanted with the Nucleus 22 who use the SPEAK strategy' (p.102).

Observations

This study reports on speech perception tests six and 12 months postoperatively, comparing two devices, the Nucleus 22 (SPEAK) and Clarion (CIS) implanted in congenitally deaf children below age 5 years.

The reported findings suggest the Clarion users outperform Nucleus users over this period. However, the pattern of individual achievement across GASP and PB-K demonstrates the spurious nature of the findings: most scores are nil on the GASP sentence test, with just two Clarion children scoring above nil at 12 months. For the PB-K test, the six-month results show just one out of 13 Nucleus children scoring above nil, against five out of 17 Clarion children, three of whom score below 10%. At 12 months, one Nucleus child achieved over 80%, while no Clarion child achieved over 30%. It is clear from the individual scores that the wide range of individual performance, and the floor effects, skewed the statistical analyses performed. Judging by the graphed individual results, the within-group individual variation might well account for greater difference than the between-group results, which would leave individual performance as the main source of variance. Given the small numbers involved especially at the 12-month interval (only six Clarion users), and the obvious inappropriateness of this level of test for the children involved (most scoring nil over the full test period on both assessments), this study's findings must, unfortunately, be regarded as flawed.

Zwolan TA, Zimmerman-Phillips S, Ashbaugh CJ, Hieber SJ, Kileny PR, Telian SA (1997) Cochlear implantation of children with minimal open-set speech recognition skills. Ear and Hearing 18(3): 240–251.

Population size

24

Population comments

2 × 12 pre-CIs

Demographics

CI device: Nucleus 22
Age at implantation: (idem)
Communication mode: (idem)

Speech processor type: Nucleus Mini Speech Processor or Spectra
Speech encoding strategy
Selection criteria
12 CIs with no open-set speech perception skills (GASP = 0%)
12 CIs with minimal open-set speech perception skills (GASP > 0%)
No other selection criteria detailed
Dependent variables
Speech recognition test battery pre-operatively and at six and 12 months after CI:
- MTS-W/S
- GASP-W/S
- WIPI
- NU-CHIPS
Independent variables
Comparison of minimal/no speech perception prior to CI implantation (GASP)
Method
Paired t-tests
Results
The scores of the borderline group improved significantly on five of six speech-recognition measures when six-month postoperative scores obtained with the implant were compared with preoperative test scores obtained with hearing aids. By the 12-month postoperative interval, the scores of the borderline group had improved significantly ($p < 0.05$) on all six measures. In contrast, scores obtained by the traditional group had improved significantly on three of six measures at both the six- and 12-month postoperative intervals. Comparison of postoperative test scores revealed that the borderline group scored significantly higher than the traditional group on three of six measures at the six-month test interval and on six of six measures at the 12-month test interval ($p < 0.05$).

At the six-month postoperative interval the mean scores of the borderline group were significantly higher than the mean scores of the traditional group on three of six measures tested: MTS-W ($p = 0.007$), MTS-S ($p = 0.005$) and the GASP-W ($p = 0.049$; Figure 6). Although the mean scores of the borderline group also were greater than those of the traditional group on the WIPI and GASP-S tests, these differences were not statistically significant.

At the 12-month postoperative interval (Figure 7), the mean scores of the borderline group were significantly higher than those of the traditional group on all six measures: MTS-W ($p = 0.012$), MTS-S ($p = 0.039$), WIPI ($p = 0.009$), NU-CHIPS ($p = 0.001$), GASP-W ($p = 0.004$) and GASP-S ($p = 0.011$).

Conclusions
The findings of this study indicate that both groups derive significant benefit from their cochlear implants. Although the mean preoperative audiograms for the implanted ears did not differ significantly for the two groups of children, members of the borderline group exhibited significantly better speech-recognition skills than the traditional group during the first year after implantation. These findings suggest that the increased auditory experience of the borderline children positively influenced their performance with a cochlear implant. The authors advocate that the selection criteria used to determine paediatric cochlear implant candidacy be broadened to include consideration of children who demonstrate minimal open-set speech-recognition skills.

Observations
The purpose of this study, as reported by the authors at outset, was to evaluate the postoperative performance of 12 children who demonstrated some open-set speech-recognition skills before receiving a Nucleus multichannel cochlear implant with a view to expanding the selection criteria for cochlear implant candidacy to include children who derive minimal benefit from amplification. Results confirm the report by Gantz et al.

(1999), which was based on a much smaller group. Both concern a candidacy issue: to implant children with pre-existing speech perception (not hitherto considered).

The comparison set up is that between 12 cochlear implant users who demonstrated no speech-perception skill before implantation (defined by a zero score on the GASP test) with 12 cochlear implant users who demonstrated some existing skill prior to implantation.

The authors report that the group with some limited speech-perception skill prior to implantation (the borderline group) derived significant benefit from the cochlear implant. Therefore they suggest that children with a greater range of scores on the GASP test prior to implantation might benefit from a cochlear implant. This contrasts with the research into levels of residual hearing as an issue in candidacy as reported by Geers (1997). The recommendation arising out of that research, in the same year, was that there were no grounds to relax the implant candidacy criteria to include those whose

'pure tone average thresholds are less than 100 dB in the better ear, regardless of their speech perception scores' (p.154).

The authors suggest that the PTA for the borderline group is consistent with that of 'silver hearing aid users,' and the PTA for the traditional group is consistent with that of 'bronze hearing aid users' based on the classification scheme of Miyamoto, Osberger, Todd, Robbins, Karasek, Dettman, Justice and Johnson (1994), a text not included in the reviews here.

The authors write that 18- and 24-month postoperative data are not yet available for all children in the study because the decision to implant borderline children was only recently implemented at their facility. These matched pairs, they go on, will be followed to see if the mean scores of the traditional group eventually catch up with those of the borderline group. It is hypothesized that this may occur at about 18 to 24 months, because several authors have reported that congenitally and early-deafened implant candidates demonstrate substantial gains in speech-recognition during this time frame.

The decision to implant children with open-set speech-recognition skills should not be taken lightly, according to the authors, while care must be exercised to verify that such children will derive more benefit from an implant than from hearing aids. The results of this study, they insist, clearly indicate that properly selected children with minimal preoperative open-set speech-recognition skills derive significant benefit from cochlear implants and that their performance may greatly exceed that achieved with hearing aids.

Chapter 4
Outcomes and factors: a discussion

Introduction

Chapter 2 showed that there has been a great deal of research into the comparatively young and complex field of paediatric cochlear implantation, and looked at the issues that have been most heavily researched up to the date of the review. The research is clear mainly in areas of audition, illustrating that paediatric cochlear implantation can be effective in terms of providing an experience of hearing to deaf children that is better than was available through hearing aids, notably in terms of offering better access to spoken language. However, as is already clear from this review, the field is complex in terms of research and this chapter will examine issues arising from the research methodology. Based on the studies reported, the chapter first discusses the outcomes and the factors influencing them. It then goes on to discuss the challenges faced by cochlear implant research, suggest areas for future research and also suggest the minimum information that needs to be provided in publications on paediatric cochlear implantation to facilitate appropriate comparisons between reports.

Outcomes

From the analysis so far, it is apparent that the various possible outcomes of implantation have received different degrees of attention in the research literature and have differing resulting levels of evidence.

The outcomes may be divided into three categories.

- **Robust outcomes** - the first are those that describe outcome measures where there are many research studies and where the evidence was robust; for example, speech recognition and production, and improved auditory performance.

- **Inconclusive or contradictory outcomes** – the second area is that category where the evidence was inconclusive, or there is contradictory evidence, such as for language development, educational placement and mode of communication.
- **Outcomes with little or no research** – the third category comprises those outcomes where there was little or no research found; for example, educational outcomes, employment, psychosocial outcomes, family life and parental perceptions, and quality of life measures.

Robust outcomes

Speech perception and production

It is not surprising that most of the research has been in the area of audition and speech, since the primary aim of implantation is to improve auditory perception, with the expected effect of improving speech perception and production. Auditory perception is included here, although it is not reported directly in many studies, as the claim that improved speech perception implies improved auditory perception would seem self-evident and thus legitimate.

As is apparent from the review, a large number of studies report improvements in speech perception and production after implantation. It seems clear that many children who, prior to the implant, could not hear speech or heard it with great difficulty, have a better chance to hear conversation and to develop intelligible speech. Chapter 2 describes the studies that provide this evidence.

However, there are two main areas of difficulty in the study of speech production and speech perception. The first area of difficulty relates to the procedures for making decisions about a child's speech perception and/or production abilities, and the second area concerns the conclusions that are drawn from such studies.

The assessment of speech perception and production is dependent on the context in which it is assessed, the person making the assessment, the procedures used and the way in which conclusions are drawn. However, in practice, only a limited number of these factors may be taken into account. Most assessments of speech production and perception take place in a clinic or other artificial environment, the person involved is one who knows the child and the procedure usually involves the use of standard tests with only a limited range of possible responses. The task may not measure the child's speech perception or production alone, if it is not linguistically appropriate for that child. With regard to the language used, it can be argued that if the assessment is of speech production and perception, only spoken language should be involved and therefore tests are usually given in spoken language only. Only spoken language is then accepted as a relevant response, regardless of the child's usual means of communication. However, if a child can only understand what is required if signs are used, or if a child expects to be understood through the use of signs together with speech, then the task for them is somewhat different than for a child who uses spoken language alone. The expertise of the tester, and their understanding of these issues, become critical in making such assessments. The experience of the tester is also important in interpreting responses; for example, is speech intelligibility measured by one who is familiar with the child, or by an unfamiliar listener?

The second issue is not the studies of speech perception and production themselves, but the conclusions that are drawn from many such studies. It is often assumed that speech production and perception are synonymous with language, and that a child who shows an improvement in these assessments is demonstrating improvement in spoken language. Before drawing this conclusion, other assessments would be necessary. In measuring speech perception and production we need to be clear that the assessment used is linguistically appropriate and within the linguistic grasp of the child, so that the level of the child's language does not become a factor in making the assessment and we can be sure that perception and/or production alone are measured. A further caution is that it is often assumed that performance in the assessment is a measure of a child's ability to communicate through speech in their usual environment. However, the assessment may be artificial because of clinical location and format, and the tester may be a single adult who has experience with deaf children. Many other factors will contribute to how well the child can communicate beyond the assessment situation, with those unfamiliar with deafness, with groups and in noisy situations for example. Very few studies attempt to assess the child's ability to perceive and produce spoken language in their day-to-day lives, after implantation, rather than in clinical tests.

Inconclusive or contradictory outcomes

Communication and language development

A major aim of cochlear implantation, particularly with young children, is to facilitate the development of spoken language, as we discussed in Chapter 1, and most studies focus on this aspect of language development. While some studies show marked development in spoken-language acquisition after implantation, the evidence as a whole remains inconclusive for a number of reasons.

As has been suggested, a major issue for cochlear implant research is that speech production and perception is often assumed to be the same as language. While there clearly can be a relationship between the two, and a child who develops good language skills is likely to demonstrate improvements in the area of speech perception and speech production, the relationship is not straightforward. This is particularly true of children who are implanted when they are older, who may develop this ability to perceive and produce words, but have limited ability in their overall language competence. Communication and language ability, while being one of the most important outcomes of implantation, can also be a factor in a child's development following an implant. This applies to older children who are language users before implantation, but some research also suggests that children with good communication abilities prior to implantation, independent of mode of communication, make better progress afterwards. Assessing these early communication abilities in young deaf children is complex, with a wide range of 'normal' behaviours, making the drawing of conclusions problematic.

With regard to the use of sign language, there are three main issues: first, sign language as a variable may be ignored; second, children's competence in it may not be assessed; and third, there may be confusion as to mode of communication (whether it is signed or spoken) and language. For example, British Sign Language is a language in its own right (as are other naturally occurring sign languages) but Sign Supported English is not. This is a significant issue for research on implantation, as some children, particularly older ones or those in educational settings or countries where sign language is promoted, will have acquired some signing skills before implantation. Sign languages are languages, therefore any comments about a child's overall language competence, or lack of it, has to state which language is being considered. The use of sign language remains an issue for cochlear implant research, as its role in the development of spoken language is not clearly researched, neither is how spoken language is best developed after cochlear implantation in a child who has previously developed some sign language. This area, while clearly important, has been the focus of little research and requires attention to the notion of the assessment of language competence discussed above.

Research programmes into cochlear implantation naturally focus on spoken language, and consideration needs to be given to the implications of presenting tasks in spoken language if a child would access them better through sign, and taking spoken answers only if the child has the ability to respond in sign but not speech. There are implications for making judgements of a child's language competence based on such assessment procedures and these have to be recognized and discussed within the studies when reported. Such rigorous testing requires very skilled and experienced testers.

There are further issues in language as an outcome of implantation and these relate to how language is assessed. Often studies focus on the use of language in a laboratory setting which, while it provides useful information, does not inform as to how useful the language is in everyday situations. Studies may use standard tests of language, which may be inappropriate for young deaf children, and not tap into the very early communication skills developed. Additionally, if a researcher wishes to look at sign language there is a further dilemma because many will not have the skills to communicate in sign language or to assess a child's signing competence; there is also a dearth of appropriate assessments of sign language.

Assessments of language vary; some, for example, measure vocabulary alone and others may tap into limited areas of language, such as measuring Mean Length of Utterance (MLU), particularly at the younger ages. Care must be taken in drawing wider conclusions from measures of one area of communication or language. Overall language development consists of a number of inter-related skills such as vocabulary, syntax, grammar and pragmatics, and inevitably its assessment is a more complex issue than may be at first anticipated.

Educational placement and communication approach

Although most research shows that children with cochlear implants are more likely to be placed in mainstream schools than in special schools for deaf pupils or other specialist provision, and that they are also more likely to use spoken language than other profoundly deaf children, the results are not robust and may appear contradictory.

In considering such results, there are a number of issues. For example, an increasing trend towards children with implants being placed in mainstream schools needs to be considered in terms of the general trend towards greater inclusion of children with disabilities in mainstream schools worldwide. It is inappropriate for studies to compare the number of pupils with implants placed in mainstream with the number of profoundly deaf children in mainstream settings in the past. Comparisons with the present situation of other deaf children, either profoundly or severely deaf, would seem more appropriate, although the possibility that children who receive implants may be those with the greater potential for spoken language development must always be borne in mind. Equally, the children who do not receive implants may include a greater proportion of those who have additional needs.

It is also important to clarify whether educational placement and communication mode are outcomes of implantation or factors in developing these outcomes. Children may be placed in mainstream settings and encouraged to use spoken language because it is felt that this will optimize their use of their implant, and thus placement becomes a factor rather than a measure of the efficacy of the implant.

Comparisons of studies in this area present a number of problems relating to comparability of samples. First, there are differences between countries and within countries in terms of their policy on educational approach, and the likelihood of mainstream placement. Deaf children may be placed in mainstream schools as a matter of local politics rather than as a response to the child's individual needs, and although mainstream placement has been viewed as an outcome, it may not be the most appropriate placement for some children. Second, countries differ in the extent of their use of sign language and the role it is seen as having in the lives of deaf children.

With regard to communication mode itself, it may also be that parents of children who are implanted are more likely to encourage spoken language than parents of other deaf children. Also, because we know that strong factors in assessing communication mode are age of implantation and length of time of use of implant, research studies that draw on different samples may have different results. This may be particularly important in assessing communication mode over time, as informal evidence indicates this is an area in which change can be observed over time, but strict attention must be paid to the groups observed to ensure true comparisons are made.

Outcomes with little or no research

Educational outcomes and employment

Ultimately, one of the main areas in which the benefit from implantation will be judged is likely to be educational outcomes and employment. Educational outcomes, and employment measures, which could be considered as more significant in terms of long-term achievements, have received relatively little consideration so far and there has been a limited focus on attainments in general. This is not surprising, as it is likely to be a long-term measure and the number of children implanted early with measurable educational outcomes is still comparatively small, and those in employment even fewer. The short period over which implantation has taken place means that relatively few pupils have reached the end of their educational life. Those who have finished their schooling may have been implanted as older children, or implanted when implant programmes were in an early stage of development and the technology was also less advanced.

In measuring the educational attainments of deaf children as a whole, evidence has generally been inconclusive (Powers 1996; Powers et al. 1998), with limited comparable information, if we wish to compare deaf children with implants with other deaf children. An additional issue to consider is which group should be the comparable group: the deaf or the hearing? Should deaf children be assessed on tests normed on hearing children?

There are signs that research into educational achievement is being investigated further. Since the review took place, two large major studies have begun reporting – the study of Geers and Moog in the US and that of the Medical Research Council's Institute of Hearing Research in the UK. These studies, in addition to smaller, more focused studies, may be able to provide more robust evidence in the area of education. For robust employment outcomes, we are likely to have to wait longer.

Psychological and social outcomes

In this section, psychological outcomes, including both emotional and cognitive consequences, are considered as well as social outcomes. Quality-of-life outcomes, because of their importance in medical research literature, are discussed separately below. There is a sense in which research in the area is inconclusive; there are few studies that pay attention to cognitive or social/emotional development. The small number of studies, the limitations of the measures used and the implicit aims of the studies to demonstrate the lack of psychological or social problems associated with implantation mean that the depth of study this topic requires is missing.

The studies addressing social and emotional issues tend to use questionnaires and structured interviews rather than make greater use of sociology research methods to promote an in-depth exploration of these complex areas. The questions as to what should be asked in such studies and who should ask the questions may influence the outcomes. As with quality-of-life studies (see below), the value of proxy responses by parents or other caregivers can be an issue in this research. Studies are usually carried out by implant teams themselves or based on data acquired by implant teams in the context of their work, but the relationship of parents with the professionals who are closely connected with the implantation process may not be ideal to explore the psychological process involved.

A further issue for such studies, as for other cochlear implant research, is the nature of the comparisons that can be made. Should comparisons be with the psychological wellbeing of other deaf children, or with hearing children? In general, studies tend to take hearing norms for comparison. However, this raises questions about the nature of the notion of psychological wellbeing of deaf and hearing people, and the concept that psychological wellbeing could be different for deaf and hearing people is not explored.

There are further notable absences from this research area. There is a clear need to look at the implications of implantation for teenagers, both of those implanted as teenagers and those who were implanted early and became teenagers. There are particular issues of identity at this age, as for all young people, but these remain relatively under-investigated for all deaf children and this group in particular. The issue of non-use of cochlear implants also remains under-researched, with little information about why some become non-users and what could be learnt from them to improve practice and hence outcomes. Further information about this group would provide valuable information about the implantation process, although there are obvious problems in such research because of the difficulty of contacting such a group, and there may be a reluctance to address the issue.

Quality-of-life measures

Health has been defined by the World Health Organisation as not only the absence of disease but also the presence of physical, mental and social wellbeing. The recognition that health is more than the absence of disease gives credence to the need for a measure of outcome that encompasses all aspects of wellbeing. Quality of life is potentially such an outcome measure. It would be incorrect to report that quality of life as a measure of outcome has been ignored in the paediatric cochlear implant literature as, to some extent, all the outcomes measured and reported in the review are measuring aspects of a child's quality of life following implantation. However, studies that focus explicitly on quality of life are very few.

In attempting to measure quality of life, the researcher is confronted with a number of issues

- Should quality of life be defined by professionals or by the individuals themselves?
- How can a child's quality of life be measured?
- What dimensions of quality of life should be included and should any negative changes to quality of life be included?
- At what point in time is it appropriate to measure quality of life following an intervention?

It is clear that if a professional defines quality of life, this definition is likely to be influenced by their own standpoint. A medical professional may only be concerned with the effect of an intervention on physical health. For example, within cochlear implantation surgeons may only be concerned with whether or not the device improves a child's hearing. In contrast, it could be argued that quality of life should be defined by the individuals whose life one is trying to assess. This would require researchers to ask each study population how they perceive quality of life, and to work within this definition. For young children, this is an unlikely goal; however, it may be possible for young people.

Measuring children's quality of life is often only possible through the use of a proxy (parent or professional) and, once more, the difficulties of using a proxy become apparent. As a result, it is the proxy's perception of the child's quality-of-life changes that are measured. Congenitally deaf children have not lost hearing, because they never had it. One might expect these children's perceptions of their quality of life to be markedly different from their parents, who can only imagine what it would be like to lose hearing. In addition, there is a developmental dimension involved in measuring a child's quality of life. That is, when measuring quality-of-life changes following an intervention one needs to know what proportion of the change would have occurred without the intervention anyway because of the child's developmental stage changing. If this is not accounted for, research will estimate the benefit of the intervention in quality-of-life terms inaccurately. It is perhaps, therefore, not surprising that few studies attempt to measure the global quality of life of children following cochlear implantation.

It is clear that the choice of domains used to define quality of life will influence the level and nature of the change detected. A global measure of quality of life would include all the domains that make up quality of life. In practice, most studies measure a component of quality of life. Therefore, it needs to be clear how quality of life is defined and how it has been measured if the results are to be interpreted in an appropriate manner. Quality of life is often perceived as a positive concept, but it is equally important to capture the negative impacts of an intervention in order to present a balanced outcome. The time at which quality of life is measured is also likely to influence what is measured. It is possible for an individual's definition of quality of life to change over time or for the level of quality of life to change.

From this brief discussion, it is clear that no consensus exists about how to define and measure quality of life in this area. Given this, if research into quality of life is to be meaningful, authors need to define what they are measuring. Authors should state explicitly whose perspective is taken, and whether they are measuring objective or subjective quality of life. It is also important to report and justify the aims and methods used in measuring quality of life, highlighting any advantages and disadvantages of the chosen approach.

To conclude, research is much needed in this underdeveloped aspect of paediatric cochlear implantation. A clear, fully operational, conceptual definition of quality of life is required if a global measure of the quality-of-life changes following paediatric cochlear implantation is to be comprehensively valued. It is important that negative changes, as well as positive, are incorporated. Using proxies is not ideal, but it may be the only option, at least until the children are old enough to talk for themselves.

Health economics

Health economics is a developing area within research looking at cochlear implantation. Currently it is limited by the small sample size of most studies and the fact that studies tend to concentrate on a small number of centres, whereas a wide range of centres and countries is required so that results can be more generalizable. This would also allow an exploration of how cost-effectiveness varies by patient characteristics; a subgroup analysis of such factors as the effect of different degrees of hearing loss, or additional disabilities, is clearly important.

The vast majority of studies reported in this book used assumed outcomes. The instruments economists use to measure the change in utility could be argued as being too narrow – since they measure health-related quality of life – to pick up the broader outcome aspects of cochlear implantation, for example the child's improved safety or the benefits for family members. The ideal economic framework to capture these wider outcomes is cost-benefit analysis, where the outcomes are also measured in monetary terms using methods such as contingent valuation. A few partial cost-benefit analyses have been undertaken but these have tended to measure outcome only in terms of the financial cost savings, for example in education, resulting from paediatric cochlear implantation. These studies should not be used in resource allocation decision making since any decisions taken would be based purely on financial cost data with no consideration of actual outcomes. Sound decisions need to consider the impact of an intervention both in terms of costs and effects. Clearly there is much scope for further work looking at the outcomes used in economic studies. In particular, it would be worth taking advantage of contingent valuation methodology to capture the wider benefits and to explore the change in outcome over time. In addition, an economic study to empirically measure outcome for this population showed that using different instruments to measure utility generated different-sized gains. It would be worth exploring why these differences occurred in order to understand what the values reflect.

To date, economic studies on paediatric cochlear implantation have focused on the question of whether or not cochlear implantation is cost-effective compared to other interventions. There is a consensus across studies that cochlear implantation is cost-effective. This would suggest a need to broaden the economic research agenda to consider how cost-effectiveness and technical efficiency could be improved, that is how the resources allocated to this intervention could best be utilized to maximize outcomes. Within this, economists could explore issues to do with the skill-mix of implant teams or how support is divided between patient subgroups, for example. It is important to realize that cost-effectiveness is not static; the cost-effectiveness of programmes is likely to change over time. For example, as technology improves, candidature criteria change or staff become more experienced. The emergence of bilateral implantation raises new economic questions; principally one needs to know if the increased cost is justified by changes to outcomes. As a result, it may be important to reassess cost-effectiveness at key stages in the history of an intervention, before developments become normal practice.

Factors influencing outcomes

Research, in addition to demonstrating the outcomes from implantation, can also indicate the various factors that contribute to outcomes. The major established factor that has been shown by the research to strongly predict the outcomes of implantation is age at implantation, where the earlier the age of implantation, the greater the likelihood of benefit. Studies have clearly shown that early implantation improves outcomes, but it is not yet established how early implantation needs to take place to optimize outcomes, and whether it is different for differing groups. The age of onset of profound deafness is less thoroughly researched, but nevertheless there is general consensus of its impact – where a child had hearing for some time before implantation, they are more like to be successful implant users.

However, there remain very many factors where there are few or no studies or the results are not clear. These factors can be grouped as follows:

- **Factors relating to the support the child receives** – these include pre-implant communication, family support, rehabilitation and educational placement, and the type of device and the effectiveness of its functioning and tuning.
- **Factors residing within the child** – these include a child's residual hearing, cognitive ability and any additional disabilities that are likely to have an impact.
- **Demographic factors** – these are relevant for many outcomes for children in many areas, and include socio-economic status, gender and ethnicity.

Established factors

Age at implantation

While there are robust findings that relate to the age at which a child is implanted, there are complications in considering these data and there are a number of issues that need to be considered carefully. Clearly there must be an interaction between age of onset of deafness, age at implantation and length of time for which a child has used an implant. Unfortunately not all studies make this clear, and combine data for age at implantation to include children born deaf and children who become deaf. It is important that these are considered separately.

Many studies have established that for the child born deaf, the earlier the age at which they are implanted, the greater the success in terms of measured outcomes. Thus children implanted between 2 and 4 years of age are likely to achieve more than those implanted later. However, care is needed in comparing outcomes for older and younger children, as most of the measures used will be affected by the developing maturity of the child, older children doing better. It is important that progress over time, in addition to actual scores at set intervals, are taken into account or the achievements of younger children may not be fully recognized. This has implications for the length of time over which outcomes from paediatric implantation should be measured: for example, some studies show older children doing better than younger children. This may be due to a short timescale, and the younger children not understanding the task or having insufficient linguistic skills to complete it. Over a longer time span the younger children are likely to overtake the older children.

While it is established that younger children have better outcomes, it is not yet clear how young it is necessary to be to achieve the best outcomes. To date, the literature reports largely on children from the age of 2 years upwards, without adequate data available to draw conclusions about children implanted below the age of 2 years. This is likely to become available in the near future as more children under the age of 2 are implanted, following earlier diagnosis and greater confidence in the implantation procedure itself and its benefits. However, such research brings problems of its own. It is difficult to assess infants in an appropriate and quantifiable way, and assessments do not always indicate whether a particular skill is absent because the child has not reached that stage of development, or is emerging and likely to occur in the near future.

In investigating early implantation, it is necessary to consider changing audiological criteria, with increasing numbers of older children who would previously have been considered successful hearing aid wearers being implanted, and those with progressive losses also receiving implants.

Age at onset of deafness

As already discussed, those with later onset of profound deafness have been found to be likely to do better than those with early onset, but the outcomes may be influenced by the cause of deafness and any other sequelae that may have followed. Having an established language base prior to implantation may seem beneficial, but late-onset deafness may be associated with other problems linked to the cause of deafness, which may have a negative effect on development.

Factors that are not established

Factors relating to the support the child receives

Pre-implant language and communication

While it is likely that the child's language and communication competence prior to implantation will be a factor in the outcome, and many implant teams will have this information as part of the prior assessment process, very few studies report the effect of early language and communication on later language competence. One study indicates that communication prior to implantation is a predictor of speech perception and production following implantation; this was found to be true whether the communication was oral or sign or gesture.

Since the major goal of implantation in young deaf children is spoken language, a particular concern is the role of sign language pre-implantation. The role of sign language for children with cochlear implants is controversial, with some assuming they are incompatible and some supporting the use of sign language. However, the evidence remains inconclusive as to the role of sign language competency as a factor in the developing use of a cochlear implant.

It may be that linguistic competence prior to implantation, however measured, is a more significant factor than presently shown by the evidence, as there are a number of children who are identified as having language problems some years after implantation which were not identified prior to implantation. The addition of some useful hearing may help to identify other linguistic difficulties that it was not possible to identify before implantation, but which may have been a significant factor in progress, or lack of it, later.

The functioning and tuning of implant

No research has been undertaken to access the impact of the functioning of the device or the quality of the tuning process on outcomes. This may reflect the complexity of trying to measure this effect while controlling for other confounding variables. While device integrity can be measured within the clinic, it may not have been documented over the time of the study. It may also be that if a device is found not to be functioning to specification in the clinic it has been functioning sub-optimally for some time, and thus may have been a factor in a child's developing outcomes.

It is also not clear what constitutes poor tuning; in reality, there is likely to be a wide range of what could be termed adequate tuning. Many adults or long-term users resist change in the tuning process, and clearly appropriate tuning is important. However, we do not know to what extent this is true of younger implanted children. Clearly this challenging area is potentially important for the outcomes of implantation and warrants further research.

Family support
This area is under-researched in relation to cochlear implantation; it may well be that family support and background influences access to implantation itself and long-term support, and hence outcomes from the intervention. Other research has shown the importance of the family in the progress that deaf children make. For example, family attitudes to deafness have been found to affect the child's psychological wellbeing and acceptance of deafness. It is also widely believed that family income may also correlate with outcomes. Together, this suggests that families play an important role in the outcomes their child achieves after implantation.

Rehabilitation – education and communication approach
Although much reference is made to rehabilitation (mostly stressing its importance to successful outcomes), none of the research has attempted to analyse its effect. There is a lack of studies that compare types of rehabilitation, for example between implant programmes, or contrast rehabilitation for children with cochlear implants with that for another group of aurally rehabilitated deaf children. This is also surprising, because some research has turned up indications that intensive rehabilitation can be a strain on family resources. It is not clear how much of an overall effect on outcomes is attributable to which factor in the combination of cochlear implantation and aural rehabilitation. This has not to date been a focus of research during the period studied.

Clear-cut comparisons of one type of training or rehabilitation with another are confounded by the education the child may be receiving prior to, and after, the implant, and by the natural course of development of the child himself. In most countries, a profoundly deaf child will be receiving the support of a teacher of the deaf and some sort of specialist teaching, to a greater or lesser degree. How this links with the rehabilitation felt appropriate by the cochlear implant clinic in the case of a child varies a great deal. In both the field of cochlear implantation and the field of deaf education there has been ongoing debate about where rehabilitation should be provided, by whom and the most effective form it should take. The literature review to date has not provided these answers, although there is some ongoing work looking at these issues, and various models are described. Various models of provision have been proposed and implemented, ranging from purely clinic-based training, through liaison with local educational services, to no rehabilitation being provided by the implant centre and the local services being required to provide it in its entirety. In some countries, cochlear implant centres have established close links with schools for the deaf, establishing special classes for children with cochlear implants, with appropriate support.

Various claims have been made in the literature about the relative merits of different types of rehabilitation or intervention; primarily whether it should be purely auditory, or by methods involving total communication or those promoting the first language of the deaf as sign language. Little evidence of the efficacy of one method over another is found in this review and evidence is mixed. Claims of the supremacy of oral methods may be met with questions of the 'chicken and egg' type: did the child do well using oral methods because of their effectiveness, or were they placed in an oral setting because they were doing well with the implant system? However, if the major goal of cochlear implantation is spoken language because of increased access to effective hearing, then it is a reasonable assumption that any rehabilitation or intervention after implantation should include an emphasis on using audition and spoken language. To what degree this is necessary and how it could be monitored has not yet been determined. The debate about whether children with implants need more or less support than those with hearing aids has also not yet been answered.

Two recent major studies, one in the US and one in the UK, may address and answer some of these issues. Geers and Kirk (2003) recently reported on the study of cochlear implants and the education of the deaf child. A total of 181 children between the ages of 8 and 9, who had been implanted under the age of 5, were investigated; they were drawn from throughout the US and Canada. All performance measures were significantly higher for children in educational settings that emphasized speaking and listening than for those in signing settings; the type of educational setting was more important than the number of hours of therapy the child received. Interestingly, this study also looked at gender, IQ and implant (tuning and device) characteristics and found them all significant; issues that have been paid little attention in the reviewed research.

In the UK, a study on support options for deaf children (including those with hearing aids and those with cochlear implants) led by Summerfield and colleagues at the Medical Research Council's Institute of Hearing Research identified 1700 children and looked at the type and amount of support received, and at educational outcomes and quality-of-life measures. This will be reported soon; an early report by Fortnum is included in the review.

Educational placement was also an inconclusive outcome and can be considered as an inconclusive factor. For example, while educational placement in the mainstream may be seen as a goal of implantation for many, it may also be a factor in progress. In mainstream education, spoken language is more likely to be encouraged; however, conversely, some children may be isolated in mainstream education with individual sign language support, and in fact receive less oral communication than in a school for the deaf.

Factors residing within the child

Residual hearing

For deaf children in general, it is accepted that greater degrees of residual hearing are correlated with more successful outcomes in terms of spoken language. Given that cochlear implants are assumed to build on existing listening and spoken-language skills, it would seem this must be a relevant factor. However, there is little evidence concerning the effect of prior residual hearing on children who are implanted, although informal evidence suggests that it is related to outcomes. The largely anecdotal evidence suggests that the greater the residual hearing, the better the outcome, and this is supported by increasing evidence from adult studies. Clearly this effect is limited because for significantly greater degrees of residual hearing only small relative gains are possible.

Further research is important in this area, particularly in view of the relevance of residual hearing in assessing candidacy, and with younger children being assessed.

Cognitive ability

There is little research into the effect of cognitive ability as a predictor of outcomes. In the past, the benefit for some children with profound learning difficulties was seen to be so limited in the measured domains as to preclude them benefiting adequately from a cochlear implant. However, increasingly, the tendency is to consider potential benefit to overall quality of life, and this is an area that will receive more attention in future.

Additional disabilities

Given that over 30% of deaf children are likely to have an additional disability, this is increasingly becoming an issue to be considered. In the early days of implantation, few children with additional disabilities were implanted, but increasingly more such children are now being assessed and the presence of an additional disability is rarely, in itself, a reason not to implant. For disabilities such as visual impairments, an implant may be seen as being able to confer particular benefits. The evidence, however, remains inconclusive, particularly in view of relatively low numbers and short timescales.

However, there are some areas where there seem to be additional concerns. These include children with specific language difficulties, children with very low cognitive ability and children with auditory nerve pathology. Autism and disabilities on the autistic continuum require particular consideration. While the presence of disabilities in addition to deafness may not be a reason to reject implantation, it may well be that the assessment and evaluation will need to be different to take into account the impact of the additional disability.

All this suggests that this is an area in need of further research, albeit of a different research design. Small samples or case study design rather than larger comparative studies may be more appropriate for these specialist groups.

Demographic factors

Socio-economic status

Socio-economic measures are taken for two main reasons: either they assist in determining the representativeness of a population sample, or they provide an indication of social class and thus its effects on outcome. Socio-economic measures are, however, problematic, because our understanding of what class is, how relevant class is and how class is to be measured is continually shifting.

Class is clearly relevant because of growing evidence that social inequality is widening, and because there is a direct correlation between inequality, patterns of economic underperformance, including most markedly patterns of migration in and out of unemployment, and social exclusion in post-industrial societies. In this context, socio-economic measures matter because deafness (especially profound deafness) is implicated in forms of social exclusion, including forms resulting in patterns of educational and later economic underperformance. In such contexts, attention to 'class' (whichever way this is formulated) seems relevant in all elements of research on cochlear implantation, including the selection of candidates, participation and performance in rehabilitation, and language and education outcomes.

Further research is needed in this area, using measures that have been found useful. For example, in the UK, a number of measures are located in the British Household Surveys. Income is probably one of the most fundamental measures taken, and doubles in much research as an indicator of poverty or deprivation in particular, in combination with information on housing and geographic location via postcode data. Some US studies take income measures from parents, largely in attempts to position the research sample in the national context, and this can be a useful indicator.

Gender

Research studies of the outcomes of cochlear implantation regularly mention the gender of subjects in their methodology, but few go on to treat it as a variable to be examined, and to assess gender effects (Fortnum et al. 2002 is a notable exception). In fact, the reporting of gender seems to be more to establish the legitimacy of the sample, or its comparability with other studies, than to reflect an interest in gender differences themselves.

This omission seems to be one that could be readily rectified, given the existence of the necessary data. Readjustment in the attention paid to gender is appropriate for two reasons: first, because life outcomes are partly defined by goals on which gender, as social experience, is a real influence. And second, because education results reveal gender-based differences in the attainments of school populations. There is a trend for girls to perform better in language-based subjects, and for boys to perform marginally better in mathematics. We should, in particular, expect that if the emergent pattern of correlation between language skills/interests and girls' achievements proves persistent over time, this may realistically result in gender-based patterns in, for example, auditory rehabilitation and the achievement of spoken-language skills following cochlear implantation. Certainly, in those studies on deaf attainment where gender is explored, differences tend to be in the same direction as those for hearing pupils; in other studies, no differences are found. It is therefore important to continue tracking changing patterns of gender differentiation in a range of outcomes over time.

Ethnicity

No research in the reviewed collection of research reports has included an assessment of ethnicity. Ethnicity nevertheless deserves a mention because (multi) ethnicity is part of the societies in which we live, and it has a number of well-known and often-investigated attributes. In particular, ethnicity is often shown as related to socio-economic measures and educational performance. This is no different for deaf populations, where, in addition, ethnicity is likely to interrelate with language preference and English language skill (Powers et al. 1998), and is therefore likely to account for some of the commonly reported individual variation in outcome. For children for whom the acquisition of spoken language is a major goal following implantation, the process may be made more complex by the number of languages they hear, if, for example, school and home language are different. Hence ethnicity may be a factor in their outcomes, and a factor in how they should be measured.

Furthermore, there is a possibility that there might be an effect of ethnicity on pre-implantation processes, such as candidacy and test performance. It may also be a factor in obtaining access to the process of implantation, as accessing the services and information may be more difficult for ethnic minority families.

Researching outcomes in paediatric cochlear implantation

Throughout the previous discussion a number of common themes have emerged from the review of the research into paediatric cochlear implantation. Before exploring them further, it is worth pointing out that this research area is itself particularly difficult for a number of reasons, and it is helpful here to review some of the issues around test effectiveness and authenticity, particularly in relation to cochlear implantation.

Are the assessments fit for their purpose?

Test effectiveness

Effectiveness concerns the extent to which a test measures a specific outcome. Single point-in-time measures may fail to recognize the nature of cochlear implantation outcomes, which are part of a process, while repeated measures at various intervals can mark progress. Effectiveness can be expressed with reference to procedures: all measurements require procedures (test design, sampling, test administration, analysis, statistical methods, grounding results in theory, for example). Measures are normally considered to be of high quality if they can withstand efforts to falsify them. The two most common tools in this process of critical assessment are validity and reliability, which are often assumed to equate with generalizability of findings.

Validity

Validity measures the extent to which a test actually measures what it is intended to measure. It might be assumed that test validity is relatively unproblematic in the majority of the research reviewed here, but this would be false. First of all, validity requires a 'gold standard' measure in order to compare any assessment method with it and conclude if the method is valid or not. 'Face validity' is a common compromise and compares the proposed assessment method with other tests or methods widely used in the literature.

Most investigations reported in the present project are of a relatively simple design: the focus is on a limited subset of outcomes (mostly spoken-language skills) and the tests, although not validated, are commonly standardized. However, this standardization has its own problems: few tests exist that have been standardized on deaf children – most have been designed for, and normed on, hearing children. This means that any description of the performance of deaf children, even where there is no comparison intended, is inherently derived from comparisons with hearing children's performance, assuming that implanted children have equal access to spoken language. This, however, is false; even a child making good use of their implant system has a unilateral loss, with a mild/moderate loss in the implanted ear unless they have bilateral implants. A child who is continuing to use sign language may be at a disadvantage. On the other hand, cochlear implantation aims to facilitate spoken language and researchers may be interested only in assessing how 'close' to hearing children the test performance of children with cochlear implants is, and the comparison is therefore valid. This, however, should be made explicit.

Some comparative research combines over-time measures in one population with a single point-in-time measure of a comparison population. Apart from the test–retest issues (see below), this approach creates difficulties with the over-time elements of the analysis. The two sets of data are not equivalent, and external variables such as maturation come into play. Moreover, most of the studies reviewed are not longitudinal and different children are assessed at the various intervals, making comparisons impossible.

However, comparing the same group of children over a long time frame is difficult. Tests should be designed to be age-appropriate for the population studied. A test design suitable for children in the bottom end of the age range is not necessarily suitable for children who are much older. Where designs use a test-battery with different tests for different age ranges, this complicates the validity of the measure; in both scenarios the internal validity of the assessment across the age range is affected. In some instances, there is a tendency to generalize test results into more general statements concerning outcome. This particularly affects language assessments, where outcome on a spoken-language measure is taken to be representative of overall language development, or where outcomes of a particular test (such as the Reynell Developmental Language Scale) is taken to have captured the overall spoken language skills of a deaf child. This is particularly salient because the tests used are most commonly administered in one-to-one situations using one administrator. Such a clinical approach may not reflect the child's everyday performance at home or school, and the perceptions of clinicians and parents may vary widely.

Research designs in which a particular test, or battery of tests, is administered and re-administered over periods of time should cover issues around test–retest habituation, the gaps between tests and the overall time frames. There is no reference made in the available research to habituation effects, and in some research the gaps between test and retest are not held constant for individuals; this issue affects comparison with other research. The overall time frames also vary, although retesting after six months or one year is a commonplace pattern. The overall time frame is particularly important for tests that have a targeted age group that is narrower than that characterizing the research population.

Reliability

Reliability addresses consistency of results, and is often linked with the replication of findings using different observers (inter-observer reliability) or at a later point in time using the same observer (intra-observer reliability). Many of the assessment methods used with implanted children have not been evaluated for both inter- and intra-observer reliability. This weakens the outcomes of those studies considerably.

However, the most obvious problem in test reliability is where tests are administered to low numbers of children with implants and results are reported as group aggregates. Results in paediatric cochlear implantation in particular are subject to wide ranges of individual performance, and even within one individual over time, test experience (habituation) and the higher co-occurrence of further disabilities among deaf children are both factors to be taken into account.

Floor and ceiling effects are common, particularly in research measuring performance over greater stretches of time, and research based on a population characterized by a wide age range. In some instances, the test used is inappropriate for the target population.

Percentage reporting is a common way of reporting findings, aggregating scores across a tested population and reflecting means. In research in which there is cause to suspect wide individual variation, the reporting of percentage scores is an issue in itself. Where the number of tested children is low, an individual's high achievement on a test may skew the overall percentage score, confounding the reported results; individual data should be given.

Most of the tests in the literature concern speech-perception tests that do not involve comparisons with hearing children and assess progress through time. However, this type of research has other problems. Reliability is very important, because it is exactly the pattern of improvement that becomes the measure of performance. What is of particular interest is tracking a population over time, i.e. the same individuals at different time intervals. Unfortunately, there will be migration out of the sample for various reasons, and the reported studies are rarely longitudinal. This results in recording different individuals at different intervals and the sample size becomes smaller and smaller. Thus, the group mean results get less and less reliable (notably more subject to individual variation) over time. Although this is methodologically less troublesome, there is a clear duty to report the numbers involved at each test interval.

Finally, a significant number of studies are lacking in demographic description. This affects the generalizability of the findings in particular, because it is not possible to assess how representative of the entire population the sample is. It also affects reliability in that no comparisons can be made with outcomes reported elsewhere, and there is no scope either to replicate the result or to recode variables to establish equivalence with other research outcomes.

Test authenticity

Test authenticity concerns the extent to which tests are able to capture core attributes of paediatric cochlear implantation outcomes. Since outcomes from cochlear implantation are processes, authenticity should be concerned with how well particular measures reflect different directions in and opportunities for cochlear-implanted children and their families. An alternative description of authenticity is that tests should ideally be 'native' to the population in which they are used and should not be incompatible with their interests or socio-cultural and linguistic background. An assessment of authenticity should therefore take into account the current variation in the experience of deafness, and the different choices made by deaf children and their families. Any formulation of aims to be targeted by outcomes research should therefore include parents, deaf pupils and deaf adults, as well as professionals.

With regard to the research reviewed, there are three major observations: first, in more general terms, proxy measures are focused on spoken language and mainstream placement. Second, although the research is, to an extent, responsive to concerns among deaf people, it addresses those concerns mostly in refuting claims. Third, very few of the tests used in the available research (and none of those that have been normed or standardized) reflect the practical language situation of deaf children.

Two common criticisms are those of item bias and test administration. Item bias captures the appropriateness of test elements; they should be appropriate for the population and sensitive to changes, as previously discussed.

Test administration, in the collection of research reviewed here, covers four main administration patterns. The first is auditory only, through a sound system; the second auditory alone with live voice, but without lipreading; the third is live voice, with spoken language only but visual clues; and the fourth is using sign language if a particular child prefers it. Each method of administration should be made entirely clear in the study.

In summary, test effectiveness, authenticity, reliability and validity allow us to determine whether the tests that are used to arrive at outcome measures are fit for their purpose. In relation to both test effectiveness and authenticity, there is a need for greater focus on outcome as a process, and an increased awareness that current measures are proxies for a much wider range of outcomes that address language performance and preferences. Finally, test design and test administration must recognize this wider pattern of possible experiences, rather than approach deafness exclusively as hearing loss. There is a need for assessment methods designed for deaf implanted children, especially the very young. Proper validation is of utmost importance. Last, but not least, these methods, their administration and their use in research need to be standardized in order to derive generalizable results.

For the future

How can cochlear implant research meet these challenges? There has been a tension throughout the study between the context in which implantation is set – a surgical intervention – and the domains in which the outcomes were measured – social, psychological and educational. Thus the aims of both the social and medical research paradigms come into play, and they may differ in their emphases. This is reflected in the journals in which the material was largely found: medical and scientific, rather than educational, linguistic or psychological.

Traditional research set in the medical domain has been characterized by recognized levels of evidence; thus, for example, evidence obtained by randomized controlled trials is held to be more valuable than that of repeated-measures studies taken over time. The research reviewed here into cochlear implantation – a medical procedure – is inevitably influenced by such values. The medical model of deafness, and the basis for implantation, asserts that not to hear is undesirable and that any restoration of hearing is positive. However, this is in contradiction to other views of deafness, particularly those held by the deaf community, which sees deafness as difference and deaf people as a minority group.

There may also be the assumption that medical intervention as opposed to non-intervention, is itself beneficial, and in this case, that to hear is always better than not hearing (Wever, 2002). Hence comparisons have largely been with non-intervention rather than with different types of non-medical or audiological intervention. Outcomes, too, may be limited in scope and more restricted to specific measures looking at how implantation works, rather than looking at wider issues of the possible value of the procedure to the child in daily life.

In addition, because of the controversy surrounding the implementation of a medical procedure in deaf children for reasons other than medical ones, the demands made on the research have been that implantation should:

- prove its efficacy
- justify and therefore legitimize its implementation
- prove its safety
- prove its economic value
- define factors that influence outcomes, to maximize benefit.

However, for cochlear implantation, these issues are complex, set as they are in a multiprofessional context, with the differing values and standpoints of those involved. In practice, much of the research into outcomes has relied on research paradigms within the field of deaf education. It is fair to point out that research into the outcomes of cochlear implantation reflects the challenges of research in deaf education in general. The difficulties here relate to the fact that linguistic, educational and social outcomes do not lend themselves to formal measure and hard data in the way that other factors do. The issues are further compounded by the low incidence of deafness in childhood, and the difficulties of establishing studies with large enough numbers to be reliable. Matched control groups are difficult to find because of the number of variables affecting progress, and the studies reported in this volume will have variously compared implanted children with hearing children, and profoundly deaf children and severely deaf children, with and without hearing aids.

The controversy surrounding the implementation of cochlear implantation in children gave rise to a comparatively large amount of research in a comparatively short space of time, given the low incidence of deafness, and hence the comparatively small numbers we are talking about. The low incidence of deafness, in addition to influencing the types of research that are possible, has also meant there is a comparatively small group of people looking at outcomes from implantation. This group largely consists of practitioners who regularly compare anecdotal evidence, with much of it never published. In addition, given that the bias in the published literature will be the recognized one of publishing positive, rather than negative, results, there may be a large pool of valuable unpublished information among those involved with children with cochlear implants that has not been tapped in this review, and is not represented in the literature. Ways of formalizing this anecdotal evidence would be helpful.

Suggestions and guidelines for future research

This review, as illustrated by its size and comprehensiveness, has shown that much progress has been made in the research literature on outcomes from cochlear implantation. The field of implantation responded to the demand for evaluation with a large number of scientific studies undertaken and published in a comparatively short time frame. However, many of the studies are carried out by companies or implant programmes and are not truly independent, and this has already been the subject of major criticism. In addition, this review has revealed an imbalance in the various areas of research into outcomes. Two areas feature heavily in the review: speech perception and age at implantation. Both of them have been researched extensively, with studies repeating the same conclusions, whereas many other relevant areas have been neglected up to the date of the review.

There are, therefore, a number of challenges remaining and there is still room for further research. A number of themes and issues emerge that should be addressed in future studies. To conclude this review, we make some recommendations for future research with regard to:

- assessment measures used
- the process of the research
- factors necessary to include and investigate
- additional areas to explore.

Assessment measures used

It is important that researchers :

- develop and use assessments that are developmentally appropriate, valid and reliable
- clarify terminology used, for example, be clear about speech and language terms
- take care with test items to ensure that they measure what is being considered and that they are sensitive to change
- be explicit about norms being used
- use tests that tap into functioning in everyday life, rather than within the clinic setting.

The research process

It is important that the research methods used are appropriate to the study. Although randomized controlled studies may be the gold standard in some areas of research, in others, dealing with smaller numbers, case study research may be the most feasible and appropriate. Qualitative research methods, taken from the sociology field, may have much to offer the field of cochlear implantation, and have been under-used so far.

In considering the research process, researchers should:

- use research processes appropriate for the objective of the study
- define clear objectives of the study at the outset
- use large sample sizes with adequate statistical power wherever feasible, to enable subgroup comparisons
- use non-clinical settings in addition to clinical settings in order to assess real-life functioning
- use longer time frames with the same groups over time, to avoid reducing numbers at different intervals
- compare identifiable groups
- accurately describe and account for the language and modal preferences of the children included in the study population
- promote collaboration in particular areas or subgroups between centres to compare and to give larger numbers for study, although this may present difficulties in terms of comparison
- recognize the influence of maturation in the child population
- be aware of the advantages and disadvantages of using proxies to participate in the study on behalf of children
- recognize that cochlear implantation is a lifelong process, and that outcomes and factors change over time
- ensure that the tester has the expertise to carry out the procedure and understand the responses
- subject the results to rigorous statistical analysis whatever the research methods used.

Factors to include and investigate

In order that comparisons can be made between research reports, it would be helpful if researchers included and made explicit in their investigations and reports:

- age of sample
- age at implant
- age at onset of deafness
- gender of subjects
- ethnicity of subjects
- details of device type, tuning and functioning of the implant system
- aetiology of deafness of the subjects
- the numbers studied at each interval
- individual raw data in addition to providing percentages.

Additional areas to explore

There are a number of areas that are currently either not explored at all, for various reasons, or that are under-researched and are worthy of further consideration. These include:

- educational attainments rather than educational placement; these are necessarily long-term outcomes
- employment issues; once more these are long-term outcomes
- social issues, including family and parental views
- quality-of-life measures, looking at the wider implications of cochlear implantation on changes in the child's quality of life
- psychological measures, looking at the effect of implantation on the developing deaf child
- everyday use of the implant system in the long term, as greater numbers of children reach the adolescent years
- non-use of the implant system; in the long term are these children choosing to wear their devices, or are they electing as they reach adolescence to be selective about their use?
- young people's views; to date what research has been done in the area of views of quality of life and everyday use of implant systems has largely been done by proxy, using parents' views. Now that there are significant numbers of young people who are able to speak for themselves, robust exploration of their views is necessary
- tuning and its effectiveness; this is an area that is likely to have more of an impact than has currently been acknowledged or explored
- device functioning; similarly, in the long term, accurate and frank exploration of the continued functioning of the devices used is necessary
- children with additional disabilities and those with complex needs; as increasing numbers of these children are being considered and implanted it is becoming realistic to research outcomes in this group further
- rehabilitation and education – the type and quantity of support offered and what is considered to be appropriate are yet to be determined, and require further exploration
- changes in outcomes over time; as significant numbers of deaf children have implants for longer periods of time, it becomes possible to consider more fully how outcomes change over long time frames.

In conclusion, cochlear implantation has been found to be an exciting and important area of research, bringing together a number of disciplines with their own areas of expertise, expectation and interest. Robust further research will contribute to our understanding and knowledge of the interaction between hearing, learning and psychosocial development of deaf children. It may also promote closer collaboration between the professionals and confirm that although cochlear implantation may begin as a medical and scientific procedure, the outcomes lie in the educational, social and psychological domains. How researchers can investigate these long-term implications of cochlear implantation for the lives of deaf children, and produce rigorous evidence of benefit, remains a challenge.

List of abbreviations

ASL	American Sign Language
BATOD	British Association of Teachers of the Deaf
BIT	Beginner's Intelligibility Test
BKB	Bench-Kowal-Bamford sentence test
BSL	British Sign Language
CAP	Categories of Auditory Performance
CASALA	Computer Aided Speech and Language Analysis
CBCL	Child Behaviour Checklist
CBA	cost-benefit analysis
CDT	Connected Discourse Tracking
CEA	cost-effectiveness analysis
CELF	Clinical Evaluation of Language Fundamentals
CHATS	Cochlear Implant, Hearing Aid, Auditory and Tactile Skills curriculum (University of Miami, US)
CHILDES	Child Language Data Exchange System
CI	cochlear implantation/child with cochlear implant
CID	Central Institute for the Deaf
CIs	children with cochlear implants
CIS	Continuous Interleaved Sampling (processor strategy)
CMA	cost-minimization analysis
CNC	Consonant-Nucleus-Consonant monosyllabic word test
CPT	Common Phrase Test
CT	computed tomography (scan)
CUA	cost-utility analysis
CVPT	Children's Vowel Perception Test
dB HL	hearing level (in decibels)
dBEHL	equivalent hearing level (in decibels)
EARS	Evaluation of Auditory Responses to Speech (test battery)
EAT	Edinburgh Articulation Test
ENT	ear, nose and throat discipline of medicine
EOWPVT	Expressive One-Word Picture Vocabulary Test
ERM	Educational Resource Matrix
ESL	English as a second language
ESPT	Early Speech Perception Test
EVT	Expressive Vocabulary Test
FDA	Food and Drug Administration (US)
GAEL	Grammatical Analysis of Elicited Language
GASP	Glendonald Auditory Screening Procedure
GRI	Gallaudet Research Institute (Gallaudet University, Washington, US)

HA	hearing aid users
HA+	'Gold' hearing aid users (PTA 90–100 dB HL)
HUI	Health Utilities Index
IMSPAC	Imitative Test of the Perception of Phonologically Significant Speech Pattern Contrasts
IPC	Interpersonal Process Code
IPSyn	Index of Productive Syntax
IOWA	Iowa Closed Set Sentence Test
IST	Iowa Sentence Test
LEA	local educational authority (UK)
LiP	Listening Progress (profile)
LNT	Lexical Neighborhood Test
MAC	Minimum Auditory Capabilities test
MAIS	Meaningful Auditory Integration Scale
ME	magnitude estimation
MLNT	Multisyllabic Lexical Neighborhood Test
MLU	mean length utterance
MLUL	mean length utterance (five longest utterances)
MRI	magnetic resonance imaging
MSP	mini speech processor
MTP	Monosyllable Trochee Polysyllable test
MTS	Monosyllable Trochee Spondee test
MTSP	Miami Tactual Screening Procedure
MUSS	Meaningful Use of Speech Scale
NH	normally hearing (control group)
NU-CHIPS	Northwestern University Children's Perception of Speech
PALS	Profile of Actual Linguistic Skills
PB-K	Phonetically Balanced Kindergarten word list
PHU	Partially Hearing Unit (school based)
PIAT	Peabody Individual Achievement Test
PIC	Peer Interaction Code
PLS	Preschool Language Scales
PPVT	Peabody Picture Vocabulary Test
PSI	Pediatric Speech Intelligibility
PTA	pure tone average (hearing loss measure expressed in decibels)
PTE	Phonetic Task Evaluation
QALY	quality-adjusted life-year
RDLS	Reynell Developmental Language Scale
RITLS	Rhode Island Test of Language Structure
SALT	Systematic Analysis of Language Transcripts
SAT-HI	Stanford Achievement Test-Hearing Impaired
SC	simultaneous communication
SCIPS	Screening Inventory of Perception Skills
SECS	Scales of Early Communication Skills for Hearing Impaired Children
SES	socio-economic status
SG	standard gamble
SIR	Speech Intelligibility Rating
SLN	Sign Language of the Netherlands
SPINE	Speech Intelligibility Evaluation
TAC	Test of Articulation Competence
TACL	Test of Auditory Comprehension of Language
TC	total communication
TTO	time trade-off
TV	tactile vocoder

VAS	visual analogue scale
VWP	Vowel Perception test
WIPI	Word Intelligibility by Picture Identification test
WISC	Wechsler Intelligence Scale

Glossary of health economic terms

Economic evaluation type

There are four types of full economic evaluation (listed below). The costing methodologies are the same for all types of economic evaluation, and therefore it is the choice of outcome measure that determines which type of evaluation is to be performed. Economic evaluation takes the difference in costs between two or more interventions and divides them by the difference in outcomes to produce an incremental cost-per-outcome ratio, which can be used to compare interventions in resource allocation decision making.

Cost-effectiveness analysis (CEA)

Outcome is measured in natural units of effect. This analysis often uses clinical indicators as outcome measures and these are often one-dimensional, in that they only measure one dimension of outcome. For example, cost per life year saved is effectively only measuring the change in mortality resulting from the introduction of a new programme/intervention. This type of evaluation is particularly suited to answering questions seeking to find the best way of allocating given resources within a medical specialty.

Cost-utility analysis (CUA)

This uses utility as a measure of outcome. Utility measures changes to wellbeing. The most commonly used measure is QALYs (quality-adjusted life-years), which are multidimensional since they measure both change to quality and length of life. Utility can be valued using four different methods:

- visual analogue scale (VAS): the VAS asks the patient or proxy (parent or professional) to rate the patient's health on a scale from 0 to 1, where 1 is perfect health and 0 the worst imaginable health state. Patients also need to indicate where death falls on the scale. By doing this, patients provide an ordinal ranking of their health status. It is cognitively easy to answer and quick to fill in. It also does not place any restrictions on what an individual includes in their own assessment of health status. However, a number of measurement biases have been found in the literature (Bleichhrodt and Johannesson 1997), such as 'end-of-the-scale bias' and 'spacing out bias', where patients avoid the ends of the scale and space out their outcomes irrespective of the scale of outcomes. VAS values may also be reflecting how optimistic or pessimistic a person is, which is more of a problem when looking at absolute values rather than relative changes. The most commonly used VAS is that used as part of the EuroQol.

- standard gamble (SG): the SG trades on an individual's preference for (un)certainty. That is, a person is presented with two alternatives. The first alternative offers the option of perfect health for t years with a probability of p or they experience immediate death with a probability $1 - p$. The second alternative offers a chronic health state for t years. The level of p is varied until the individual becomes indifferent between the two alternatives and p represents the individual's value. It has been widely used to value health states but has a few limitations. It may be unrealistic to ask someone with a chronic condition, which cannot cause death, to consider a scenario involving death. For such conditions you can substitute death with the worst chronic health state possible. There is also evidence that people's attitudes to risk affect their valuations and that people find the cognitive demands of using probabilities high.

- time trade-off (TTO): the TTO trades using time as the unit of measurement. The individual is given two alternatives. The first is a suboptimal health state for time t, then death and the second perfect health for time x, where x is less than t, then death. x is varied until the participant is indifferent between the two options and at this stage the individual's value is given by x divided by t.

- magnitude estimation (ME): respondents are asked to rate the magnitude of one health state to another in terms of a ratio, e.g. five times as much.

These measures are quite cognitively demanding for respondents and, therefore, economists have developed a range of multi-attribute utility scales which ask respondents to tick the level which best describes their health for each health domain. The various measures are detailed in Table 5.1. Underlying utility values are then attached to the levels respondents report. These utility values were estimated during the development of the instrument using a sample of the general population's values from TTO, VAS, SG, ME or a mix of these. The measures have been found to elicit different utility values for the same health states, which suggests that they are either measuring or valuing the same health states differently. As a result, economists should always justify their choice of instrument with relation to the question/intervention being addressed. CUA aids resource allocation decisions concerning how to divide up a budget between different medical specialities.

Cost-benefit analysis (CBA)

This measure attaches a monetary value to outcomes using either stated preference techniques such as contingent valuation methods (one such method asks respondents their hypothetical willingness to pay for the intervention based on a contingent or hypothetical market) or revealed preference methods such as travel cost method (this measures the patient's travel and time costs associated with receiving the intervention as a proxy for their value of the benefit. If they did not value the programme they would not be willing to pay these costs). Since costs and outcomes are commensurate, the advantage of this method is that interventions from across different sectors of the economy can be compared, even where health is not a major domain of outcome. So, for example, it becomes possible to compare the economic value of a school building programme to a cancer screening programme directly. CBA can also measure the non-health benefits of health programmes, for example process utility and non-user values. Process utility refers to the benefit patients get from attending a healthcare programme, such as the value of information gained in the session which may not directly affect the health outcome. Non-user values refer to the benefits to others of someone else receiving healthcare; for example if someone has a vaccination this has benefits for others in society in terms of the risk of catching the condition vaccinated against.

Cost-minimization analysis (CMA)

CMA is a special form of CEA where the benefits of two or more interventions are the same. Therefore, a cost analysis is all that needs to be performed in order to see which intervention should be adopted (i.e. the cheapest).

Study perspective

The choice of study perspective will depend on many factors:

- who is sponsoring the study/ purpose of the study
- available data/resources
- study question
- how important (how large) various cost components are likely to be.

Decisions made by Government require a societal perspective to be taken, since they should represent the interests of all those affected by the implementation of a policy. A societal perspective should include the costs incurred by the health sector, any other sector of the economy affected, e.g. social services, education, etc., and patient costs. The benefits should also not be restricted to patient benefits but valued by the general population. Studies that focus on the patient perspective or payers' perspective are of interest, but in a nationally funded healthcare scheme such as the UK NHS they should not be used to make resource allocation decisions.

Comparator intervention

Economists are interested in the incremental or marginal effect of introducing a new intervention compared to an existing intervention - that is, what is the difference in costs and effects between the old and the new intervention? Decisions made on the basis of average cost-effectiveness (the new intervention compared to a do-nothing option, that is total costs divided by total outcome) can lead to misallocation. Therefore, it is important for studies to compare the new intervention to current practice. In the case of cochlear implantation, the comparator should be hearing aids, although some authors choose to use a do-nothing comparator because they claim the cost of hearing aids is negligible.

Source of effectiveness data

The ideal source is an estimate from primary research within the study, usually eliciting respondents' values or using effectiveness data from clinical records. However, this is not always possible and, therefore, recourse to published data or assumed values may have to be made.

Direct costs

All costs incurred in the provision of the intervention or in dealing with a side effect.

Indirect costs

Correctly defined (Gold et al., 1996, p. 399), this term refers to the productivity costs involved in illness or death. However, many of the economic studies included in this review mistakenly state other direct costs, such as education costs, as indirect costs. They have, therefore, been reported as the authors report them, despite this being technically incorrect.

Discount rate

The interest rate used to discount future values into present values. This rate reflects society's rate of time preference for consumption or health today. As an example, if you were asked whether you would prefer £100 today or £100 in one year's time, which would you choose? Most people would opt for the former, knowing that they could place the £100 in a bank account and earn interest on it over the year such that the value of the £100 today would be worth more than £100 in one year's time.

Outcome measure

See under 'Economic evaluation type' above (effectiveness, utility and monetary).

Currency and price year

This refers to the currency used to present results and the year the results relate to. It is important to know this in order to be able to adjust values to reflect current values or to compare cost-per-outcome ratios in a common price year.

Sensitivity analysis

Sensitivity analysis involves a range of techniques designed to test the uncertainty surrounding key variables in an economic model/analysis. It is standard practice to include sensitivity analysis in order to test how meaningful and robust the results are.

Table 5.1 Description of preference-based health status measurement instruments

Preference-based instrument	Domains/Attributes	Levels of severity	Number of health states	Valuation/sample
Rosser classification	Disability Distress	8 4	29	ME*/70, selected, London, UK and later a representative 140 UK citizens
EQ-5D (EuroQol 5 dimensions)	Mobility Self-care Usual activities Pain/discomfort Anxiety/depression	3 3 3 3 3	243	TTO and VAS/3395 representative UK citizens
QWB (quality of well being index)	Mobility Physical activity Social functioning and 27 symptoms, e.g. tiredness	3 3 3 2	1170	VAS/866 people from San Diego, USA
SF-6D (short form 6 dimensions, adapted from the SF-36)	Physical functioning Role limitations Social functioning Pain Mental health Vitality	6 4 5 6 5 5	18 000	SG/836 representative UK sample
HUI-II (Health Utilities Index version 2)	Sensory Mobility Emotion, Cognitive Self-care Pain Fertility	4 5 5 4 4 5 3	24 000	VAS transformed into SG/203 parents in Hamilton, Canada
HUI-III (Health Utilities Index version 3)	Vision Speech Hearing Ambulation Dexterity Emotion Cognition Pain	6 5 6 6 6 5 6 5	972 000	VAS transformed into SG/504 representative Hamilton citizens, Canada

*ME = magnitude estimation, which involves eliciting individuals' ratios of disutility between health states. Adapted from Brazier et al 1999.

Papers reviewed

Allen C, Nikolopoulos T, O'Donoghue GM (1998) Speech intelligibility in children following cochlear implantation. American Journal of Otology 19: 742-746. — 48

Allen SE, Dyar D (1997) Profiling linguistic outcomes in young deaf children after cochlear implantation. American Journal of Otology 18: s127-s128. — 49

Allum JH, Greisiger R, Straubhaar S, Carpenter MG (2000) Auditory perception and speech identification in children with cochlear implants tested with the EARS protocol. British Journal of Audiology 34(5): 293-303. — 49

Archbold SM, Lutman ME, Gregory S, O'Neill C, Nikolopoulos TP (2002) Parents and their deaf child: their perceptions three years after cochlear implantation. Deafness and Education International 4(1): 12-40. — 51

Archbold SM, Nikolopoulos T, Lutman ME, O'Donoghue GM (2002) The educational settings of profoundly deaf children with cochlear implants compared with age-matched peers with hearing aids: implications for management. International Journal of Audiology 41(3): 157-161. — 52

Archbold SM, Nikolopoulos TP, O'Donoghue GM, Lutman ME (1998) Educational placement of deaf children following cochlear implantation. British Journal of Audiology 32: 295-300. — 53

Archbold SM, Nikolopoulos TP, Tait M, O'Donoghue GM, Lutman ME, Gregory S (2000) Approach to communication, speech perception and intelligibility after paediatric cochlear implantation. British Journal of Audiology 34(4): 257-264. — 55

Archbold S, Robinson K, Hartley D (1998) UK teachers of the deaf - working with children with cochlear implants. Deafness and Education 22(2): 24-30. — 57

Bat-Chava Y, Deignan E (2001) Peer relationships of children with cochlear implants. Journal of Deaf Studies and Deaf Education 6(3): 186-199. — 58

Baumgartner WD, Pok SM, Egelierler B, Franz P, Gstöttner W, Hamzavi J (2002) The role of age in pediatric cochlear implantation. International Journal of Pediatric Otorhinolaryngology 62(3): 223-228. — 60

Beadle EA, Shores A, Wood EJ (2000) Parental perceptions of the impact upon the family of cochlear implantation in children, Annals of Otology, Rhinology and Laryngology 185: s111-s114. — 61

Bichey BG, Hoversland JM, Whynne MK, Miyamoto RT (2002) Changes in quality of life and the cost-utility associated with cochlear implantation in patients with large vestibular aqueduct syndrome. Otology and Neurotology 23: 323-327. — 62

Blamey PJ, Sarant JZ, Paatsch LE, Barry JG, Bow CP, Wales RJ, Wright M, Psarros C, Rattigan K, Tooher R (2001) Relationships among speech perception, production, language, hearing loss, and age in children with impaired hearing. Journal of Speech, Language and Hearing Research 44(2): 264-285. — 63

Boothroyd A (1997) Auditory capacity of hearing-impaired children using hearing aids and cochlear implants: issues of efficacy and assessment. Scandinavian Audiology Supplement 26(46): s17-s25. — 66

Boothroyd A, Eran O (1994) Auditory speech perception capacity of child implant   67
    users expressed as equivalent hearing loss. Volta Review 96(5): 151-168.

Bosco E, D'Agosta L, Ballantyne D (1999) 'Small group' rehabilitation in adolescent   69
    cochlear implant users: learning experiences. International Journal of Pediatric
    Otorhinolaryngology 47(2): 187-190.

Brinton J (2001) Measuring language development in deaf children with cochlear   70
    implants. International Journal of Language and Communication Disorders 36:
    s121-s125.

Carter R, Hailey D (1999) Economic evaluation of the cochlear implant. International   71
    Journal of Technology Assessment in Health Care 15(3): 520-530.

Cheng AK, Grant GD, Niparko JK (1999) Meta-analysis of pediatric cochlear implanta-   72
    tion literature. Annals of Otology, Rhinology and Laryngology 108(4/2): 124-128.

Cheng AK, Rubin HR, Powe NR, Mellon NK, Francis HW, Niparko JK (2000) Cost-utility   73
    analysis of the cochlear implant in children. Journal of the American Medical
    Association 284: 850-856.

Chin SB, Finnegan KR, Chung BA (2001) Relationships among types of speech intelligi-   74
    bility in pediatric users of cochlear implants. Journal of Communication Disorders
    34(3): 187-205.

Chmiel R, Sutton L, Jenkins H (2000) Quality of life in children with cochlear   76
    implants. Annals of Otology, Rhinology and Laryngology 185: s103-s105.

Cleary M, Pisoni DB, Geers AE (2001) Some measures of verbal and spatial working   77
    memory in eight- and nine-year-old hearing-impaired children with cochlear
    implants. Ear and Hearing 22(5): 395-411.

Coerts J, Mills AE (1995) Spontaneous language development of young children with a   79
    cochlear implant. Annals of Otology, Rhinology and Laryngology 166: s385-s387.

Cowan RS, DelDot J, Barker EJ, Sarant JZ, Pegg P, Dettman S, Galvin KL, Rance G,   80
    Hollow R, Dowell RC, Pyman B, Gibson WP, Clark GM (1997) Speech perception
    results for children with implants with different levels of preoperative residual
    hearing. American Journal of Otology 18(6 Suppl): s125-s126.

Crosson J, Geers A (2000) Structural analysis of narratives produced by young cochlear   81
    implant users. Annals of Otology, Rhinology and Laryngology 109(12): s185: 118-119.

Crosson J, Geers A (2001) Analysis of narrative ability in children with cochlear   82
    implants. Ear and Hearing 22(5): 381-394.

Cullington H, Hodges AV, Butts SL, Dolan-Ash S, Balkany TJ (2000) Comparison of   84
    language ability in children with cochlear implants placed in oral and total com-
    munication educational settings. Annals of Otology, Rhinology and Laryngology
    185: s121-s123.

Davids L, Brenner C, Geers A (2000) Predicting speech perception benefit from loud-   86
    ness growth measures and other map characteristics of the Nucleus 22 implant.
    Annals of Otology, Rhinology and Laryngology 109 (12): s185: 56-58

Dawson PW, Blamey SJ, Dettman LC et al. (1995) A clinical report on speech   86
    production of cochlear implant users. Ear and Hearing 16: 551-561.

Dawson PW, McKay CM, Busby PA, Grayden DB, Clark GM (2000) Electrode   89
    discrimination and speech perception in young children using cochlear implants.
    Ear and Hearing 21(6): 597-607.

Dawson PW, Nott PE, Clark GM, Cowan RS (1998) A modification of play audiometry   90
    to assess speech discrimination ability in severe-profoundly deaf 2- to 4-year-old
    children. Ear and Hearing 19(5): 371-384.

Daya H, Ashley A, Gysin C, Papsin BC (2000) Changes in educational placement and   91
    speech perception ability after cochlear implantation in children. Journal of
    Otolaryngology 29(4): 224-228.

Diller G, Graser P, Schmalbrock C (2001) Early natural auditory-verbal education of   93
    children with profound hearing impairments in the Federal Republic of Germany:
    results of a 4 year study. International Journal of Pediatric Otorhinolaryngology
    60(3): 219-226.

Dorman MF, Loizou PC, Kemp LL, Kirk KI (2000) Word recognition by children listen-   94
ing to speech processed into a small number of channels: data from normal-
hearing children and children with cochlear implants. Ear and Hearing 21(6):
590-596.

Easterbrooks SR, Mordica JA (2000) Teachers' ratings of functional communication   96
in students with cochlear implants. American Annals of the Deaf 145(1): 54-59.

Eilers RE, Cobo-Lewis AB, Vergara KC, Oller D et al. (1996) A longitudinal evaluation   97
of the speech perception capabilities of children using multichannel tactile
vocoders. Journal of Speech and Hearing Research 39(3): 518-533.

Filipo R, Bosco E, Barchetta C, Mancini P (1999) Cochlear implantation in deaf   99
children and adolescents: effects on family schooling and personal well-being.
International Journal of Pediatric Otorhinolaryngology 49s1: s183-s187.

Fortnum HM, Marshall DH, Bamford JM, Summerfield AQ (2002) Hearing-impaired   101
children in the UK: Education setting and communication approach. Deafness
and Education International 4(3): 123-141.

Francis HW, Koch ME, Wyatt JR, Niparko JK (1999) Trends in educational placement   102
and cost-benefit considerations in children with cochlear implants. Archives of
Otorhinolaryngology, and Head and Neck Surgery 125: 499-505.

Frisch SA, Pisoni DB (2000) Modeling spoken word recognition performance by   104
pediatric cochlear implant users using feature identification. Ear and Hearing
21(6): 578-589.

Fryauf-Bertschy H, Tyler RT, Kelsay DM et al. (1997) Cochlear implant use by prelin-   105
gually deafened children: The influences of age at implant and length of device
use. Journal of Speech, Language and Hearing Research 40(Feb): 183-199.

Gantz BJ, Rubinstein JT, Tyler RS, Teagle HFB, Cohen NL, Waltzman SB, Miyamoto   107
RT, Kirk KI (1999) Long-term results of cochlear implants in children with
residual hearing. Annals of Otology, Rhinology and Laryngology (Supplement)
184: s33-s36.

Gantz BJ, Tyler RS, Woodworth GG, Tye-Murray N, Fryauf-Bertschy H (1994) Results   108
of multichannel cochlear implants in congenital and acquired prelingual deafness in children: five-year follow-up. American Journal of Otology 15-S: 1-7.

Geers AE (1997) Comparing implants with hearing aids in profoundly deaf children.   109
Otolaryngology - Head and Neck Surgery 117(3/1): 150-154.

Geers AE (2004) Factors affecting the development of speech, language and   111
literacy in children with early cochlear implantation. Education and Cochlear
Implantation

Geers A, Brenner C (1994) Speech-perception results: audition and lipreading   112
enhancement. Volta Review 96(5): 97-108.

Geers A, Brenner C, Nicholas J, Uchanski R, Tye-Murray N, Tobey E (2002)   113
Rehabilitation factors contributing to implant benefit in children. Annals of
Otology, Rhinology and Laryngology 189: s127-s130.

Geers A, Moog J (1994) Spoken language results: vocabulary, syntax and communi-   115
cation. Volta Review 96(5): 131-148.

Geers A, Nicholas J, Tye-Murray N, Uchanski R, Brenner C, Davidson L, Torretta G   116
(2000) Effects of communication mode on skills of long-term cochlear implant
users. Annals of Otology, Rhinology and Laryngology 109(12)s185: 89-91.

Gfeller K, Witt SA, Spencer LJ, Stordahl J, Tomblin B (1998) Musical involvement   118
and enjoyment of children who use cochlear implants. Volta Review 100(4):
213-233.

Gordon KA, Daya H, Harrison RV, Papsin BC. (2000) Factors contributing to limited   120
open-set speech perception in children who use a cochlear implant.
International Journal of Pediatric Otorhinolaryngology 56(2): 101-111.

Gstöttner W, Hamzavi J, Egerlierler B, Baumgartner WD (2000) Speech perception   121
performance in prelingually deaf children with cochlear implants. Acta Oto-
Laryngologica 120: 209-213.

Hamzavi J, Baumgartner WD, Egelierler B, Franz P, Schenk B, Gstöttner W (2000)   122
Follow up of cochlear implanted handicapped children. International Journal of
Pediatric Otorhinolaryngology 56(3): 169-174.

Harrigan S, Nikolopoulos TP (2002) Parent interaction course in order to enhance   124
communication skills between parents and children following pediatric cochlear
implantation. International Journal of Pediatric Otorhinolaryngology 66: 161-166.

Harrison RV, Panesar J, El-Hakim H, Abdolell M, Mount RJ, Papsin B (2001) The   125
effects of age of cochlear implantation on speech perception outcomes in
prelingually deaf children. Scandinavian Audiology 30(53): s73-s78.

Hildesheimer M, Teiltelbaum R, Segal O, Tenne S, Kishon-Rabin L, Kronenberg Y,   126
Muchnik C (2001) Speech perception results - the first 10 years of a cochlear
implant program. Scandinavian Audiology 30(52): s39-s41.

Hodges AV, Dolan Ash M, Balkany TJ, Schloffman JJ, Butts SL (1999) Speech per-   127
ception results in children with cochlear implants: contributing factors.
Otolaryngology - Head and Neck Surgery 121(1): 31-34 .

Huang WH, Huang TS (1997) Speech perception performance of prelingually deaf-   128
ened children and adolescents with Nucleus 22-channel cochlear implant.
Advances in Oto-Rhino-Laryngology 52: 224-228.

Hutton J, Politti C, Seeger T (1995) Cost-effectiveness of cochlear implantation of   130
children: a preliminary model for the UK. Advances in Oto-Rhino-Laryngology
50: 201-206.

Illg A, von der Haar-Heise S, Goldring JE, Lesinski-Schiedat A, Battmer RD, Lenarz T   130
(1999) Speech perception results for children implanted with the Clarion
cochlear implant at the Medical University of Hanover. Annals of Otology,
Rhinology and Laryngology 108: 93-98.

Incesulu A, Vural M, Erkam U (2003) Children with cochlear implants: parental   132
perspective. Otology and Neurotology 24(4): 605-611.

Inscoe J. (1999) Communication outcomes after paediatric cochlear implantation.   133
International Journal of Pediatric Otorhinolaryngology 47(2): 195-200.

Kelsay DMR, Tyler RS (1996) Advantages and disadvantages expected and realised by   134
paediatric cochlear implant recipients as reported by their parents. American
Journal of Otology 17: 866-873.

Kiefer J, Gall V, Desloovere C, Knecht R, Mikowski A, von Ilberg C (1996) A follow-up   136
study of long-term results after cochlear implantation in children and
adolescents. European Archives of Oto-Rhino-Laryngology 253(3): 158-166.

Kirk KI (1998) Assessing speech perception in listeners with cochlear implants: the   137
development of the Lexical Neighborhood Tests. Volta Review 100(2): 63-85.

Kirk KI, Hay-McCutcheon M, Sehgal ST, Miyamoto RT (2000) Speech perception in   139
children with cochlear implants: effects of lexical difficulty, talker variability, and
word length. Annals of Otology, Rhinology and Laryngology 109(12): 79-81.

Kluwin TN, Stewart DA (2000) Cochlear implants for younger children: a preliminary   140
description of the parental decision process and outcomes. American Annals of
the Deaf 145(1): 26-32.

Knutson JF, Boyd RC, Goldman M, Sullivan PM (1997) Psychological characteristics of   142
child cochlear implant candidates and children with hearing impairments. Ear
and Hearing 18(5): 355-363.

Knutson JF, Boyd RC, Reid JB, Mayne T, Fetrow R (1997) Observational assessments   144
of the interaction of implant recipients with family and peers: preliminary
findings. Otolaryngology - Head and Neck Surgery 117(3/1): 196-207.

Knutson JF, Wald RL, Ehlers SL, Tyler RS (2000) Psychological consequences of   145
pediatric cochlear implant use. Annals of Otology, Rhinology and Laryngology
185: s109-s111.

Koch ME, Wyatt JR, Francis HW, Niparko JK (1997) A model of educational resource   146
use by children with cochlear implants. Otolaryngology - Head and Neck
Surgery 117(3/1): 174-179.

Lachs L, Pisoni DB, Kirk KI (2001) Use of audiovisual information in speech perception by prelingually deaf children with cochlear implants: a first report. Ear and Hearing.22(3): 236-251.   147

Lea RA, Hailey DM (1995) The cochlear implant: a technology for the profoundly deaf. Medical Progress through Technology 21: 47-52.   149

Lenarz T, Lesinski-Shiedat A, von der Haar-Heise S, Illg A, Bertram B, Battmer RD (1999) Cochlear implantation in children under the age of two: the MHH experience with the Clarion cochlear implant. Annals of Otology, Rhinology and Laryngology 108: 44-49.   150

Lesinski A, Battmer RD, Bertram B, Lenarz T (1997) Appropriate age for cochlear implantation in children: experience since 1986 with 359 implanted children. In: Honjo I, Takahashi H (eds) Cochlear Implant and Related Sciences Update: Advances in Oto-Rhino-Laryngology 52: 214-217.   151

Lesinski A, Hartrampf R, Dahm MC, Bertram B, Lenarz T (1995) Cochlear implantation in a population of multihandicapped children. Annals of Otology, Rhinology and Laryngology 104(166): s332-s334.   152

Lesinski A, von der Haar-Heise S, Battmer RD, Cords S, Goldring J, Lenarz T (2000) Performance of German-speaking children with the Clarion cochlear implant. In: Waltzman SB, Cohen NL (eds) Cochlear Implants. New York, USA: Thieme (art.11e), pp. 215-216.   153

Lutman ME, Tait DM (1995) Early communicative behaviour in young children receiving cochlear implants: factor analysis of turn-taking and gaze orientation. Annals of Otology, Rhinology and Laryngology 104: 397-399.   153

McConkey Robbins AM, Bollard PM, Green J (1999) Language development in children implanted with the CLARION® cochlear implant. Annals of Otology, Rhinology and Laryngology (Supplement) 177: s113-s118.   155

McConkey Robbins AM, Green J, Bollard P (2000) Language development in children following one year of Clarion implant use. Annals of Otology, Rhinology and Laryngology (Supplement) 185: s94-s95.   157

McConkey Robbins AM, Kirk KI, Osberger MJ et al. (1995) Speech intelligibility of implanted children. In: Clark, Cowan (eds) International Cochlear Implant, Speech and Hearing Symposium, pp. 399-401.   158

McConkey Robbins AM, Osberger MJ, Miyamoto RT, Kessler KS (1995) Language development in young children with cochlear implants. Advances in Oto-Rhino-Laryngology. 50: 160-166.   159

McConkey Robbins AM, Svirsky M, Kirk KI (1997) Children with implants can speak, but can they communicate? Otolaryngology - Head and Neck Surgery 117(3): 155-160.   160

McDonald Connor C, Hieber S, Arts HA, Zwolan TA (2000) Speech, vocabulary, and the education of children using cochlear implants: oral or total communication? Journal of Speech, Language, and Hearing Research 43(5): 1185-1204.   161

Meyer TA, Svirsky MA, Kirk KI, Miyamoto RT (1998) Improvements in speech perception by children with profound prelingual hearing loss: effects of device, communication mode, and chronological age. Journal of Speech, Language, and Hearing Research 41(4): 846-858.   164

Meyer V, Hertram B, Lenarz T (1995) Performance comparisons in congenitally deaf children with different ages of implantation. Advances in Oto-Rhino-Laryngology 50: 129-133.   166

Miyamoto RT, Kirk KI, Svirsky MA, Sehgal ST (1999) Communication skills in pediatric cochlear implant recipients. Acta Oto-Laryngologica 119(2): 219-224.   167

Miyamoto RT, Kirk KI, Todd MA, Robbins AM, Osberger M (1995) Speech perception skills of children with multichannel cochlear implants or hearing aids. Annals of Otology, Rhinology and Laryngology 104: 334-337.   169

Miyamoto RT, Svirsky MA, Robbins AM (1997) Enhancement of expressive language in prelingually deaf children with cochlear implants. Acta Oto-Laryngologica 117(2): 154-157.   170

Molina M, Huarte A, Cervera-Paz FI, Manrique M, Gracia-Tapia R (1999) Development   172
of speech in two-year-old children with cochlear implants. International Journal
of Pediatric Otorhinolaryngology 47(2): 177-179.

Mondain M, Sillon M, Vieu A, Tobey E, Uziel A (1997) Speech perception skills and speech   173
intelligibility in prelingually deafened French children using cochlear implants.
Archives of Otorhinolaryngology, and Head and Neck Surgery 123: 181-184.

Moog JS, Geers AE (1999) Speech and language acquisition in young children after   174
cochlear implantation. Otolaryngologic Clinics of North America 32(6): 1127-1141.

Nakisa MJ, Summerfield AQ, Nakisa RC, McCormick B, Archbold S, Gibbin KP,   175
O'Donoghue GM (2001) Functionally equivalent ages and hearing levels of
children with cochlear implants measured with pre-recorded stimuli. British
Journal of Audiology 35(3): 183-199.

Nevins ME, Chute PM (1995) Success of children with cochlear implants in   177
mainstream educational settings. Annals of Otology, Rhinology and Laryngology
104: s100-s102.

Nikolopoulos T, Archbold S, Lutman ME, O'Donoghue GM (2000) Prediction of   178
auditory performance following cochlear implantation of prelingually deaf
young children. In: Waltzman SB, Cohen NL (eds) Cochlear Implants. New York,
USA: Thieme (art.11f), pp. 216-217.

Nikolopoulos TP, Archbold SM, O'Donoghue GM (1999) The development of auditory   179
perception in children following cochlear implantation. International Journal of
Pediatric Otorhinolaryngology 49-s1: 189-191.

O'Donoghue G, Nikolopoulos TP, Archbold SM (2000) Determinants of speech   180
perception in children after cochlear implantation. Lancet 356(9228): 466-468.

O'Neill C, Archbold S, O'Donoghue GM, McAlister DA, Nikolopoulos TP (2001) Indirect   181
costs, cost-utility variations and the funding of paediatric cochlear implantation.
International Journal of Pediatric Otorhinolaryngology 58: 53-57.

O'Neill C, O'Donoghue GM, Archbold S, Normand C (2000) A cost-utility analysis of   182
pediatric cochlear implantation. Laryngoscope 110: 156-160.

Osberger MJ, Fisher L, Zimmerman-Phillips S, Geier L, Barker MJ (1998) Speech   182
recognition of older children with cochlear implants. American Journal of
Otology 19(2): 152-157.

Osberger MJ, Geier L, Zimmerman-Phillips S, Barker MJ (1997) Use of a parent   183
report scale to assess benefit in children given the Clarion cochlear implant.
American Journal of Otology 18: s79-s80.

Osberger MJ, McConkey Robbins AM, Todd SL, Riley AI (1994) Speech intelligibility of   184
children with cochlear implants. Volta Review 96(5): 169-180.

Osberger MJ, McConkey Robbins AM, Todd SL, Riley AI, Miyamoto R (1994) Speech   186
production skills of children with multichannel cochlear implants. In: Hochmair-
Desoyer IJ, Hochmair ES (eds) Advances in Cochlear Implants. Vienna, Austria:
Manz, pp. 503-508.

Paganga S, Tucker E, Harrigan S, Lutman M (2001) Evaluating training courses for   186
parents of children with cochlear implants. International Journal of Language
and Communication Disorders 36: s517-s522.

Parisier SC, Chute PM, Popp AL, Suh GD (2001) Outcome analysis of cochlear implant   187
reimplantation in children. Laryngoscope 111(1): 26-32.

Perrin E, Berger-Vachon C, Topouzkhanian A, Truy E, Morgon A (1999) Evaluation of   189
cochlear implanted children's voices. International Journal of Pediatric
Otorhinolaryngology 47(2): 83-98.

Pisoni D, Geers A (2000) Working memory in deaf children with cochlear implants: 190
correlations between digit span and measures of spoken language processing.
Annals of Otology, Rhinology and Laryngology 109(12): s185.

Preisler G, Ahlstrom M, Tvingstedt AL (1997) The development of communication and   192
language in deaf preschool children with cochlear implants. International
Journal of Pediatric Otorhinolaryngology 41(3): 263-272.

Purdy SC, Chard LL, Moran CA, Hodgson SA (1995) Outcomes of cochlear implants   193
    for New Zealand children and their families. Annals of Otology, Rhinology, and
    Laryngology (Supplement) 166: 102-105.

Pyman B, Blamey P, Lacy P, Clark G, Dowell R (2000) The development of speech   195
    perception in children using cochlear implants: effects of etiologic factors and
    delayed milestones. American Journal of Otology 21(1): 57-61.

Quittner AL, Smith LB, Osberger MJ, Mitchell TV et al. (1994) The impact of audition   196
    on the development of visual attention. Psychological Science 5(6): 347-353.

Rose DE, Vernon M, Pool AF (1996) Cochlear implants in prelingually deaf children.   199
    American Annals of the Deaf 141(3): 158-261.

Schulze-Gattermann H, Illg A, Schoenermark M, Lenarz T, Lesinski-Schiedat A (2002)   200
    Cost-benefit analysis of pediatric cochlear implantation: German experience.
    Otology and Neurotology 23: 674-681.

Shea JJ, Domico EH, Lupfer M (1994) Speech perception after multichannel cochlear   201
    implantation in the pediatric patient. American Journal of Otology 15: 66-70.

Smith LB, Quittner AL, Osberger MJ, Miyamoto RT (1998) Audition and visual atten-   202
    tion: the developmental trajectory in deaf and hearing populations.
    Developmental Psychology 34(5): 840-850.

Spencer LJ, Tye-Murray N, Tomblin JB (1998) The production of English inflectional   204
    morphology, speech production and listening performance in children with
    cochlear implants. Ear and Hearing 19(4): 310-318.

Spencer L, Tomblin JB, Gantz BJ (1997) Reading skills in children with multichannel   206
    cochlear-implant experience. Volta Review 99(4): 193-202.

Summerfield AQ, Marshall DH (1999) Pediatric cochlear implantation and health-   207
    technology assessment. International Journal of Pediatric Otorhinolaryngology
    47: 141-151.

Summerfield AQ, Marshall DH, Archbold SM (1997) Cost-effectiveness considerations   208
    in pediatric cochlear implantation. American Journal of Otology 18: s166-s168.

Svirsky MA, Meyer TA (1999) Comparison of speech perception in pediatric   209
    CLARION® cochlear implant and hearing aid users. Annals of Otology, Rhinology
    and Laryngology (Supplement) 177: 104-109.

Szagun G (2001) Language acquisition in young German-speaking children with   210
    cochlear implants: Individual differences and implications for conceptions of a
    'sensitive phase'. Audiology and Neuro-Otology 6(5): 288-297.

Tait DM, Lutman ME (1994) Comparison of early communicative behaviour in young   212
    children with cochlear implants and with hearing aids. Ear and Hearing 15:
    352-361.

Tait DM, Lutman ME (1997) The predictive value of measures of pre-verbal communica- 214
    tion behaviours in young deaf children with cochlear implants. Ear and Hearing
    18(6): 472-478.

Tait DM, Lutman ME, Robinson K (2000) Preimplant measures of preverbal commu-   215
    nicative behaviour as predictors of cochlear implant outcomes in children. Ear
    and Hearing 21(1): 18-24.

Tobey EA, Geers AE, Douek BM, Perrin J, Skellet R, Brenner C, Toretta G (2000)   216
    Factors associated with speech intelligibility in children with cochlear implants.
    Annals of Otology, Rhinology and Laryngology 109(12): 28-30.

Tomblin JB, Spencer L, Flock S, Tyler R, Gantz B (1999) A comparison of language   217
    achievement in children with cochlear implants and children using hearing aids.
    Journal of Speech, Language and Hearing Research 42: 497-511.

Truy E, Lina-Granade G, Jonas AM, Martinon G, Maison S, Girard J, Porot M, Morgon   219
    A (1998) Comprehension of language in congenitally deaf children with and
    without cochlear implants. International Journal of Pediatric
    Otorhinolaryngology 45(1): 83-89.

Tye-Murray N, Spencer L, Gilbert Bedia E (1995) Relationships between speech pro-   220
    duction and speech perception skills in young cochlear-implant users. Journal of
    the Acoustical Society of America 98(5/1): 2454-2460.
Tye-Murray N, Spencer L, Gilbert Bedia E, Woodworth G (1996) Differences in   221
    children's sound production when speaking with a cochlear implant turned on
    and turned off. Journal of Speech and Hearing Research 39(3): 604-610.
Tye-Murray N, Spencer L, Woodworth GG (1995) Acquisition of speech by children   223
    who have prolonged cochlear implant experience. Journal of Speech and
    Hearing Research 38(2): 327-337.
Tyler RS, Fryauf H, Gantz BJ, Kelsay DMR, Woodworth GG (1997) Speech perception   225
    in prelingually implanted children after four years. In: Honjo I, Takahashi H (eds)
    Cochlear Implant and Related Sciences Update. Advances in Oto-Rhino-
    Laryngology 52: 187-192.
Tyler RS, Fryauf-Bertschy H, Kelsay DMR, Gantz BJ, Woodworth GP, Parkinson A   226
    (1997) Speech perception by prelingually deaf children using cochlear implants.
    Otolaryngology - Head and Neck Surgery 117(3/1): 180-187.
Tyler RS, Gantz BJ, Woodworth GG, Fryauf-Bertschy H, Kelsay DMR (1997)   227
    Performance of 2- and 3-year-old children and predictions of 4-year from 1-year
    performance. American Journal of Otology 18: s157-s159.
Tyler RS, Kelsay DMR, Teagle HFB, Rubinstein JT, Gantz BJ, Christ AM (2000) 7-year   228
    speech perception results and the effects of age, residual hearing and preim-
    plant speech perception in prelingually deaf children using the Nucleus and
    Clarion cochlear implants. In: Kim CS, Chang SO, Lim D (eds) Updates in
    Cochlear Implantation. Advances in Oto-Rhino-Laryngology 57: 305-310.
Tyler RS, Rubinstein JT, Teagle H, Kelsay DMR, Gantz BJ (2000) Pre-lingually deaf   229
    children can perform as well as post-lingually deaf adults using cochlear
    implants. Cochlear Implants International 1(1): 39-44.
Tyler RS, Teagle HFB, Kelsay DMR, Gantz BJ, Woodworth GG, Parkinson AJ (2000)   229
    Speech perception by prelingually deaf children after six years of cochlear
    implant use: effects of age at implantation. Annals of Otology, Rhinology and
    Laryngology (Supplement) 185: s82-s84.
Uziel AS, Reuillard-Artieres F, Sillon M et al. (1995) Speech perception performances   230
    in prelingual deafened children with the Nucleus multichannel cochlear implant.
    Advances in Oto-Rhino-Laryngology 50: 114-118.
Vermeulen A, Hoekstra C, Brokx J, van den Broek P (1999) Oral language acquisition   231
    in children assessed with the Reynell Developmental Language Scales.
    International Journal of Pediatric Otorhinolaryngology 47(2): 153-155.
Wald RL, Knutson JF (2000) Deaf cultural identity of adolescents with and without   233
    cochlear implants. Annals of Otology, Rhinology and Laryngology 185: s87-s89.
Waltzman SB, Cohen NL, Gomolin RH, Green J, Shapiro W, Brackett D, Zara C (1997)   234
    Perception and production results in children implanted between 2 and 5 years
    of age. Advances in Oto-Rhino-Laryngology 52: 177-180.
Waltzman SB, Cohen NL, Gomolin RH, Green JE, Shapiro WH, Hoffman RA, Roland JT   235
    (1997) Open-set speech perception in congenitally deaf children using cochlear
    implants. American Journal of Otology 18(3): 342-349.
Wang HL, Toe D (1998) The development of communicative competence in adoles-   236
    cents with cochlear implants. Caedhh Journal/La Revue Acesm 24(1): 27-45.
Young NM, Gorhne KM, Carrasco VN, Brown C (1999) Speech perception of young   237
    children using nucleus 22-channel or CLARION® cochlear implants. Annals of
    Otology, Rhinology and Laryngology 108(4): 99-103.
Zwolan TA, Zimmerman-Phillips S, Ashbaugh CJ, Hieber SJ, Kileny PR, Telian SA   238
    (1997) Cochlear implantation of children with minimal open-set speech recogni-
    tion skills. Ear and Hearing 18(3): 240-251.

Additional references

Bleichhrodt H, Johannesson M (1997) An experimental test of the theoretical foundation for rating-scale valuations. Medical Decision Making 17(2): 208–216.

Brazier J, Deverill M, Green C, Harper R, Booth A (1999) A review of the use of health status measures in economic evaluation. Health Technology Assessment 3(9): 1–164.

Dauman R, Debruge E, Carbonniere B, Lautissier Berger S, Bouye J, Soriano V (1996) Development of capacities of communication and socialization in young deaf children: utility of a common assessment protocol for implanted or hearing aid equipped children. Acta Oto-Laryngologica 116(2): 234–239.

Geers A, Kirk IK (2003) Ear & Hearing 24(1).

Powers S (1996) Deaf pupils' achievement in ordinary schools. Journal of British Associatiopon of Teachers of the Deaf 20(4): 11–123.

Powers S, Gregory S, Thoutenhoofd ED (1998) The Educational Achievements of Deaf Children. Research Report RR65. London: Department for Education and Employment.

Wever C (2002) Parenting Deaf Children in the Era of Cochlear Implantation. PhD thesis, University of Nijmegen.

Further reading

Allum DJ (1996) Cochlear Implant Rehabilitation in Children and Adults. London: Whurr.

Chute PM, Nevins ME (2002) The Parents' Guide to Cochlear Implants. Washington, DC: Gallaudet University Press.

Clark GM, Cowan RSG, Dowell RC (eds) (1997) Cochlear Implantation for Infants and Children. San Diego, CA: Singular Publishing Group.

Drummond MF, O'Brien B, Stoddart GL, Torrance (1997) Methods for the economic evaluation of health care programmes, 2nd edn. Oxford: Oxford University Press.

Gallaway C, Young A (eds) (2003) Deafness and Education in the UK: research perspectives. London: Whurr.

Gregory S, Knight P, McCracken W, Powers S, Watson L (eds) (1998) Issues in Deaf Education. London: David Fulton.

McCormick B, Archbold S (2003) Cochlear Implants for Young Children, 2nd edn. London: Whurr.

Miyamoto RT, Chin SB (2003) Speech and language benefits of cochlear implantation. Volta Review 102(4).

Nevins ME, Chute PM (1996) Children with Cochlear Implants in Educational Settings. San Diego, CA: Singular Publishing Group.

Niparko JK, Iler Kirk K, Mellon NK, Robbins AM, Tucci DL, Wilson BS (eds) (2000) Cochlear Implants: principles and practice. Philadelphia, PA: Lippincott Williams & Wilkins.

Powers S, Gregory S, Lynas W, McCracken W, Watson L, Boulton A, Harris D (1999) Good Practice in the Education of Deaf Children. London: RNID.

RNID (2003) Working with Children with Cochlear Implants: educational guidelines project. London: RNID.

Robinson Colin (2001) Real World Research. Oxford: Blackwell.

Spencer PE, Marschark M (2003) Cochlear Implants, Issues and Implications. In: Marschark M, Spencer PE (eds) Deaf Studies, Language and Education. New York: Oxford University Press.

Tyler RS (ed.) (1993) Cochlear Implants Audiological Foundations. London: Whurr.

Waltzman S, Cohen N (eds) (2000) Cochlear Implants. New York: Thieme.

Index

An asterisk (*) before a page number indicates an entry in the glossary of health economic terms. The abbreviation PCI is used in the index for paediatric cochlear implantation

abbreviations 269-71
age at implantation
  influencing outcome 251-2
  speech production and 31-2
  speech recognition and 20-2
age at onset of deafness
  congenital/acquired deafness 23
  influencing outcome 252
  medical/linguistic 23
  prelingual/postlingual 23-4
  speech production and 32
  speech recognition and 23-4
assessment
  of hearing 3
  of language 245
  of outcomes 12
  for PCI 6-7
  surgical 6-7
audiological issues
  candidacy issues 4-5
  choice of ear 5
  developing technology 2-3
  discrimination of sounds 4
  hearing assessment 3
  implant performance 5-6
  tuning the system 3-4
audiometric guidelines 4
auditory nerve pathology 257
auditory stimulation 5
autism 257

British Sign Language (BSL) 11, 244

candidacy
  audiological issues 4-5
  speech recognition and 27
central nervous system, stimulation 5
children, deaf
  with additional disabilities/needs 4, 7,
    256-7
  of deaf parents 10

development of language and
    communication 9-10
  educational issues 10-11
  family life 10
  of hearing parents 10
  quality of life 10
  social life 10
  very young 7-8
  see also schools
cognitive ability
  affecting outcome 256
  very low 257
cognitive outcome, little or no research 247
cognitive outcome measures 44
  reviewed material 44
communication
  pre-implant, affecting outcome 253
  simultaneous 11, 32
  total communication 11, 36, 40, 40-1
communication approach 39-40
  affecting outcome 254-6
  inconclusive/contradictory outcomes
    245-6
  outcomes 40-1
  reviewed material 41
communication development 9-10, 37-9
  inconclusive/contradictory outcomes
    243-5
communication mode, and speech
  intelligibility 36
congenital deafness 4, 4-5, 23
contingent valuation 45
cost analysis 45
cost-benefit analysis (CBA) 45, 250, *274
cost-effectiveness analysis (CEA) 45-6,
  *272
cost effectiveness of PCI 250-1
cost-minimization analysis (CMA) 45, *274
cost-utility analysis (CUA) 45, *272-4
costs, direct/indirect *276
craniofacial syndromes 7

criteria for PCI 4
currency *276

deafness
    acquired 23
    age at onset, *see* age at onset of
        deafness
    in children 9-11
    congenital 4, 4-5, 23
    disability or difference? 2, 10, 13, 263
    medical *v.* educational/sociological model
        13
    prelingual/postlingual 23-4
demographic factors, affecting outcome 251,
    257-9
development of PCI 1-2
    audiological issues 2-3
direct costs *276
disabilities, additional 4, 7, 256-7
discount rate *276
discrimination of sounds 4

ear, choice of, for PCI 5
economic evaluation outcomes 45-6
    reviewed material 46
economic evaluation type *272
education approach, affecting outcome
    254-6
educational issues 10-11
    sign *v.* spoken language 2, 9, 11
    see also schools
educational outcomes, little or no research
    246-7
educational placement 11, 39-40
    affecting outcome 255-6
    inconclusive/contradictory outcomes
        245-6
    outcomes 40
    reviewed material 41
    speech production and 33-4
    speech recognition and 28
effectiveness data, source of *275
emotional issues, little or no research 247
employment outcomes, little or no research
    246-7
equivalent hearing loss 26, 27
ethnicity, affecting outcome 258-9
EuroQol 5 dimensions (EQ-5D) *277
experience of cochlear implants, speech
    recognition and 23

factors influencing outcomes 251-9
    demographic 251, 257-9

established 251-2
not established 253-6
relating to support received by child
    251, 253-6
residing within the child 251,
    256-7
families
    family/social life 10
    income 254, 257
    quality of life 10
family support, affecting outcome 254
follow-up care 8
further reading 288

gender, affecting outcome 255, 258

health, WHO definition 248
health economics
    glossary of terms *272-7
    little or no research 250-1
health status, preference-based
    measurement instruments *277
Health Utilities Index *277
hearing
    assessment 3
    discrimination of sounds 4
    residual 5, 256
    threshold levels, aided 3, 4
hearing aids 5
    comparisons with PCI
        speech intelligibility 35
        speech production 33
        speech recognition 26-7
    simultaneous use of PCI and 5

implantable devices 2-3
    functioning and tuning, lack of research
        253-4
    multi-channel 2-3
    performance 5-6
implantation
    aim of 19
    bilateral 5
    candidacy for, *see* candidacy
    criteria for 4
    multidisciplinary approach 6, 7
    of very young 7-8
income, of family 254, 257
indirect costs *276
IQ, affecting outcome 255

journals 14-15
knowledge, incidental 9

language
    assessment in everyday situations 245
    pre-implant, affecting outcome 253
    tone languages 29
    see also sign language; spoken
        language
language development 9-10, 37
    inconclusive/contradictory outcomes
        243-5
    speech perception/production and
        243-4
    see also spoken language
literacy skills development 9
long-term findings
    speech intelligibility 35
    speech production 32-3
    speech recognition 24-6

magnitude estimation (ME), for measuring
    utility *273, *277
manually coded English (see Sign
    Supported English)
medical issues 6-8
meningitis 3, 4, 8

outcomes of PCI 241-51
    assessment, purposes of 12
    categories 241-2
    differing perspectives of 12-13
    evaluation 12-13
    factors influencing, see factors
        influencing outcomes
    inconclusive/contradictory 242, 243-6
    with little or no research 242, 246-51
    measures of 19-47
    miscellaneous 46-7
        reviewed material 47
    outcome measure (economic) *276
    primary 12
    relative importance of 13
    researching, see review of research on
        PCI outcomes
    robust 241, 242-3
    secondary 12-13
    see also individual outcome measures

parents
    deaf 10
    decision on PCI 7, 12
    hearing 10
    income 254, 257
    role 7
    stress levels in 43

parents' perspectives 42-3
    reviewed material 43
performance of implant 5-6
proxies 247, 249
psycho-social outcomes 41-2
    little or no research 247-8
    proxy responses 247
    reviewed material 42

quality of life
    deaf children and families 10
    defining 248, 249
    little or no research 248-9
    use of proxy 249
quality of well-being index (QWB) *277

reading ability 11
references, additional 287
rehabilitation, affecting outcome 254-6
research studies
    anecdotal evidence 264
    criticism of 13
    face validity 259
    for the future 263-4, 265-8
        additional areas 267
        assessment methods 265
        factors for inclusion 266
        research process 265-6
    item bias 262
    percentage reporting 261
    test administration 262-3
    test authenticity 262-3
    test design 263
    test effectiveness 259, 263
    test reliability 261-2
    test validity 259-61
residual hearing 5
    affecting outcome 256
review of research on PCI outcomes 1
    concerns and measures 17-18
    database search 17
    key journals 14-15
    literature search 14
    papers reviewed (detail) 48-240
    papers reviewed (list) 279-86
    search restrictions 16

schools
    mainstream v. specialist 11
    see also educational entries
selection for PCI, see candidacy
sensitivity analysis *276
short form 6 dimensions (SF-6D) *277

sign language
  inconclusive/contradictory outcomes 244, 245
  outcomes 39
  reviewed material 39
  v. spoken language 2, 9, 11
Sign Supported English 11, 244
simultaneous communication 11, 32
social life 10
social outcomes, see psycho-social outcomes
socio-economic status, affecting outcome 257
sound discrimination 4
speech intelligibility 35
  communication mode and 36
  comparisons with other aided populations 35
  long-term findings 35
  miscellaneous factors and 36
  placement measures and 36
  reviewed material 36-7
  speech perception and 35, 36
  speech production and 31
speech perception
  language development and 243-4
  robust outcomes 242-3
  speech intelligibility and 35, 36
speech production
  age at implantation and 31-2
  age at onset of deafness and 32
  comparisons with other aided populations 33
  educational placement and 33-4
  language development and 243-4
  long-term findings 32-3
  miscellaneous factors and 34
  reviewed material 34-5
  robust outcomes 242-3
  speech intelligibility and 31
speech recognition 19-20
  age at implantation and 20-2
  age at onset of deafness and 23-4
  candidacy and 27

cochlear implant experience and 23
  comparisons with other aided populations 26-7
  educational placement and 28
  long-term findings 24-6
  miscellaneous factors and 28-9
  reviewed material 29-31
  variation in individual performance 19-20
spoken language
  development 31-2
  outcomes 37-8
  reviewed material 38-9
  v. sign language 2, 9, 11
standard gamble (SG), for measuring utility *273, *277
stimulation, auditory 5
study perspective *275
support for child, influencing outcome 251, 253-6
surgical issues 6-8
  assessment 6-7
  children with additional needs 7
  complications 8
  minimally invasive surgery 8
  multidisciplinary approach 6, 7
  very young children 7-8

technology
  developing 2-3
  see also implantable devices
teenagers, little or no research 247-8
threshold levels, aided hearing 3, 4
time trade-off (TTO), for measuring utility *273, *277
tone languages 29
total communication 11, 36, 40, 40-1

utility
  methods of measurement *272-4, *277
  see also cost-utility analysis

visual analogue scale (VAS), for measuring utility *273, *277